T0248766

Breast Cancer: Tumor Microenvironment and Biology

Breast Cancer: Tumor Microenvironment and Biology

Edited by **Sandra Lekin**

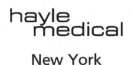

New York

Published by Hayle Medical,
30 West, 37th Street, Suite 612,
New York, NY 10018, USA
www.haylemedical.com

Breast Cancer: Tumor Microenvironment and Biology
Edited by Sandra Lekin

International Standard Book Number: 978-1-63241-068-9 (Hardback)

Printed in the United States of America.

Contents

Preface   VII

Part 1   Breast Cancer Cell Lines, Tumor Classification,
          In Vitro Cancer Models   1

Chapter 1 **Breast Cancer Cell Line Development
          and Authentication**   3
          Judith C. Keen

Chapter 2 **Insulin-Like-Growth Factor-Binding-Protein 7:
          An Antagonist to Breast Cancer**   21
          Tania Benatar, Yutaka Amemiya,
          Wenyi Yang and Arun Seth

Chapter 3 ***In Vitro* Breast Cancer Models as
          Useful Tools in Therapeutics?**   51
          Emilie Bana and Denyse Bagrel

Chapter 4 **Breast Cancer: Classification Based on Molecular
          Etiology Influencing Prognosis and Prediction**   69
          Siddik Sarkar and Mahitosh Mandal

Chapter 5 **Breast Cancer from Molecular Point of View:
          Pathogenesis and Biomarkers**   85
          Seyed Nasser Ostad and Maliheh Parsa

Chapter 6 **Remarks in Successful Cellular Investigations
          for Fighting Breast Cancer Using Novel
          Synthetic Compounds**   109
          Farshad H. Shirazi, Afshin Zarghi, Farzad Kobarfard,
          Rezvan Zendehdel, Maryam Nakhjavani, Sara Arfaiee,
          Tannaz Zebardast, Shohreh Mohebi, Nassim Anjidani,
          Azadeh Ashtarinezhad and Shahram Shoeibi

Part 2   Breast Cancer and Microenvironment   127

Chapter 7   **Novel Insights Into the Role of Inflammation
in Promoting Breast Cancer Development**   129
J. Valdivia-Silva, J. Franco-Barraza,
E. Cukierman and E.A. García-Zepeda

Chapter 8   **The Role of Fibrin(ogen) in Transendothelial Cell
Migration During Breast Cancer Metastasis**   165
Patricia J. Simpson-Haidaris, Brian J. Rybarczyk and Abha Sahni

Chapter 9   **Interleukin-6 in the Breast Tumor Microenvironment**   191
Nicholas J. Sullivan

Chapter 10   **Hyaluronan Associated Inflammation and Microenvironment
Remodelling Influences Breast Cancer Progression**   209
Caitlin Ward, Catalina Vasquez, Cornelia Tolg,
Patrick G. Telmer and Eva Turley

Part 3   Breast Cancer Stem Cells   235

Chapter 11   **Breast Cancer Stem Cells**   237
Fengyan Yu, Qiang Liu, Yujie Liu, Jieqiong Liu and Erwei Song

Chapter 12   **The Microenvironment of Breast Cancer Stem Cells**   253
Deepak Kanojia and Hexin Chen

Chapter 13   **Involvement of Mesenchymal Stem Cells in
Breast Cancer Progression**   263
Jürgen Dittmer, Ilka Oerlecke and Benjamin Leyh

Permissions

List of Contributors

Preface

Every book is initially just a concept; it takes months of research and hard work to give it the final shape in which the readers receive it. In its early stages, this book also went through rigorous reviewing. The notable contributions made by experts from across the globe were first molded into patterned chapters and then arranged in a sensibly sequential manner to bring out the best results.

The causes of cancer are diversified. Cancer is the principal reason of death in the majority of countries and it results in enormous financial, societal and mental burden. Breast cancer is the most diagnosed kind of cancer and the foremost reason of death due to cancer amongst women. This book deals with various aspects of breast cancer. It discusses topics related to breast cancer cell lines, classification of tumors and stem cells. It also elucidates the microenvironment of breast cancer. It intends to help students and experts in gaining more knowledge regarding the topic.

It has been my immense pleasure to be a part of this project and to contribute my years of learning in such a meaningful form. I would like to take this opportunity to thank all the people who have been associated with the completion of this book at any step.

Editor

Part 1

Breast Cancer Cell Lines, Tumor Classification, *In Vitro* Cancer Models

Breast Cancer Cell Line Development and Authentication

Judith C. Keen

University of Medicine and Dentistry of New Jersey
USA

1. Introduction

Inarguably, the development of cell culture and the ability to grow human cells *in vitro* has revolutionized medicine and scientific research. In the nearly sixty years since the first successful culture of immortalized human tumor cells in the lab in 1952, new fields of research have emerged and new scientific industries have been launched. Without cell lines, medicine would not be as advanced as it is today. Modern techniques that allow for manipulation of cell have allowed for a more complete understanding of the of fundamental basics of cellular and molecular biology and the biological system as a whole.

Different types of cell lines exist. Lines are maintained as continuous cultures, are established as primary cultures for transient studies, are created as explants of tumor or tissue samples, or cultivated from a single individual cell. Cell lines, especially cancer cell lines, are ubiquitous and are used for everything. By using cell lines, our understanding of cells and genes, how they function or malfunction, and how they interact with other cells has increased the pace of discovery and fundamentally changed how science is conducted. Cell lines have been established as a model of specific disease types. Individual cell lines have been derived from specific disease states and therefore possess specific characteristics of that disease state. Therefore, they are exceptionally useful to gain insight into normal physiology and how that physiology changes with onset of disease. Novel treatments and therapeutic strategies are investigated in cell lines in order to gain a fundamental detailed understanding of how a cell will react. Initial protocols are developed and tested in cell lines prior to use in animal models or testing in humans. This has enormous implications in discovery and reducing unintended side effects.

The first breast cancer cell line was established in 1958. Today, lines modeling the varied types of breast cancer help to develop targeted therapy and to provide a molecular signature of gene expression. Cell lines of estrogen/progesterone receptor (ER/PR) positive, ER/PR negative, triple negative (ER/PR/Her2), normal mammary epithelium, metastatic disease, and more are so widely used that it is nearly impossible to identify a recent discovery that hasn't used cell line models at some point during development.

Unfortunately, significant shortcomings of the use of cell lines exist. Cell lines are a model system. They do not always predict the outcome in humans and therefore, do not replace use of whole organisms. They are grown and tested in isolation, therefore the influence of neighboring cells or organs is non-existent in cell culture systems. Over time, cells can differentiate resulting in a change in phenotype from the original culture. Cell lines can become contaminated by infectious agents such as mycoplasma or even by other cell lines. Such contamination may not be readily detectable and can result in dramatically different results leading to false or irreproducible data. Some of these issues can be addressed to thwart the waste of reagents, money, and time. This includes testing and authenticating cell lines while they are actively grown and in use in the lab. Companies exist that can test for mycoplasma infection or DNA fingerprinting of cell lines to authenticate a particular cell line. Other shortcomings are merely inherent to this model system and must simply be identified and addressed.

2. A brief history of cell culture

Since the first successful establishment of a human cancer cell line in 1952, cell lines have been the backbone of cancer research. They have provided the understanding of systems at the molecular and cellular levels. Cell lines are used in the vast majority of research labs to understand the fundamentals of basic mechanisms as well as the translation to clinical settings.

Modern tissue culture techniques were made possible through the contributions of many scientists across the world whose attempts to understand physiology and to establish a source of tissue to study lead to fundamental changes in our understanding of biology and medicine. Among the contributions include those of Sydney Ringer at the University College London, who determined the ion concentrations necessary to maintain cellular life and cell contractility, and ultimately created Ringers Solution. Through his seminal work in the 1880s, Ringer described the concentrations of calcium, potassium and sodium required to maintain contraction of a frog heart and began the steps towards modern day cell culture (Miller, 2004; Ringer, 1882, 1883). In 1885, Wilhelm Roux at the Institute of Embryology in Germany cultured chicken embryonic tissue in saline for several days. This was followed by the work of Ross Harrison at the Johns Hopkins University in 1907, who was the first to successfully grow nerve fibers in vitro from frog embryonic tissues. While this was the outgrowth of embryonic tissue, these tissue cultures were successfully maintained *ex vivo* for 1 - 3 weeks (Skloot, 2010)(Ryan, 2007b). In 1912, Alex Carrel at the Rockefeller Institute for Medical Research successfully cultured the first mammalian tissue, chicken heart fragments. He claimed to maintain beating chicken heart fragments in culture for over 34 years and outliving him by one year (Ryan, 2007a). Although controversy as to whether these cultures were authentic or supplemented with fresh chicken hearts still remains (Skloot, 2010). This controversy may have slowed progress towards the establishment of cell lines in culture to some degree, it did not prevent work to create a source of material and model systems to allow for testing *in vitro*.

It would be another 40 years before the establishment of the first continuously growing human cell line, however steady advances towards that goal were ongoing. Carrel, working with Charles Lindbergh, worked to create novel culturing techniques that included use of pyrex glass. This glass could be heated and sterilized to reduce, or preferably eliminate, bacterial contamination. This led to the creation of the D flasks in the 1930s which improved cell culturing conditions by reducing contamination (Ryan, 2007c).

Tissue culture took another leap forward in 1948 when Katherine Sanford at Johns Hopkins was the first to culture single mammalian cells on glass plates in solution to produce the first continuous cell line (Earle et al., 1943; Sanford et al., 1948). Prior to this, tissues were attached to coverslips, inverted and grown in droplets of blood or plasma.

Her work set the stage for modern practices of growing cells in media on plates or flasks (Sanford et al., 1948).

2.1 Establishment of the HeLa cell line and cell line production

Indoubtedly, the most important factor to change biomedical research and our understanding of disease at the cellular and molecular levels was the establishment of the first continuously growing human cell line, the HeLa cell (Gey et al., 1952). In 1952, Henrietta Lacks was a patient with adenocarcinoma of the cervix treated at the Johns Hopkins Hospital. A portion of her tumor was used in the laboratory of George Gey at Johns Hopkins University and the revolution of modern biomedical research began. These cells were grown in roller flasks in specialized medium containing serum developed by Evans and Earle et al. and continued to proliferate (Evans et al., 1951). Almost 60 years later, these cells are still proliferating in laboratories across the globe and used to increase our understanding of cellular mechanisms from cell signaling, to the implications of weighlessness/zero gravity on cellular aging, and everything in between. The implications of establishing this cell line have been tremendous and is still ongoing. HeLa cells have not stopped growing and neither has the vast amount of knowledge gleened from them.

In 1953, Gey demonstrated that HeLa cells could be infected with the polio virus and therefore were a useful tool for testing the efficacy of the polio vaccine that was under development. This set the stage for the mass production of cell lines for distribution and use worldwide. The National Science Foundation established the first production lab at the Tuskegee Institute in 1953 that would provide HeLa cells to scientists involved in the development of the polio vaccine (Brown and Henderson, 1983). The goal was to ship at least 10,000 cultures per week. At the peak of production, 20,000 cultures were shipped per week and a total of 600,000 cultures were shipped in the two years the lab was in existence (Brown and Henderson, 1983). This, along with the Lewis Coriell's development of the laminar flow hood to reduce contamination of cell cultures and methods to freeze and recover cell lines (Coriell et al., 1958; McGarrity and Coriell, 1973, 1974)(Coriell and McGarrity, 1968; Greene et al., 1964; McAllister and Coriell, 1956; Silver et al., 1964), led to the establishment of cell repositories to house and distribute cells. It also led to the development of tumor specific cancer cell lines that created models of different types of human cancer and to an explosion of understanding of how cells work without the influence or perturbation of other cells. These models were also an ideal system to test novel therapeutics and treatment strategies without use of whole animals or humans.

2.2 Culturing cells

The terms tissue culture and cell culture are used interchangeably, but in reality they are two distinct entities. While both methods are derived from specific cells isolated from the whole organism, the cultures established are quite different and used for different endpoints (Freshney, 2010a).

Tissue, or primary, cultures are established from isolated tissue or organ fragment, most commonly from tumor slices (McAteer and Davis, 2002). These primary cultures can be used either for immediate experimentation to determine how primary cells operate or to establish a continuous cell line. Generally, primary cultures are established through placing an organ explant into culture media and allowing for outgrowth of cells or by digesting the tissue fragment using enzymatic or mechanical digestion. By definition, these cultures are transient. Primary culture refers to the period of time the primary tissue/organ fragment is kept in culture *in vitro* prior to the first passage or subculturing of cells, at which time they are referred to as a cell culture. This could range from days to a few weeks at most (MacDonald, 2002).

Cell lines are primary cultures that have been subcultured or passaged and can be clonal, terminal or immortalized cells (McAteer and Davis, 2002). Clonal cell cultures are created by selecting a single cell that will proliferate to establish a single population. Terminal cell lines are able to grow in culture for a few generations before senescence occurs and the cell line can no longer survive in culture media. Immortalized cell lines are able to grow in culture forever. These immortalized cell lines can occur naturally, such as HeLa cells, or through transformation events, such as Epstein-Barr Virus transformation. All types of *in vitro* cell cultures are used in breast cancer research.

3. The establishment of human breast cancer cell lines

The first human breast cancer cell line, BT-20, was established by Lasfargues and Ozzello in 1958 from an explant culture of a tumor slice from a 74 year old caucasian woman (Lasfargues and Ozzello, 1958). These cells are estrogen receptor alpha (ER) negative, progesterone receptor (PR) negative, Tumor Necrosis Factor alpha (TNF-α) positive, and epidermal growth factor receptor (EGFR) positive (Borras et al., 1997). While BT-20 is the oldest established breast cancer cell line, it is not the most commonly used line. By far, the most widely used breast cancer cell line worldwide is the MCF-7 cell line (Table 1 and Figure 1)(Burdall et al., 2003). Established in 1973 by Soule and colleagues at the Michigan Cancer Foundation, from where it derives its name, MCF-7 cells were isolated from the plural effusion of a 69 year old woman with metastatic disease (Soule et al., 1973). Since its establishment, MCF7 has become the model of ER positive breast cancer (Lacroix and Laclercq, 2004). Establishment of other cell lines has followed, including ones from other breast cancer types such as BRCA mutant, triple negative, HER2 overexpressing, and those derived from normal mammary epithelial cells such as MCF-10A cells (Soule et al., 1990) (Table 2).

Cell line use in labs is ubiquitous and continues to increase. From 2000 - 2010, the publication of manuscripts using the 10 most commonly used cell lines has almost tripled (2.8% increase) (Figure 2). Clearly demonstrating that the importance of, need for, and use of breast cancer cell lines will not diminish in the near future. Evaluation of the existing lines indicates that most breast cancer cell lines in use are derived from metastatic cancer and not other breast cancer phenotypes (Borras et al., 1997). Indeed, the overall success rate of establishing a cell line is only 10%. Most of the cell lines that exist today have been derived from pleural effusion instead of from primary tumors and are primarily ER - lines (Table 2 and reviewed in (Lacroix and Laclercq, 2004). This is surprising since ER - breast cancer is detected in only 20 - 30% of all primary tumors, whereas ER + tumors are detected 55-60% of the time (Ali and Coombes, 2000; McGuire et al., 1978). The reason for this discrepancy remains unknown, however it has been postulated that this could be because ER - cells are easier to establish in culture than ER + or that as cells are grown in culture, the epithelial like phenotype is lost while more mesenchymal traits are retained, therefore cells in culture appear to undergo a endothelial to mesenchymal transition (EMT) *in vitro* which is associated with the ER - phenotype (Lacroix and Laclercq, 2004). This suggests that culture systems are a model of metastatic disease that can grow in isolation and not a model the wide heterogeneity of disease that is detected clinically. Although current cell lines are derived form only a subset of primary cancers, overall these lines are a reliable model to study the fundamental questions concerning cell growth, death, and the basic biology of breast cancer. Indeed, many advances in breast cancer biology have been made using cell culture systems and should not be dismissed because of these concerns.

Cell line	No of publications 1/1/2000 to 12/31/2010	origin
BT-20	79	breast
MCF7	11813	pleural effusion
MDA-MB-231	3489	pleural effusion
MDA-MB-435 *	719	pleural effusion
MDA-MB-468	486	pleural effusion
SkBr3	372	pleural effusion
T47D	1168	pleural effusion
ZR75.1	96	ascites
BT474	251	pleural effusion
MCF-10A	451	subcutaneous mastectomy
* not a breast cancer cell line		

Table 1. List of commonly used cell lines, the number of citations and their origin

3.1 Breast cancer cell lines as models of primary tumors

Using breast cancer cell lines clearly hold advantages over use of animal or human models. Beyond the ethical implications of animal or human use, the advantages to using cell lines include the ease of obtaining cell lines (can be purchased from commercial sources), the ease of harvesting large numbers of cells (can be grown in culture for long periods of time to accumulate the necessary concentration), and the ability to test an individual cell type without confounding parameters such as other cell types or local microenvironment (to date, no two cell lines can grown simultaneously in culture for extended periods). Conversely, much debate has circulated concerning the applicability of the data derived from isolated cell lines to the predicted outcomes in humans. One area that this debate has been most contentious has been regarding the importance of the immune system in cancer development. Clearly, the microenvironment and infiltrating immune cells contribute to development and progression of disease, therefore individual cells grown in isolation will lack the influence of other neighboring cells (Voskoglou-Nomikos et al., 2003). Genetic, epigenetic and cytotoxicity studies that focus on outcomes in breast cells clearly benefit from use of cell culture systems. The fundamental understanding of the underlying genetic or molecular pathways involved in breast cell growth and its response to cytotoxic agents are best understood in isolated cell culture systems (Voskoglou-Nomikos et al., 2003).

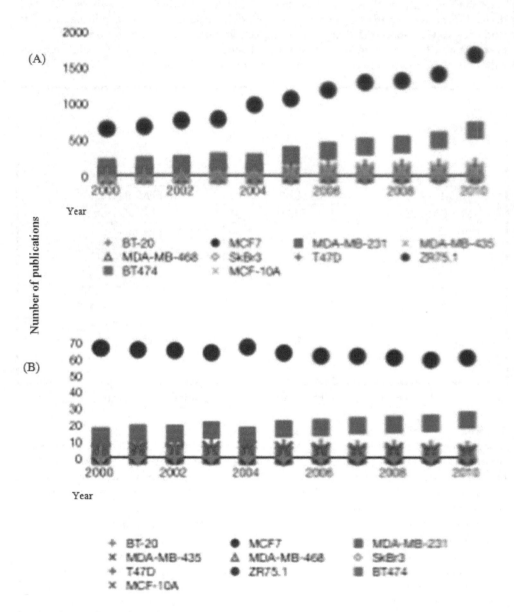

Fig. 1. The total number of publications per breast cancer cell line from 2000 through 2010. The most commonly used cell line is the ER+ MCF7 cell line, followed by ER - MDA-MB-231 cell lines. Many other cell lines are in use, however the number of publications using these models is quite small. A. Total number of publications using breast cancer cell lines. B. Each breast cancer cell line as a percentage of the total breast cancer cell lines used per year.

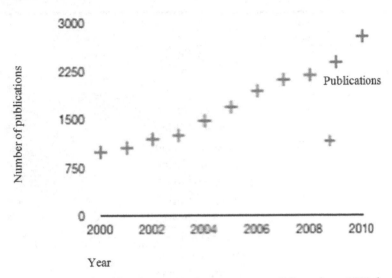

Fig. 2. The total number of publications using breast cancer cell lines from 2000 through 2010. Use of breast cancer cell lines has steadily been rising since 2000.

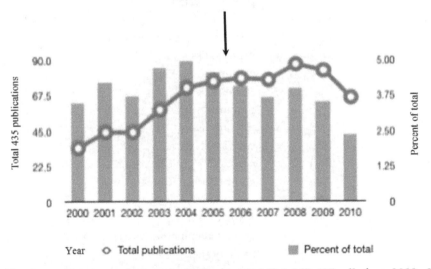

Fig. 3. Number and percent of papers published using MDA-MB-435 cells from 2000 - 2010. The tumor type that gave rise to MDA-MB-435 cells has been controversial since 2000. In 2004, STR profiling confirmed that MDA-MB-435 was not a breast cell line but rather has been contaminated with the M4 melanoma cell line. There has been a subsequent drop in the use and publication of these cells. Shown is the total number of papers published using MDA-MB-435 cells (green bars) and the percent of the total number of publications use MDA-MB-435 cells (blue circles). Arrow denotes when MDA-MB-435 were identified as M14 melanoma cells.

cell line	year established	origin	ER/PR status
BT-20	1958	primary tissue	-/?
SK-Br-3	1970	pleural effusion	+/+
SW13	1971	?	?
MDA-MB-134-VI	1973	pleural effusion	+/-
MDA-MB-157	1973	pleural effusion	?
MDA-MB-175-VII	1973	pleural effusion	?
MDA-MB-231	1973	pleural effusion	-/-
MDA-MB-361	1973	brain metastasis	?
MDA-MB-330	1973	pleural effusion	?
MDA-MB-415	1973	pleural effusion	?
MDA-MB-436	1973	pleural effusion	?
MDA-MB-453	1973	pleural effusion	-/-
MDA-MB-468	1973	pleural effusion	-/-
MDA-MB-157	1974	pleural effusion	?
MCF7	1974	primary tissue	+/+
CAMA-1	1975	pleural effusion	?
SW527	1977	?	?
Hs578Bst	1977	non-tumorigenic breast tissue	-/-
Hs578T	1977	primary tissue	-/-
ZR-75-1	1978	ascites	+/+
ZR-75-30	1978	ascites	?
BT483	1978	primary tissue	?
DU4475	1979	primary tissue	?
T47D	1979	pleural effusion	+/+
MCF10A	1984	non-tumorigenic breast tissue	-/-
MCF10F	1984	non-tumorigenic breast tissue	-/-
MCF10-2A	1984	non-tumorigenic breast tissue	-/-
184A1	1985	normal mammoplasty (transformed)	?
184B5	1985	normal mammoplasty (transformed)	?
UACC-812	1986	primary tissue	-/-
UACC-893	1987	primary tissue	-/-
HCC38	1992	primary tissue	-/-
HCC70	1992	primary tissue	-/-
HCC202	1992	primary tissue	-/-
HCC1008	1994	lymph node	-/-
HCC1143	1994	primary tissue	-/-
HCC1187	1994	primary tissue	?/-

cell line	year established	origin	ER/PR status
HCC1395	1994	primary tissue	-/-
HCC1419	1994	primary tissue	-/-
HCC1428	1995	pleural effusion	?
HCC1500	1995	primary tissue	+/+
HCC1569	1995	primary tissue	-/-
HCC1806	1995	primary tissue	-/-
HCC1937	1995	primary tissue	-/-
HCC1954	1995	primary tissue	+/+
HCC2157	1995	primary tissue	-/+
HCC2158	1996	primary tissue	-/?
HCC1599	1998	primary tissue	-/-
AU565	1998	pleural effusion	?

Table 2. Commercially available cell lines, their establishment date, and hormonal receptor status

Debate has also centered on whether cell lines grown in culture maintain the same genotypic/phenotypic changes that are detected in the primary tissues from which they are derived. Characterization of breast cancer cell lines has been ongoing since their establishment in 1958. In general, breast cancer cell lines are representative models of the primary breast tumors they are derived from (Kao et al., 2009). Initial characterization including karyotyping and comparative genomic hybridization (CGH) demonstrate that, when created and propagated in culture, cell lines maintain the same mutations and chromosomal abnormalities as their primary tumor samples (Lacroix and Laclercq, 2004). While new mutations and chromosomal instability develop in cultured cell lines, overall the genotype remains generally consistent between primary cells and cell lines (Lacroix and Laclercq, 2004). Due to differences in the *in vitro* environment, lack of surrounding naturally occurring microenvironment, and selection pressures, differentiation in culture can occur (Kao et al., 2009; Lacroix and Laclercq, 2004; Voskoglou-Nomikos et al., 2003). Because cancer cells are inherently unstable, differences between same cell line grown in different labs under different environments, even if the growth conditions are the same, are evident (Lacroix and Laclercq, 2004; Osborne et al., 1987). This impacts experimentation as data derived from one lab may not be reproducible in another lab, even is using the same cell line. Caution must be taken when relying on one or two cell lines to draw conclusions.

Use of more modern molecular techniques to characterize cell lines has revealed that while differences between primary cells and cell lines do exist. These techniques do confirm, however, that cell lines maintain the molecular distinction found the primary tumors. Gene expression changes detected in primary tumors are not dramatically different to those found in culture systems, even when cultures are grown directly on plastic in 2D cultures or in reconstituted 3D cultures (Vargo-Gogola and Rosen, 2007). Direct comparison of primary tissue to cultured cells revealed "close similarities" between molecular profiles (Dairkee et al., 2004). Indeed, even epigenetic changes found in primary cancers are similarly detected in cell lines (Lacroix and Laclercq, 2004). This suggests that cell lines are an appropriate model of primary disease and, depending on the research focus, cell lines will faithfully reflect the processes of primary tissues.

Since cell lines generally remain faithful in terms of the molecular and genetic profiles of the primary tumor from which they are derived, it is critical to consider the correct model system. While ER/PR status of primary tumors leans predominantly toward ER+ expression (55-60%), most breast cancer cell lines have been derived from ER - tumors or pleural effusions (McGuire et al., 1978)(Table 2). Therefore it is of utmost importance to select the proper model to answer the experimental question. A detailed analysis of the applicability of cell lines to accurately model primary breast tumors revealed that overall breast cancer cell lines as a whole do model primary tumors, however on an individual basis, one specific cell line does not accurately mirror a primary breast tumor, even with the same gene expression profile. Since variability in cell lines exist, it is generally thought that to more accurately predict outcomes in primary tissue, a panel of breast cancer cell lines rather than just 1 or 2 individual lines should be tested. Using panels more accurately reflects primary breast tumors and will help translate findings from *in vitro* studies to *in vivo* therapeutic options (Dairkee et al., 2004).

Microarray analysis clearly defined primary breast tumors and breast cancer cell lines at the genetic level. Perou and others have conducted detailed studies using microarray platforms and determined a molecular signature of gene expression changes found in primary breast cancer tumors (Alizadeh et al., 2001; Perou et al., 1999b; Perou et al., 2000b; Ross et al., 2000; Sorlie et al., 2001). These signatures are used to understand the molecular basis of breast cancer and to define different subtypes of cancer that occur naturally in humans. It was also developed as a diagnostic tool to detect breast cancer tumors earlier and to facilitate proper treatment based on a gene signature. Based on these studies, 5 molecular signatures and types of primary breast tumors have been identified. These are luminal A, luminal B, basal-like, HER2+, and normal-like profiles (Perou et al., 1999a; Perou et al., 2000a; Ross et al., 2000; Sorlie et al., 2001). Prior to establishment of these molecular signatures, diagnosis was determined by receptor expression status, i.e. ER/PR/HER2, and treatment regimes assigned accordingly. Using this molecular approach, luminal A and luminal B tend to also be ER + expressing tumors, basal-like encompasses ER - tumors, HER2+ incorporate those HER2+ expressing tumors, and normal-like have similar expression patterns to non-cancerous cells (Perou et al., 1999a; Perou et al., 2000a; Ross et al., 2000; Sorlie et al., 2001). Such molecular characterization will lead to providing more personalized therapy to patients. Efficacy of drugs in different subtypes will be easily determined and accurately assigned to patients expressing a similar molecular profile. While such personalized medicine may be still in the future, some current breast cancer treatment options that exist today are based on the molecular profile of the tumor. For example, tumors expressing the estrogen receptor are treated with selective estrogen receptor modulator (SERM) or other similar anti-estrogen compound whereas tumors lacking ER do not receive the same therapy. Similarly, HER2+ tumors are susceptible to trastuzumab because of HER2 expression. In the future as molecular characterization improves and new chemotherapeutics are developed, more personalized options will be available.

Do cell lines reflect the molecular signature of primary tumors? In a direct comparison of the molecular profiles from cell lines and primary tumors, Kao et. al. found that instead of the 5 breast cancer subtypes identified in primary breast tumors, cell lines can be divided into three main groups, luminal, basal A, or basal B phenotypes (Kao et al., 2009). Luminal cells contained all ER + cell lines, both Basal A and B consisted of all ER - cell lines. HER2+ cell lines were grouped into the luminal. Basal A contained the HCC cells and BRCA1 mutant cells, whereas basal B genotype contained non-tumorigenic lines including MCF10A cells (Kao et al., 2009). This highlights that breast cancer cell lines are a model of disease.

Cell lines are merely a model of breast disease that aim to provide clinical predictability of outcomes in humans. To directly test the applicability of breast cancer cell lines, xenograft cancer models, and mouse breast cancer models to clinical outcome, Voskoglou-Nomikos et. al. compared outcomes *in vitro* to those in xenograft models, to mouse models and phase II clinical trails (Voskoglou-Nomikos et al., 2003). In these comparisons, a general correlation between relative risk (predictive value of a drug in cell line) and the phase II human trial (tumor/control ratio) existed for *in vitro* cell lines. A general predictive value when using xenograft models to predict outcome to chemotherapy was detected, however this was dependent on the drug tested and the grade/type of tumor analyzed (Voskoglou-Nomikos et al., 2003). Overall, Vaskoglou-Nomikos et. al. concluded that cell lines and xenograft models were good predictors of clinical phase II trial outcomes, but are reliable predictors only when testing cytotoxic drugs and when using the correct model system. These models generally were not predictive of human outcomes when testing non-cytotoxic drugs (Voskoglou-Nomikos et al., 2003). Taken together, these studies emphasize the critical need to establish more breast cancer cell lines that model the heterogeneity of breast cancer and to employ many *in vitro* and xenograft model systems using multiple cell lines per experiment to reliably predict clinical outcome.

4. Contamination

Overt contamination of cell lines, such as bacterial, fungal or yeast infections, is readily detectable merely by altered appearance of the culture and can be rectified without impacting the quality or reproducibility of the data. Less overt contamination, such as mycoplasma and cell line cross-contamination, can occur undetected and can seriously jeopardize experimental findings. While it is well recognized that periodic testing for mycoplasma is a necessary requirement when using cell lines, cross-contamination with other cell lines is less recognized as a problem and therefore and cell authentication practices are not routine.

Cell line cross-contamination is most evident in the case of MDA-MB-435 cells. When Ross et. al. published the molecular profiles of breast cancer cell lines in 2000, the MDA-MB-435 cell line consistently fell outside the range of profiles of the other breast cancer cell lines and clustered with melanoma cell lines (Ross et al., 2000). This sparked great debate about the authenticity of the this line. Derived in 1976 from the pleural effusion of a 31 year old patient with metastatic adenocarcinoma of the breast, initial debate suggested that this was still a breast cancer cell line, but had been derived from a patient who may have also had undiagnosed melanoma (Cailleau et al., 1978). Data indicating that MDA-MB-435 cells expressed a mixture of both melanoma and epithelial markers fueled this debate, however the overwhelming belief was the these were indeed breast cancer cells (Chambers, 2009; Sellappan et al., 2004)(Figures 2 and 3). Indeed, early characterization of the cell line indicated that they were highly metastatic and secrete milk proteins, findings consistent with those of breast cancer cells (Howlett et al., 1994; Price, 1996; Price et al., 1990; Price and Zhang, 1990; Sellappan et al., 2004; Suzuki et al., 2006; Welch, 1997). Confusingly, MDA-MB-435 cells also expressed the melanocyte markers tyrosinase, melan A and S100 (Ellison et al.,

2002; Sellappan et al., 2004). Because of such conflicting results, these data just propagated the debate instead of satisfactorily squelching it as intended. MDA-MB-435 cells were still used and published as a breast cancer cell line (Figure 3).

Finally in 2007, DNA fingerprinting, or short tandem repeat (STR) analysis, in conjunction with SNP analysis, cytogenetic analysis, and comparative genomic hybridization using the earliest stocks of MDA-MB-435 cells revealed that these cells were identical to the M14 human melanoma cells and were melanoma rather than breast cancer cells (Garraway et al., 2005)(Rae et al., 2007). Rae et. al., who conducted the analysis, concluded that at some point early in passage, MDA-MB-435 cells were contaminated with M14 melanoma cells which took over the colony, leading to the establishment of a M14 melanoma cell line rather than a breast cancer line (Rae et al., 2007). This change was never detected. Stocks were unknowingly mislabeled, marked as MDA-MB-435 cells and distributed. Still, after the molecular characterization was published, debate as to whether MDA-MB-435 were really M14 melanoma cells or if M14 were really MDA-MB-435 breast cell still existed (Chambers, 2009). Ultimately, it was determined that MDA-MB-435 cells were really M14, based on the original 1974 publication that initially characterized the morphology, growth and tumorigenicity of MDA-MB-435 cells. In the original paper, MDA-MB-435 cells were reportedly non-tumorigenic in nude mice. After the initial creation in 1974, the MDA-MB-435 cells were not extensively used for testing until the 1990s when Price et. al. used these cells. At this time, MDA-MB-435 cells were characterized as a tumorigenic cell line (Cailleau et al., 1978; Price, 1996; Price et al., 1990; Price and Zhang, 1990).

While impossible to reconstruct that actually happened, this indirect evidence suggests that the MDA-MB-435 cells were contaminated with M14 melanoma cells and the original breast cancer cells died off. Subsequent frozen stocks were of the contaminating M14 cell lines, although they were labeled as MDA-MB-435 cells. No one was aware of this misidentification. Therefore, M14 cells were masquerading as MDA-MB-435 cells and used as a model of breast cancer until 2007. A total of 1803 PubMed indexed articles using MDA-MB-435 cells were published over that period (Figure 3). Since 2007, however, the number of publications using MDA-MB-435 cells has diminished, indicating that it is generally accepted that these cells are clearly not breast cancer cells and therefore should not be used as such.

4.1 Authentication

Cell line cross-contamination is hardly a new problem in tissue culture studies, although it still remains largely ignored. When HeLa were the only human cell line and few scientists studied them, cross-contamination was not a concern(Buehring et al., 2004; Skloot, 2010). Now, it is estimated that 20 - 30% of all cell lines are inadvertently contaminated (Alston-Roberts et al., 2010; Buehring et al., 2004; Gartler, 1968; Rojas and Steinsapir, 1983). Gartler et. al, was the first to highlight the problem in 1967 at the Second Decennial Review Conference on Cell, Tissue and Organ culture (Gartler, 1968). He was the first to demonstrate that many cultures from many labs were contaminated with other cell lines, primarily by HeLa cells. This meant that a significant amount of research was incorrectly interpreted because it was conducted in a different cell line and therefore the data were false. His findings were largely ignored. Over the years, others, including MacLeod, Freshney, Nardone, Alston-R, Buehring and Capes-Davis, have also documented contamination with HeLa and other cell lines, including cross-species contamination, however this issue has rarely been adequately addressed (Alston-Roberts et al., 2010; Bartallon et al., 2010; Buehring et al., 2004; Capes-Davis et al., 2010; Freshney, 2008; MacLeod et al., 2008; MacLeod et al., 1999; SDO et al., 2010). Recent efforts have again been made to increase awareness of this problem and many calls for action have been published (Buehring et al., 2004; Capes-Davis et al., 2010; Freshney, 2008, 2010b; Lichter et al., 2010; MacLeod et al., 2008; MacLeod et al., 1999; SDO et al., 2010). A group of concerned scientists gathered and created the ATCC Standard Development Organization (ATCC SDO) to develop standards for cell authentication and with maintaining databases of STR profiles.

Eliminating contamination has an easy solution. Cell line authentication using a standardized technique, Short Tandem Repeat Analysis (STR), can provide an unique DNA fingerprint of the cell line (Azari et al., 2007; Bartallon et al., 2010; Masters et al., 2001; Nims et al., 2010; Parson et al., 2005). STR is inexpensive, standardized, and provides proven methodology to produce cell line identities that is reproducible between labs. An aliquot of DNA can be analyzed and compared with known STR profiles to authenticate the cell line. STR profiles for the most commonly used cell lines are freely available and STR services are available at many universities or companies. According to the standards developed by the ATCC-SDO, cells in active use should be authenticated by STR every 2 months (SDO et al., 2010). The ATCC-SDO also recommends that such documentation of authenticity be provided with grant applications and with manuscript submission. Many funding agencies and journals agree with this idea and suggest that scientists provide such documentation prior to acceptance of a manuscript, however at this time, this is merely a recommendation.

5. Future directions

Use of breast cancer cell lines as models of breast disease will not diminish in the near future. These cell lines are an excellent resource to test novel hypotheses and to gain greater understanding about how cells work and how breast cancer can be treated. On the whole, the established cell lines are a good model for disease, however additional cell lines should be created. The addition on new lines, especially those derived from various forms of breast cancer will only strengthen the data gleaned from them. Likewise, cell authentication should become a routine part of experimental procedures. By periodically ensuring the cell lines being tested are truly the correct lines will eliminate the generation and publication of false data. Authentication will save money and potentially careers if done of a routine basis.

6. References

Ali, S., and Coombes, R.C. (2000). Estrogen receptor alpha in human breast cancer: occurence and signficance. J Mammary Gland Biol Neoplasia 5, 271-281.

Alizadeh, A., Ross, D., Perou, C.M., and van de Rijn, M. (2001). Towards a novel classification of human malignancies based on gene expression patterns. J Pathol 195, 41-52.

Alston-Roberts, C., Barallon, R., Bauer, S., Butler, J., Capes-Davis, A., Dirks, W., Elmore, E., Furtado, M., Kerrigan, L., Kline, M., *et al.* (2010). Cell line misidentification: the beginning of the end. Nat Rev Cancer *10*, 441-448.

Azari, S., Ahmani, N., Tehrani, M., and Shokri, F. (2007). Profiling and authetication of human cell lines using short tandem repeat (STR) loci: Report from the National Cell Bank of Iran. Biologicals *35*, 195-202.

Bartallon, R., Bauer, S., Butler, J., Capes-Davis, A., Dirks, W., Elmore, E., Furtado, M., Kline, M., Kohara, A., Los, G., *et al.* (2010). Recommendation of short tandem repeat profiling for authenticating human cell lines, stem cells, and tissues. In Vitro Cell Dev Biol Anim *46*, 727-732.

Borras, M., Lacroix, M., Legros, N., and Leclercq, G. (1997). Estrogen receptor-negative/progesterone receptor-positive Evsa-T mammary tumor cells: a model for assessing the biological property of this peculiar phenotype of breast cancers. Cancer Lett *120*, 23-30.

Brown, R., and Henderson, J. (1983). The mass production and distribution of HeLa cells at Tuskegee Institute, 1953-55. J History of Med and Allied Sciences *38*, 415-431.

Buehring, G., Eby, E., and Eby, M. (2004). Cell line cross-contamination: How aware are mammalian cell culturists of the problem and how to monitor it? In Vitro Cell Dev Biol Anim *40*, 211-215.

Burdall, S., Hanby, A., Lansdown, M., and Speirs, V. (2003). Breast cancer cell lines: friend or foe? Breast Cancer Res *5*, 89-95.

Cailleau, R., Olive, M., and Cruciger, Q. (1978). Long-term human breast carcinoma cell lines of metastatic origin: preliminary characterization. In Vitro *14*, 911-915.

Capes-Davis, A., Theodossopoulos, G., Atkin, I., Drexler, H., Kohara, A., MacLeod, R., Masters, J., Nakamura, Y., Reid, Y., Reddel, R., *et al.* (2010). Check your cultures! A list of cross-contaminated or misidentified cell lines. Int J Cancer *127*, 1-8.

Chambers, A.F. (2009). MDA-MB-435 and M14 cell lines: identical but not M14 melanoma? Cancer Res *69*, 5292-5293.

Coriell, L., McAllister, R., Wagner, B.L., Wilson, S., and Dwight, S. (1958). Growth of primate and non-primate tissue culture cell lines in x-irradiated and cortisone-treated rats. Cancer *11*, 1236-1241.

Coriell, L., and McGarrity, G. (1968). Biohazard hood to prevent infection during microbiological procedures. Appl Microbiology *16*.

Dairkee, S., Ji, Y., Ben, Y., Moore, D., Meng, Z., and Jeffrey, S. (2004). A molecular 'signature' of primary breast cancer culture; patterns resembling tumor tissue. BMC Genomics *5*, 47.

Earle, W., Schillig, E., Stark, T., Straus, N., Brown, M., and Shelton, E. (1943). Production of malignancy in vitro; IV: The mouse fibroblast cultures and changes seen in the living cells. J Natl Cancer Inst *4*, 165-212.

Ellison, G., Klinowska, T., Westwood, R., Docter, E., French, T., and Fox, J. (2002). Further evidence to support melanocyte origin of MDA-MB-435 cells. Mol Path *55*, 294-299.

Evans, V., Earle, W., Sanford, K., Shannon, J., and Waltz, H. (1951). The preparation and handling of replicate tissue cultures for quantiative studies. J Natl Cancer Inst *11*, 907-927.

Freshney, R. (2008). Authentication of cell lines: ignore at your peril! Expert Rev Anticancer Ther *8*, 311-314.

Freshney, R. (2010a). Culture of Animal Cells, Vol Sixth Edition (Hoboken, NJ, John Wiley & Sons).

Freshney, R. (2010b). Database of misidentified cell lines. Int J Cancer *126*, 302-303.

Garraway, L., Widlund, H., Rubin, M., Getz, G., Berger, A., Ramaswamy, S., Beroukhim, R., Milner, D., Granter, S., Du, J., *et al.* (2005). Integrative genomic analyses identify MITF as a lineage survival oncogene amplified in malignant melanoma. Nature *436*, 117-122.

Gartler, S. (1968). Apparent Hela cell contamination of human heteroploid cell lines. Nature *217*, 750-751.

Gey, G., Coffman, W., and Kubicek, M. (1952). Tissue culture studies of the proliferative capacity of cervical carcinoma and normal epithelium. Cancer Res *4*, 264.

Greene, A., Silver, R., Krug, M., and Coriell, L. (1964). Preservation of cell cutlures by freezing in liquid nitrogen vapro. Proc Soc Exp Biol Med *116*, 462-467.

Howlett, A., Peterson, O., Steeg, P., and Bissell, M. (1994). A novel function for the nm23-1 gene: overexpression in human breast carcinoma cells leads to the formation of basement membrane and growth arrest. J Natl Cancer Inst *86*, 1838-1844.

Kao, J., Salari, K., Bocanegra, M., Choi, Y.-L., Girard, L., Gandhi, J., Kwei, K., Hernandez-Boussard, T., Wang, P., Gazdar, A.F., *et al.* (2009). Molecular profiling of breast cancer cell lines defines relevant tumor models and provides a resource for cancer gene discovery. PLoS One *4*, e6146.

Lacroix, M., and Laclercq, G. (2004). Relevance of breast cancer cell lines as models for breast tumours: an update. Breast Cancer Res and Treatment *83*, 249-289.

Lasfargues, E., and Ozzello, L. (1958). Cultivation of human breast cancer carcinomas. J Natl Cancer Inst *21*, 1131-1147.

Lichter, P., Allgayer, H., Bartsch, H., Fusenig, N., Hemminki, K., von Knebel Doeberitz, M., Kyewski, B., Miller, A., and zur Hausen, H. (2010). Obligation for cell line authentication: appeal for concerted action. Int J Cancer *126*, 1.

MacDonald, C. (2002). Primary culture and the establishment of cell lines (Oxford, England, Oxford Press).

MacLeod, R., Dirks, W., and Drexler, H. (2008). One falsehood leads easily to another. Int J Cancer *122*, 2165-2168.

MacLeod, R., Dirks, W., Matsuo, Y., Kaufmann, M., Milch, H., and Drexler, H. (1999). Widespread intraspecies cross-contamination of human tumor cell lines arising at source. Int J Cancer *83*, 555-563.

Masters, J., Thomson, J., Daly-Burns, B., Reid, Y., Dirks, W., Packer, P., Toji, L., Ohno, T., Tanabe, H., Arlett, C., *et al.* (2001). Short tandem repeat profiling provides an international reference standard for human cell lines. PNAS *98*, 8012-8017.

McAllister, R., and Coriell, L. (1956). Cultivation of human epithelial cells in tissue culture. Proc Soc Exp Biol Med *91*, 389-394.

McAteer, J., and Davis, J. (2002). Basic cell culture technique and the maintenance of cell lines. (Oxford, England, Oxford Press).

McGarrity, G., and Coriell, L. (1973). Mass airflow cabinet for control of airborne infection of laboratory rodents. Appl Microbiology 26, 167-172.

McGarrity, G., and Coriell, L. (1974). Modified laminar flow biological safety cabinet. Appl Microbiology 28, 647-650.

McGuire, W., Zava, D., Horwitz, K., and Chamness, G. (1978). Steroid receptors in breast tumors -- current status. Curr Top Exp Endocrinol 3, 93-129.

Miller, D. (2004). Sydney Ringer: physiologial saline, calcium and the contraction of the heart. J Physiol 555, 585-587.

Nims, R., Sykes, G., Cotrill, K., Ikonomi, P., and Elmore, E. (2010). Short tandem repeat profiling: part of an overall strategy for reducing the frequency of cell misidentification. In Vitro Cell Dev Biol Anim 46, 811-819.

Osborne, C.K., Hobbs, K., and Trent, J. (1987). Biological differences among MCF-7 human breast cancer cell lines from different laboratories. Breast Cancer Res and Treatment 9, 111-121.

Parson, W., Kirchebner, R., Muhlmann, R., Renner, K., Kofler, A., Schmidt, S., and Kofler, R. (2005). Cancer cell line identification by short tandem repeat profiling: power and limitations. FASEB J 19, 434-436.

Perou, C., Jeffrey, S., van de Rijn, M., Rees, C., Eisen, M., Ross, D., Pergamenschikov, A., Williams, C., Zhu, S., Lee, J., et al. (1999a). Distinctive gene expression patterns in human mammary epithelial cells and breast cancers. Proc Natl Acad Sci U S A 96, 9212-9217.

Perou, C., Sorlie, T., Eisen, M., van de Rijn, M., Jeffrey, S., Rees, C., Pollack, J., Ross, D., Johnsen, H., Akslen, L., et al. (2000a). Molecular portrait of human breast tumors. Nature 406, 747-752.

Perou, C.M., Jeffrey, S., van de Rijn, M., Rees, C., Eisen, M., Ross, D., Pergamenschikov, A., Williams, C., Zhu, S., Lee, J., et al. (1999b). Distinctive gene expression patterns in human mammary epithelial cells and breast cancer. PNAS 96, 9212-9217.

Perou, C.M., Sorlie, T., Eisen, M., van de Rijn, M., Jeffrey, S., Rees, C., Pollack, J., Ross, D., Johnsen, H., Akslen, L.A., et al. (2000b). Molecular portraits of human breast tumors. Nature 406, 747-752.

Price, J. (1996). Metastasis from human breast cancer cell lines. Breast Cancer Res and Treatment 39, 93-102.

Price, J., Polyzos, A., Zhang, R., and Daniels, L. (1990). Tumorigenicity and metastasis of human breast carcinoma cell lines in nude mice. Cancer Res 50, 717-721.

Price, J., and Zhang, R. (1990). Studies of human breast cancer metastasis using nude mice. Cancer Metastasis Rev 8, 285-297.

Rae, J.M., Creighton, C., Meck, J., Haddad, B., and Johnson, M. (2007). MDA-MB-435 cells are derived from M14 melanoma cells -- a loss for breast cancer, but a boon for melanoma research. Breast Cancer Res and Treatment 104, 13-19.

Ringer, S. (1882). Regarding the action of hydrate of ammonia, and hydrate of potash on the ventricle of the frog's heart. J Physiol 3, 380-393.

Ringer, S. (1883). A further contribution regarding the influence of the different constituents of the blood on the contraction of the heart. J Physiol 4, 29-42.

Rojas, A.M., and Steinsapir, J. (1983). Multiple mechanisms of regulation of estrogen action in the rat uterus: effects of insulin. Endocrinology 112, 586-591.

Ross, D., Scherf, U., Eisen, M., Perou, C.M., Rees, C., Spellman, P., Iyer, V., Jeffrey, S., van der Rijn, M., Waltham, M., et al. (2000). Systemic variation in gene expression patterns in human cancer cell lines. Nature Genetics 24, 227-235.

Ryan, J. (2007a). Carrel and the early days of tissue culture. Corning www.corning.com.

Ryan, J. (2007b). Cell Culture Solves a Problem. Corning www.corning.com.

Ryan, J. (2007c). Charles Lindbergh - Aviator and cell and organ culturist. Corning wwwcorningcom.

Sanford, K., Earle, W., and Likely, G. (1948). The growth in vitro of single isolated tissue cells. J Natl Cancer Inst 9, 229-246.

SDO, A., Alston-Roberts, C., Barallon, R., Bauer, S., Butler, J., Capes-Davis, A., Dirks, W., Elmore, E., Furtado, M., Kerrigan, L., et al. (2010). Cell line misidentification: the beginning of the end. Nat Rev Cancer 10, 441-448.

Sellappan, S., Grijalva, R., Zhou, X., Yang, W., Eli, M., Mills, G., and Yu, D. (2004). Lineage infidelity of MDA-MB-435 cells: expression of melanocyte proteins in a breast cancer cell line. Cancer Res 64, 3479-3485.

Silver, R., Lehr, H., Summers, A., Greene, A., and Coriell, L. (1964). Use of dielectric heating (shortwave diathermy) in thawing frozen suspensions of tissue culture cells. Proc Soc Exp Biol Med 115, 453-455.

Skloot, R. (2010). The Immortal Life of Henrietta Lacks.

Sorlie, T., Perou, C., Tibshirani, R., Aas, T., Geisler, S., Johnsen, H., Hastie, T., Eisen, M., van de Rijn, M., Jeffrey, S., et al. (2001). Gene expression patterns in breast carcinomas distinguish tumor subclasses with clinical implications. Proc Natl Acad Sci U S A 98, 10869-10874.

Soule, H., Maloney, T., Wolman, S.R., Peterson, W.J., Brenz, R., McGrath, C., Russo, J., Pauley, R., Jones, R., and Brooks, S. (1990). Isolation and characterization of a spontaneously immortalized human breast epithelial cell line, MCF10. Cancer Res 50, 6075-6086.

Soule, H., Vazquez, J., Long, A., Albert, S., and M, B. (1973). A human cell line from a pleural effusion derived from a breast carcinoma. J Natl Cancer Inst 51, 1409-1416.

Suzuki, M., Mose, E., Montel, V., and Tarin, D. (2006). Dormant cancer cells retrieved from metastasis-free organs regain tumorigenic and metastasis potency. Am J Pathol 169, 673-681.

Vargo-Gogola, T., and Rosen, J. (2007). Modelling breast cancer: one size does not fit all. Nature Reviews Cancer 7, 659-672.

Voskoglou-Nomikos, T., Pater, J., and Seymour, L. (2003). Clinical predictive value of the in vitro cell line, human xenograft, and mouse allograft preclinical cancer models. Clin Cancer Res 9, 4227-4239.

Welch, D. (1997). Technical considerations for studying cancer metastasis in vivo. Clin Exp
    Metastasis, 272-306.

2

Insulin-Like-Growth Factor-Binding-Protein 7: An Antagonist to Breast Cancer

Tania Benatar, Yutaka Amemiya,
Wenyi Yang and Arun Seth
Division of Molecular and Cellular Biology, Sunnybrook Research Institute,
Department of Anatomic Pathology, Sunnybrook Health Sciences Centre,
Department of Laboratory Medicine and Pathobiology,
University of Toronto, ON,
Canada

1. Introduction

1.1 The insulin-like growth factor (IGF) system

The insulin-like growth factor (IGF) system has been shown to have an integral role in normal growth and development, and in the pathophysiology of various cancers. The IGF system is comprised of a series of circulating ligands (IGF-1, IGF-2), transmembrane receptor tyrosine kinases (IGF-1R, IGF-2R, and the insulin receptor (IR), high affinity ligand-binding proteins (IGFBP1-6), IGFBP proteases, and several low affinity IGFBP-related proteins (IGFBP-rp1 to 10) that work in unison to regulate cell growth [1].

There are two key circulating ligands, IGF-1 and IGF-2, which share approximately 50% structural homology with insulin[2]. IGF-1 is produced primarily in the liver in response to circulating levels of growth hormone(GH) [3]. IGF-1 and IGF-2 are highly homologous small peptide hormones of approximately 7 kDa molecular mass, which are important mitogens that affect cell growth and metabolism [2]. IGFs interact with specific cell surface receptors, designated type I and type 2 IGF receptors, and can also interact with insulin receptor (IR).

The type I IGF receptor (IGF-1R) is a transmembrane heterotetramer consisting of 2 extracellular alpha subunits and two intracellular beta subunits linked by disulfide bonds (fig 1). The intracellular component of IGF-1R has intrinsic tyrosine kinase activity that requires ligand binding for activation [4]. The IGF-1R and the IR share approximately 60% homology which allows them to form hybrid receptors [5]. As a result of this homology, IGF-1R can be activated not only by IGF-1 but also IGF-2 and insulin, although the affinity of IGF-1R for IGF-2 and insulin is approximately 10 fold and 1000 fold lower than for IGF-1, respectively [6]. The type 2 IGF receptor (IGF-2R), which is identical to the cation-independent mannose-6-phosphate receptor, binds IGF-2 with 500 fold increased affinity over IGF-1[7]. IGF-2R does not bind insulin. Most of the biological activity of IGF-2 is thought to be mediated through binding IGF-1R[7]. IGF-2 is known to function primarily as a scavenger receptor, regulating circulating IGF-II levels through internalization and degradation [7].

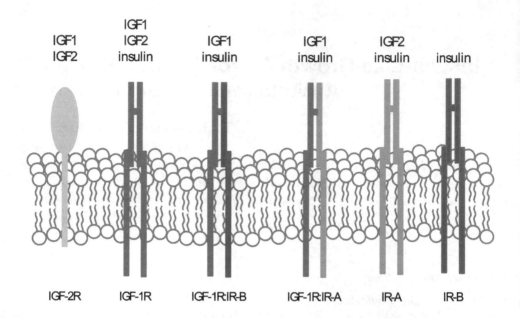

Fig. 1. Cell surface receptors for IGFs and insulin. Illustration of the different transmembrane receptors and ligands of the IGF system. Purple represents the alpha and beta subunit of IGF-1R; red represents the alpha and beta subunit of the IR-B; orange represents the alpha and beta subunit of the IR-A ; green represents the IGF-2R. The potential ligand(s) is shown above the respective receptor.

Two distinct insulin receptor isoforms have been identified and are known to hybridize with IGF-1R. The insulin receptor isoform A (IR-A), the IR fetal isoform, is generated by alternative splicing through the deletion of exon 11 of the insulin receptor gene whereas the insulin receptor isoform B (IR-B) retains exon 11 [8]. IR-A is the predominant isoform expressed in fetal tissues and cancers with ubiquitous expression, whereas IR-B appears in postnatal life within insulin-target tissues, such as muscle, adipose tissue and kidney [9,10,11]. Data obtained from murine 32D hemopoietic cells demonstrated that IR-A preferentially induces mitogenic and anti-apoptotic signals, whereas IR-B predominantly induces cell differentiation signals [12]. IR-A, but not IR-B, binds IGF-II with high affinity and operates as a second physiological receptor for this growth factor [13]. The two IR isoform half receptors (composed of one alpha and one beta subunit) can heterodimerize, resulting in the formation of either homologous IR-A/IR-A or IR-B/IR-B receptors as well as the hybrid IR-A/IR-B insulin receptors [14](fig 1). Heterodimers can also form between IGF-1R and IR, resulting in the hybrid IGF-1R/IR-A and hybrid IGF-1R/IR-B. Hybrid IGF-1R/IR receptors are believed to mostly bind IGF-1, although they can also bind insulin but with a much lower affinity [15]. The IGF system is also regulated by a group of at least six high affinity ligand-binding proteins, the insulin-like binding proteins (IGFBPs), as well as low affinity ligand-binding proteins (IGFBP-rp1 to 10).

2. The IGFBP superfamily

Unlike insulin, IGFs circulate in biological fluids complexed to a family of structurally related binding proteins, called IGF-binding proteins (IGFBPs). The IGFBP superfamily can be subdivided into two groups: the high affinity IGFBPs (IGFBP1 to 6) and the low-affinity IGFBPs (IGFBP7 to 10, and IGFBP-rP5 to 10). [16].

High affinity binding proteins (IGFBPs)

There are, to date, six well characterized mammalian IGFBPs, designated IGFBP-1 through - 6. IGFBPs are capable of binding IGF-1 and IGF-2 with higher affinity than their interactions with the IGF-1R, but do not bind to insulin. Some IGFBPs compete for activity of IGFs at the receptor level and antagonize IGF signaling, while others (eg. IGFBP2 and IGFBP5) appear to amplify IGF signaling [17]. Therefore, IGFBPs function not only as carriers of IGFs, thereby prolonging the half-life of the IGFs, but also act as modulators of IGF availability and activity[18]. Apart from their ability to inhibit or enhance IGF actions, all the IGFBPs have been reported to exert distinct biological actions such as cell proliferation, differentiation, migration, angiogenesis and apoptosis through an IGF/IGF-1R-independent manner [19,20,21,22,23].

All six IGFBPs share approximately 35% sequence identity with each other. The primary structures of mammalian IGFBPs appear to contain three distinct domains of roughly similar sizes: the conserved N-terminal domain, the highly variable midregion, and the conserved C-terminal domain. Within their N-terminal domain, all IGFBPs share a common conserved cysteine-rich domain termed IGFBP motif (GCGCCXXC) (fig 2). The IGFBP motif is encoded by a single exon, has overall similar topology and is only present in vertebrates [19]. Ten to 12 of the 16-20 cysteines found in the prepeptides are located within this domain. In IGFBP1-5 these 12 cysteines are fully conserved, whereas 10 of the 12 cysteines are invariant in IGFBP6 [19]. The midregion is believed to act structurally as a hinge between the N and C terminal domains. Posttranslational modifications (glycosylation, phosphorylation) of the IGFBPs has been found only in the midregion so far. The C-termini of IGFBPs, like the N-terminal domain, are highly conserved, and contain the remaining 6 of the total 16-20 cysteines. The primary sequence of all members of the IGFBP family surrounding the last 5 cysteines is strikingly similar (~40%), implying that the tertiary structure of the C-terminal domain should be almost identical. Interestingly, the amino acid sequences embracing these last 5 cysteines share 37% similarity with the thyroglobulin-type-1 domain, a structural motif occasionally employed as an inhibitor of proteases [19,24]. It has been hypothesized that the N and C-terminal domains are capable of acting independently of each other based on the fact that the cysteines within each of the conserved regions are even numbered, and that proteolytic cleavage products of IGFBPs contain either the C or N-terminal regions. Indeed, disulphide linkages have been shown to form typically within each conserved domain, rather than between domains[25,26]. All the IGFBPs are encoded by 4 exons, except IGFBP3 which has an extra exon, exon 5, that is not translated. The striking observation is the correlation between these IGFBP exons and the three protein domains of IGFBPs. The N-terminal domain is encoded within exon 1 in all of the IGFBPs, as is the 5' untranslated region and a few amino acids of the midregion. Exon 2 encodes the nonconserved midregion. Both exons 3 and 4 encode for the conserved C-terminal domain. The containment of the N-terminal domain within one exon, combined with the ability to bind IGFs, supports the concept of an IGFBP superfamily [27,19].

```
IGFBP-1    MSEV-----PVAR-VWLVLL-LLTVQVGVT------AG-----AP--WQ-----------CA-PC---SAEKL-ALC-PP--------VSA-------SCS-EVTR--SAGCGCCPM--CALPLGAACG  72
IGFBP-2    MLPRVGCPALPLPPPPLPLLPLLLLLLGAS-----GGGGGARAEVLFR-----------CP-PC---TPERL-AACGPPRVAPPAAVAAVAGGARMPCA-ELVR--EPGCGCCSV--CARLEGEACG 102
IGFBP-3    MQRA--------RPTLWAAALTLLVLLRGPPVAR--AGASSGGLG-PVVR-----------CE-PC---DARAL-AQCAPP--------PAV---------CA-ELVR--EPGCGCCLT--CALSEGQPCG  82
IGFBP-4    ML----------PLCLVAAL-LLA--AGP--------GPS--LGDEAIH-----------CP-PC---SEEKL-ARCRP--------FVG---------CE-ELVR--EPGCGCCAT--CALGLGMPCG  68
IGFBP-5    M-----------VLLTAVLLLAAYAGP---------AQS--LG-SFVH-----------CE-PC---DEKAL-SMCPPS-------PLG--------C--ELVK--EPGCGCCMT--CALAEGQSCG  68
IGFBP-6    MT----------PHRLLPLLLLLALLLAAS------PG----G-ALAR-----------CP-GC---GQGVQ-AGC-PG--------G---------CV-EEEDGGSPABGCAEAEGCLRREGQECG  72

IGFBP-7    M------ERPSLRALLLGAAGLLLLLL--P----LSSSSSS---D----------T----CG-PC---EP----ASCPPL-------PPLG--------CLLGETR--DACGCCPM--CARGEGEPCG  72
IGFBP-8    M-TAASMG-PVR---VAFV-VLLALC-----------------SRPAVGQN--------CSGPC-RCPDEPAPRCPA----------G--------VS--LVL--DGGCGCCRV--CAKQLGELCT  69
IGFBP-9    MQSVQSTSFCLRKQCLCLTFLLLHLL----------GQVAATQR-----------CPPQCPGRCPATP-PTCAP----------G--------VR--AVL--DGCSCCLV--CARQRGESCS  76
IGFBP-10   M-SSR-IA---R--ALALVVTLLHL-----------TRLALST-----------CPAAC--HCPLEA-PKCAP----------G--------VG--IVR--DGCGCCKV--CAKQLNEDCS  65
IGFBP-rP5  MQIP----------RAALLPLLLLLLAAPASAQ------LSRAGRSAPLAAG-------CPDRC---EP----ARCPPQ------PEH--------CEGGRAR--DACGCCEV--CQAPEGAACG  77
IGFBP-rP6  MKSV----------LLLTTLLVPAHLVAAW----------SNNYAVD----------CPQHC---DS----SECKSS-------PR--------CK-RTVL--DDCGCCRV--CAAGRGETCY  66
IGFBP-rP7  MRGTPKTH------LLAFS--LLCLL---------------SKVR-TQL----------CPTPC--TCPWPP-PRCPL--------G--------VP--LVL--DGCGCCRV--CARRLGEPCD  65
IGFBP-rP8  MRWFLPWT-LAAV-TAAAASTVLATALSPAPTTMDFTPAPLEDTSSRPQF---------CKWPC--ECPPSP-PRCPL--------G--------VS--LIT--DGCECCKM--CAQQLGDNCT  88
IGFBP-rP9  MQGLLFSTLLLAG-LAQFCCRVQGTG--PLDTTPEGRRGEVSDAPQRKQF---------CHWPC--KCPQQK-PRCPP--------G--------VS--LVR--DGGCGCCKI--CAKQPGEICN  87
IGFBP-rP10 MLPP-----PRPAA-ALALPVLLLLLVVLTPP--PTGARPSPGPDYLRRGWMRLLAEGEGCA-PC---RP----EECA--------APRG-------CLAGRVR--DACGCCWE--CANLEGQLCD  91

IGFBP-1    ---VA-TA---RCAR--GLSCRALPGEQQP-LHALTRGQ----G-ACVQES -----DAS---AP-HAAEAGSPESPESTEITEEEL-LDNFHLMA---------------P 143
IGFBP-2    ---VY-TP--RCGQ--GLRCYPHPGSELP-LQALVMGE---G-TCEKRR -----DAEYGASPEQVADNGDDHS-EG-GLVENHV-DSTMNMLGGGGSAG-RR------P 183
IGFBP-3    ---IY-TE--RCGS--GLRCQPSPDEARP-LQALLDGR---G-LCVNAS AVSRLRAYLLPAPPAPGNASESEEDRSAGSVESPS-VSSTHRVSD--PK--FH------P 167
IGFBP-4    ---VY-TP--RCGS--GLRCYPPRGVEKP-LHTLMBGQ---G-VCMELA EI---EAIQESLQ--PSDKDEGDHPMNS-------------F--S---P----C-----S 132
IGFBP-5    ---VY-TE--RCAQ--GLRCLPRQDEEKP-LHALLHGR---G-VCLNE- -----KSYREQVK-IERDSREHEEPTTSEMAEE------TY--S---PKI-FR------P 139
IGFBP-6    ---VY-TP--NCAP--GLQCHPPKDDEAP-LRALLLGR---G-RCLPAR -----------AP-AVAEENPKESKPQAGTAR----------------------P 129

IGFBP-7    GGGAG-RG--YCAP--GMECVKSRKRRRAGAAAGGPGVSG-VCVCKS ----------RYP--VCGSDGTTYPSGCQLRAASQ-----RAES--------R------G 144
IGFBP-8    ----E-RD--PCDPHKGLFCDFGS-PANRKIGVCT-AK--DGAPCIFGG ----------TVYR--SGESFQSSCKYQCTCLDGAVGCMPLCSMDVRLPSP-DC-------P 149
IGFBP-9    ---D-LE--PCDESSGLYCDRSADPSN-VBGIGT-AV--EGDNCVFDG ----------VIYR--SGEKFQPSCKFQCTCRDGQIGCVPRCQLDVLLPEP-NC-------P 156
IGFBP-10   ----K-TQ--PCDHTKGLECNFGA-SSTALKGICR-AQS-EGRPCEYNS ----------RIYQ--NGESFQPNCKHQCTCIDGAVGCIPLCPQELSLPNL-GC-------P 146
IGFBP-rP5  ----LQ-RG--PCGE--GLQCVVPFGVPAS-ATVRRRAQ--AG-LCVCAS ----------SEP--VCGSDANTYANLCQLRAASRRSERLHRPPVIVLQRGACGQGQGEDP 162
IGFBP-rP6  ----------MKCGP--GLRCQPSNGEDF--FGEEF------G-ICKD-- ----------CP---YGTFGMDCRETCNCQSG----------------------G 120
IGFBP-rP7  ----Q-LH--VCDASQGLVCQPGAGPGG-RGALCLLAE--DDSSCEVNG ----------RLYR--EGETFQPHCSIRCRCDEGGFTCVPLCSEDVRLPSW-DC-----S 146
IGFBP-rP8  ----E-AA--ICDPHRGLYCDYSGDRPRYAIGVCAQVV---GVGCVLDG ----------VRYN--NGQSFQPNCKYNCTCIDGAVGCTPLCLR-VRPPRL-WC-----P 168
IGFBP-rP9  ----E-AD--LCDPHRGLYCDYSVDRPRYETGVCAYLV---AVGCEFNQ ----------VHYH--NGQVFQPNPLFSCLCVSGAIGCTPLFI-----PKL-AG------S 163
IGFBP-rP10 LDPSAHFYG-HCGE---QLEC---R-LDTG--GDLSRGE-VPEPLCACRS ----------QSP--LCGSDGHTYSQICRLQEAA------RA---------R------P 156
```

Fig. 2. Partial amino acid sequence alignment of human IGFBP-1 to 10, and IGFBP-rP5-rP10. The consensus IGFBP motif which relates all of these sequences as a family is boxed. Consensus cysteine residues are shown in red. The matriptase consensus site sequence for cleavage is indicated in blue. Alignment was performed using the Clustalw2 sequence alignment program (European Bioinformatics Institute; http://www.ebi.ac.uk/Tools/msa/clustalw2/). Small gaps were introduced to optimize alignment. Nomenclature for the IGFBP7-IGFBP15, IGFBP-rPs: IGFBP7, IGFBP-rP1;mac25/TAF/PSF1; IGFBP8, IGFBP-rP2, CTGF; IGFBP-rP3,NovH; IGFBP-rP4, Cyr61; IGFBP-rP5, L56/HtrA; IGFBP-rP6, ESM-1; IGFBP-rP7, WISP-2/CTGF-L; IGFBP-rP8, WISP-1; IGFBP-rP9, WISP-3; IGFBP-rp10, Bono1.

Low affinity binding proteins (IGFBP-rPs)

Upon comparison of the IGFBP N-terminus in other cysteine-rich proteins, another group of proteins that were structurally related to the IGFBP family were identified, IGFBP-related proteins (IGFBP-rPs). Based on sequence alignment, the N-terminal domains of the IGFBP-rPs have significant similarities to the IGFBPs (40-57%) within their N-terminal domains, conserving all of the 12 cysteines within the N-terminal domain, including the consensus IGFBP motif. Past the N-terminus, the similarities decrease significantly to less than 15%. Unlike the IGFBPs, the IGFBP-rPs do not contain the thyroglobulin-type 1 domain at the C-terminus [28]. Their low affinity for IGFs together with their conserved structural homology to the IGFBP family suggested that these IGFBPs may have unique biological properties independent of their capacity to bind IGF. The first protein proven to be functionally related to the IGFBPs was IGFBP-rP1(IGFBP7)[29,30]. A group of highly related, cysteine-rich proteins were subsequently identified as part of the IGFBP-like family, termed the CCN family of proteins, including connective tissue growth factor (CTGF)[16], *nov* (nephroblastoma overexpressing) oncogene [31],*cyr61* [32], and three genes (WISP-1, WISP-2, and WISP-3) that are upregulated in Wnt-1-transformed cells and are aberrantly expressed in human colon tumors [33]. HtrA (IGFBP-rP5) refers to a family of serine proteases who's main functions are protein quality control, and have been implicated in tumour suppression and in the control of proliferation, migration and neurodegeneration (reviewed in [134]). IGFBP-rP10 (Bono1), the most recently identified member of the IGFBP family, with the highest homology to IGFBP7 at the amino acid level (42.2%), has been shown to be involved in the proliferation of osteoblasts during bone formation and bone regeneration [135]. This chapter will preferentially focus on IGFBP7.

IGFBP7 overview

The gene for human IGFBP7 is localized to chromosome 4q12-13 [34]. The mouse homolog shares 87.5% nucleotide identity and 94.4% similarity with human IGFBP7 [35]. IGFBP7 amino acid sequence has an overall 40-45% similarity and 20-25% identity to IGFBPs. The protein is produced as a precursor of 282 amino acids, which is processed to a mature 27 kD protein of 256 amino acids with one N-glycosylation site resulting in a secreted mature protein of 33 kD [16,30,27]. Structurally, the region of similarity of IGFBP7 to IGFBPs is confined to the N-terminal domain, encompassing the common IGFBP motif in a region containing 11 out of the 12 conserved cysteines [36](fig 2). Another domain found within the

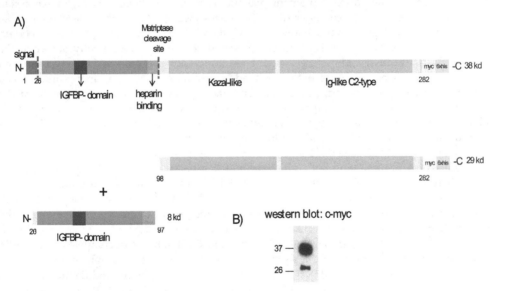

Fig. 3. Processing of recombinant IGFBP7 protein. A)Full length IGFBP7 protein is shown beginning with the signal sequence in red, which is cleaved off upon secretion from the cell. The N terminal contains the consensus IGFBP domain (dark purple), and the heparin binding domain (light purple). Kazal-like motif is shown in yellow and the Ig-like C2 domain is indicated in green. As a result of overexpression through the pSec-Tag2B plasmid, the protein is tagged in our system with *myc* and *his* at the C terminal, as shown in light pink and blue, respectively. Matriptase cleavage site is C terminal to the heparin binding domain between amino acid 97 and 98. Cleavage results in the production of 2 fragments, the N terminal portion (8 kd) and the C terminal 29 kd fragment. B) Western blotting of conditioned medium from MDA-MB-468 overproducing breast cancer cell line with anti-myc antibodies produces 2 bands, corresponding to the predominant large 38 kd protein, and the minor 29 kd cleaved protein.

N-terminus is a heparin sulfate binding site, consisting of 20 amino acid residues including 7 basic amino acids, which allows weak cell adhesion by interacting with cell surface-associated heparin sulfate proteoglycans [37](fig 3). Immediately adjacent to the N terminal domain is a stretch of 30-45 amino acid residues that has 30% similarity to the Kazal family of serine proteinase inhibitors, including the human pancreatic secretory trypsin inhibitor [38]. This domain, known as a KI domain, is also found in follistatin, leading to the hypothesis that IGFBP7 was a follistatin-like protein [35]. IGFBP7 can be proteolytically cleaved to a two-chain form by the type II membrane-bound serine proteinase, matriptase [39](fig 3). Cleavage occurs between K(Lys)97 and A(Ala)98, resulting in a 26 kD protein comprised of the C-terminal domain, and an 8 kD peptide corresponding to the N-terminal domain [40](fig 2,3). Cleavage results in almost a complete loss of both insulin/IGF-1 binding activity, while increasing cell adhesion activity [40].

IGFBP7-interacting proteins

Four groups independently identified the human IGFBP7 protein. One of these groups cloned the mac25 cDNA from normal leptomeningial and mammary epithelial cells, with expression of IGFBP7 decreased in the corresponding tumor cells [36,34]. The protein was shown to be able to bind IGFs, albeit with much lower affinity than IGFBPs [30]. During that same period, two other proteins were purified and characterized that were subsequently shown to be identical to the protein encoded by *mac*25. First, tumor adhesion factor (TAF) was isolated from the conditioned media of a human bladder carcinoma cell line, and promoted cell adhesion activity [41]. Second, prostacyclin-stimulating factor (PSF) was isolated from the conditioned media of human dipoid fibroblasts [42]. It was so termed due to its ability to stimulate prostacyclin production in endothelial cells, but not in patients with diabetes mellitus [43,44]. Finally, T1A12 was identified by subtractive cDNA cloning using RNAs from a normal breast epithelial cell line Hs578Bst and the breast cancer cell line Hs587T [45].

The ability of IGFBP7 to bind both IGF-1 and IGF-2, albeit with lower affinity than IGFBPs, led to its renaming as IGFBP7 [30]. However, IGFBP7 is unique amongst its family members in that it can bind insulin with high affinity, whereas IGFBPs 1-6 can only bind insulin with low affinity. This ability of IGFBP7 is due to the exposure of the insulin binding site at the amino terminal region due to lack of conserved cysteine residues in the C-terminal end, which are important for IGF binding by IGFBPs [46,47]. IGFBP7 can compete with insulin receptors for binding of insulin, thus preventing insulin-stimulated autophosphorylation of the insulin receptor β subunit[47]. IGFBP7 also contains a 'follistatin module' in its protein sequence, and has been shown to bind activin, a member of the TGF-β superfamily of growth factors [48]. Activin and its receptors are associated with growth modulation in glandular organs. Specifically, when activin signaling is disrupted or lost in normal mammary cells, malignant progression is potentiated, as demonstrated by the global decrease in the abundance of activin and its receptors in high grade breast cancer [49].

Another binding partner is type IV collagen. IGFBP7 co-localizes with type IV collagen in the vascular basement membrane [29]. IGFBP7 also can bind to cell surface-associated heparin sulfate proteoglycans, specifically, syndecan-1[40]. IGFBP7 has also been shown to bind certain CC chemokines, specifically, RANTES, SLC, and the CXC chemokine, IP-10 [50].

Expression

IGFBP7 is found in some biological fluids, such as serum, urine, CSF and amniotic fluid [51]. In normal human adult sera, the median IGFBP7 was 21.0 µg/liter. IGFBP7 is expressed in a variety of normal tissues including heart, spleen, ovary, small intestine and colon [52]. Immunohistochemistry performed on normal human tissues showed a ubiquitous intense staining of peripheral nerves, smooth muscle cells, including those from blood vessel walls, gut, bladder, breast and prostate. Cilia from the respiratory system, epididymis, and fallopian tube also demonstrated intense positive staining. Most endothelial cells were seen to be positive, whereas fat cells, plasma cells and lymphocytes were negative. Specific IGFBP7 expression was limited to certain cell types in the kidney, adrenal gland and skeletal muscle [52]. IGFBP7 has also been shown to play a role in endometrial physiology. IGFBP7 expression is increased in the receptive versus prereceptive endometrium, and rises sharply again in late luteal phase. The protein was localized at the apical part of the luminal and glandular epithelium, as well as in stromal and endothelial cells [53]. Strong expression of IGFBP7 has also been seen in high endothelial vessels (HEV)[50].

Oncogene induced senescence

Normal cells have a limited proliferative lifespan, after which they enter a state of irreversible growth arrest. This process, originally observed by Hayflick and Moorhead and called replicative senescence, is believed to result in human cells from telomere shortening as a consequence of cell division [54,55]. This was thought to be a failsafe mechanism preventing the expansion of aged cells[56]. Almost three decades ago, it was observed that normal cells are refractory to oncogene transformation [57]. Ectopic expression of the oncogene H-RAS^{G12V} in normal fibroblasts induced senescence that was later shown to be telomere-independent, representing another type of senescence triggered by oncogenes, called oncogene-induced senescence (OIS)[58,59]. OIS, together with oncogene-induced apoptosis, has been suggested to act as a true barrier to cancer, once cellular damage is inefficiently repaired[56,60]. OIS can be triggered by activated oncogenes like BRAF^{E600} or RAS^{V12} or by the loss of tumor suppressor proteins, like PTEN or NF1[61,62,63]. OIS is often characterized by the upregulation of the CDK inhibitors p15^{INK4B},p16^{INK4A}, and p21^{CIP1}, as well as by an increase in senescence-associated β-galactosidase (SA-β-Gal) activity [64,65]. Acute inactivation of certain genes, such as Rb or p53, can reverse OIS [66,67,68]. A typical example of OIS occurs in melanocytic nevi, which are benign skin lesions that rarely progress to melanoma [69,70]. Nevi are growth arrested and display classical hallmarks of senescence, including expression of SA-β-Gal, and the cell cycle inhibitor, p16^{INK4A} [62,71,72]. Activating BRAF mutations account for up to 82% of melanocytic nevi [73]. Senescent cells secrete a broad spectrum of factors, primarily involved in IGF and TGF-β signaling, ECM remodeling and inflammation [74,75,76,77,78]. Together, these secreted factors are referred to as the Senescence-Messaging Secretome (SMS) or the Senescence-Associated Secretory Phenotype (SASP) [79,78]. IGFBP7 has been identified as one of these factors responsible for the establishment and/or maintenance of OIS [34,75].

3. IGFBP7 as tumor suppressor in various cancers

IGFBP7 has been shown to be a tumor suppressor in a variety of solid cancers (summarized in Table 1). Its expression is lost upon progression to more aggressive cancer types. Loss of expression is associated with poor prognoses. Reexpression or exposure of cancer cell lines to IGFBP7 results in either senescence or apoptosis, and when these IGFBP7-expressing cell lines are xenografted in mice, tumor growth is inhibited.

Breast cancer

IGFBP7 has been shown to be a tumor suppressor in breast cancer. IGFBP7 was identified as one of the genes overexpressed in senescent human mammary epithelial cells (HMEC) (10 fold higher than quiescent cells of the same origin), and which was upregulated in normal mammary epithelial cells by all-*trans*-retinoic acid [34,80]. We cloned the gene for IGFBP7 by subtractive hybridization from the Hs568T breast cancer cell line and found IGFBP7 to be downregulated in primary breast cancer tissues. In normal breast tissue, IGFBP7 protein expression is concentrated in the cytoplasm of luminal epithelial cells, in ducts and acini of normal and benign primary breast tissues as well as other luminal, normal human cellular structures, suggesting an important role for IGFBP7 in the maintenance of normal breast and tissue architecture in general [45].

Cancer type		Down-regulated	Up-regulated	IGFBP7 Introduction	Effect	Reference
Breast	MCF-7			Overexpressed	G0-G1 arrest Senescence	[86]
	MDA-MB-468	pERK1/2		Overexpressed	↓ Tumour-genicity	[85]
	Xenograft-MDA-MB-468			Overexpressed	↓Growth and migration	[85]
	MDA-MB-231		pp38 p53, p21	Exogenous Protein	↓Cell growth ↑Senescence ↑Apoptosis	Manuscript submitted
Colorectal	SW620, COLO205, HT29			5-Aza-dc	↓Cell migration/invasion	[93]
	RKO, CW2	E-cadherin B-catenin pRB	p53	Overexpressed	G1 arrest Senescence	[95]
	DLD-1				↓Anchorage independent growth ↑Cell adhesion	[98]
	Xenograft-DLD-1			Overexpressed	↓ Tumour-genicity	[98]
	Xenograft-HT29, SW620			Exogenous protein	↓ Tumour-genicity	[89]
Hepatocellular	PLC/PRF/5	SMARCB1 BNIP3L p27	pERK1/2 cyclin D1 cyclin E	shRNA targeting IGFBP7 mRNA	IFNα resistance ↑ Cell growth ↓Apoptosis	[106,117]
Melanoma	Nevi	pERK1/2	RKIP	Exogenous protein	Senescence	[75]
	Cell line		BNIP3L		Apoptosis	[75]
	Xenograft				Apoptosis	[75]
	Metastatic			Intervenous protein injection	Growth inhibition	[89]
	Murine metastatic	VEGF	Caspase-3	Intra-tumoral plasmid injection	Apoptosis	[90]

Cancer type	Down-regulated	Up-regulated	IGFBP7 Introduction	Effect	Reference
Prostate	M12			Overexpressed	↑ Doubling time ↓Apoptosis sensitivity Epithelial Morphology change ↓ Colony formation	[102]
	M12 xenograft			Over-expressed	↓ Tumour size	[102]
Thyroid	N1M1	pERK1/2	p53 p21 cleaved PARP	Over-expressed	Apoptosis ↓Cell migration	[105]
	N1M1			Over-expressed	Reduced tumour growth	[105]

Table 1. IGFBP7 as a tumor suppressor in various cancer models. Summarized data from six different cancers, showing the effect of overexpression or inhibition of IGFBP7 on cancer cell growth both in vivo and in vitro, as well as signaling pathways affected.

Expression of IGFBP7 decreases with breast cancer progression. Normal breast tissues had very high IGFBP7 protein levels, such as luminal epithelial cells of normal lobules and ducts, as well as in benign proliferation of ducts consistent with fibroadenoma [45]. By immunohistochemical staining, IGFBP7 expression was detected in all normal and benign patient samples examined, with particularly strong staining in luminal epithelial cells of normal ducts, and acini or endothelial cells of blood vessels [81]. Intermediate to weak IGFBP7 staining was evident in hyperplastic breast tissue and DCIS specimens [81]. In addition, IGFBP7 was significantly upregulated in low grade ductal carcinoma in situ (DCIS) relative to high grade DCIS, as judged by CDNA microarray analysis. In invasive breast tumors, immunohistochemical analysis revealed that IGFBP7 is downregulated at the protein level [45]. IGFBP7 is downregulated in some breast tumors by loss of heterozygosity (LOH), and is also reduced by promoter methylation, both of which lead to increased tumor incidence and poor overall survival [45,82,83]. When DNA extracted from microdissected breast tissues was used with a microsatellite marker based method to determine allelic loss of the IGFBP7 locus in paired normal and invasive breast tissues, 50% of the informative samples from 30 matched pairs of normal and breast tumor tissues showed allele-specific LOH suggesting that the IGFBP7 gene was inactivated by deletions in at least a portion of each tumor [45]. A thoroughly characterized group of 106 invasive breast samples was surveyed using the tumor tissue microarray technique and immunohistochemistry [84]. Approximately 40% of tumors have low or no IGFBP7 staining suggesting that the gene or gene product was inactivated in a subset of invasive breast cancer samples [84]. Low IGFBP7 was associated with high cyclin E expression, retinoblastoma protein (pRb) inactivation, poorly differentiated tumors and higher stage. There was a significantly impaired prognosis for patients with low IGFBP7-expressing tumors. IGFBP7 also showed an inverse correlation with proliferation (Ki-67) in ER- tumors [84].

IGFBP7 expression was examined in 32 primary patient breast tumors and matched metastatic counterparts (fig 4). Low levels of IGFBP7 expression were found in 25/32 primary tumors. Approximately half of these tumors had lower levels of IGFBP7 in their metastatic tumors compared to the matched primary tumor, indicating that loss of IGFBP7 confers a selective growth advantage for metastatic lesions [85].

In order to investigate the growth of human breast cancers in an in vivo model, 7 human primary tumors were implanted into human bone grafts under the right flank of human-bone NOD/SCID mice. Only triple negative breast tumors grew in these mice (table 2). One of the triple negative primary breast tumors was serially transplanted more than five times. Each serial transplant resulted in increased tumor uptake and shorter growth rate. The tumor latency was decreased by approximately half after the first re-implantation. Examination of IGFBP7 expression revealed that each serial transplant resulted in lower levels of IGFBP7 expression by qRT-PCR [85](fig 4). Comparing the xenografted tumor to the original primary patient tumor revealed an increase in the anti-human specific proliferation marker, Ki67 (42.03 ± 8.87 to 53.3 ± 3.6). These results again confirmed an inverse correlation between IGFBP7 expression and breast tumor growth as well as aggressiveness of the tumor.

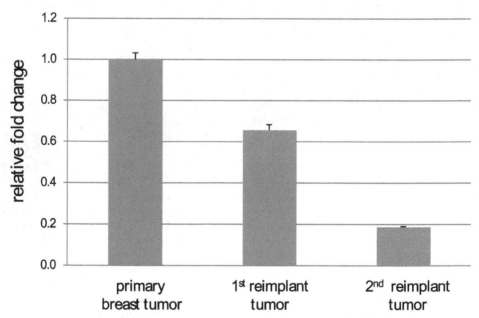

Fig. 4. Expression of IGFBP7 in primary and xenografted patient breast tumors by qRT-PCR. Quantitative PCR of IGFBP7 expression in primary and successively xenografted human breast tumors derived from first and second implantation into NOD/SCID mice. The data represent average values and standard error measurement from two triplicate samples, normalized against β-actin mRNA levels. The relative fold changes of the selected genes are obtained by dividing the expression levels of the re-implanted tumors by the expression levels in the primary patient tumors.

Patient	Age (Years)	Histo-pathological diagnosis	Grading	Estrogen /Progesterone receptor expression	ErB-2 expression	Node invasion (number positive/ number harvested)	Growth in hu-bone NOD/ SCID mice
HuP-1	67	Invasive ductal carcinoma	II/III	+/-	+	1/12	-
HuP-2	35	Metaplastic carcinoma	III	-/-	-	0/23	+
HuP-3	40	Invasive ductal carcinoma	II/III	+/+	+	0/2	-
HuP-4	48	Invasive ductal carcinoma	III	-/-	-	0/17	+
HuP-5	81	Invasive ductal carcinoma	II	+/-	-	0/1	-
HuP-6	50	Invasive and In-situ duct carcinoma	II	+/+	-	0/16	-
HuP-7	75	Invasive ductal carcinoma	I	+/+		4/15	-

Table 2. Characteristics of the human patient breast tumor tissues engrafted in hu-bone NOD/SCID mice.

The major traits of the engrafted human patient breast tumor samples (patient age, histopathological diagnosis, grading, estrogen/progesterone receptor expression, ErB-2 expression, node invasion) are indicated. The table also shows if the patient tumor samples were able to grow in the hu-bone NOD/SCID mouse model.

In order to transcriptionally characterize the colonization and aggressive behavior of engrafted patient breast tumors, microarray gene expression profiling was performed on breast tumors that were serially transplanted in the human-bone NOD/SCID mice. Genes were identified that were differentially expressed in the xenografted tumors by at least 1.5 fold compared to the primary patient tumors. There were 205 genes found to be differentially regulated in both HuP-2 and HuP-4 bone residing-breast tumors. Of the 129 known genes, 97 were expressed at higher levels and 32 at lower levels in the patient breast tumors colonized in bone. To narrow the spectrum of genes, 14 up-regulating and 18 down-regulating genes with bone colonization potentials are displayed (Table 3). Many of these gene identified have been previously associated with cancer function or metastatic activities such as cell viability, apoptosis and oncogenic transformation. IGFBP7 was identified as one of the genes that were downregulated in the xenografted tumors.

Gene	Fold Differences		Description	Identified cancer involvements
	HuP-2	HuP-4		
Down-regulated				
MTBP	7.11	1.94	Mdm2, transformed 3T3 cell double minute 2, p53 binding protein	p53 regulator, Metastasis and cell proliferation suppressor
PARK7	5.30	3.14	Parkinson disease (autosomal recessive, early onset) 7	Negative regulator of PTEN, cell survival & aggressiveness
TOB1	1.79	6.12	Transducer of ERBB2, 1	Anti-proliferative protein
SDCBP	2.01	5.64	Syndecan binding protein (syntenin)	Cell adhesion & protein trafficking
CD24	2.12	11.29	CD24 molecule	Breast cancer stem cell marker & associated with bone metastasis
IL1R1	4.27	2.44	Interleukin 1 receptor, type I	Mediate cytokine induced immune & inflammatory response
PDLIM5	2.60	1.70	PDZ and LIM domain 5	Negative factor of oncogenic activity in neural tumor
HLA-DRA	2.15	6.33	Major histocompatibility complex, class II, DR alpha	Tumor immunosurveillance
PRKACB	3.11	3.93	Protein kinase, cAMP-dependent, catalytic, beta	Cell proliferation & differentiation
UBE2I	5.55	1.63	Ubiquitin-conjugating enzyme E2I	Suppressing p53 functions via RPA2 activity
IGFBP7	3.82	2.00	Insulin-like growth factor binding protein 7	Tumor suppressor & cell proliferation
ITM2B	1.94	2.28	Integral membrane protein 2B	Cell survival
ADAMTS12	1.61	3.43	ADAM metallopeptidase with thrombospondin type 1 motif, 12	Prevents tumorigenic effect of HGF
SPIN	1.56	3.35	Spindlin	Cell cycle regulation
PTPRF	1.86	2.32	Protein tyrosine phosphatase, receptor type, F	Regulation of epithelial cell-cell contact and cell growth
UHRF1BP1L	2.54	2.34	UHRF1 (ICBP90) binding protein 1-like	Regulate VEGF gene expression & tumor angiogenesis
TRMT5	2.20	1.87	TRM5 tRNA methyltransferase 5 homolog	Methylation
NR3C1	1.62	2.29	Nuclear receptor subfamily 3, group C, member 1)	Signaling and transduction
Up-regulated				
EIF5A	2.78	1.79	Eukaryotic translation initiation factor 5A	Cell viability & senescence
PCNXL2	2.81	1.79	Pecanex-like 2	Tumorigenesis in colorectal carcinoma
CD1C	3.11	1.54	CD1c molecule	Mediate immune responses to tumors
CSF1R	3.71	5.70	Colony stimulating factor 1 receptor	Metastasis & cell invasiveness
RPS5	1.99	1.99	Ribosomal protein S5	Cell differentiation and apoptosis
GOT2	2.10	1.74	Glutamic-oxaloacetic transaminase 2, mitochondrial	Serum GOT correlated with cancer and metastatic disease
RABL4	3.95	1.64	RAB, member of RAS oncogene family-like 4	Ras-related putative GTP-binding protein
RPS14	2.39	2.02	ribosomal protein S14	Haploinsufficiency disease gene
KLF8	1.57	1.53	Kruppel-like factor 8	Oncogenic transformation & EMT, downstream of FAK
DGKQ	1.82	2.28	Diacylglycerol kinase, theta 110kDa	Signal transduction pathways
AP2S1	3.23	1.60	Adaptor-related protein complex 2, sigma 1 subunit	Clathrin adaptor complex associated with plasma membranes

PALM	1.58	1.83	Paralemmin	Cell shape control
RPS8	1.87	1.76	Ribosomal protein S8	Up-regulated in astrocytoma and pancreatic cancer
POLR2J	3.61	2.07	DNA directed RNA polyermase II	Enzyme & transcription

Table 3. Schematic representation of microarray analysis from xenografted tumors compared to primary tumors. To identify genes with bone colonization potential, xenografted tumor tissues were harvested for microarray analysis. Fold changes are obtained by dividing the gene expression levels in the xenografted tumors by the expression levels in the primary patient tumors. 205 genes are at least 1.5 fold differentially expressed in both HuP-2 and HuP4 bone residing breast-tumors compared with their primary patient breast tumors. A representation of genes whose expressions in xenografted tumors were at least 1.5 fold down-regulated from primary patient tumors (18 of 157 genes), or upregulated from primary patient tumors (14 of 48 genes) are shown.

The increased expression of IGFBP7 in senescent versus proliferating normal HMECs [34], prompted the evaluation of potential antiproliferative capabilities of IGFBP7 in breast cancer cells. In order to test this theory, IGFBP7 was overexpressed by retroviral vector in the ER/PR+ IGFBP7- MCF-7 breast cancer cell line. IGFBP7-transduced MCF-7 breast cancer cells showed a significant reduction in cell growth compared to parental IGFBP7 negative MCF-7 cells. When further analyzed, cells had arrested at the G0-G1 phase of cell cycle upon IGFBP7 expression. IGFBP7 was found to induce senescence rather than apoptosis [86].

ER/PR-negative breast cancers are the most aggressive and hardest to treat. In order to examine whether restoration of IGFBP7 could inhibit triple negative breast cancer cell growth, IGFBP7-overexpressing cells were engineered using a pSec-Tag2 plasmid in MDA-MB-468, a triple negative breast cancer line with barely detectable levels of endogenous IGFBP7, that is also tumorigenic in mice [87]. The vector contained a C-terminal c-*myc* epitope for detection with an anti-*myc* antibody, and a polyhistidine (6x*his*) tag for rapid purification with nickel-chelating resin and detection with an anti-*his*(C-term) antibody (fig 3). Western blots of conditioned medium from stable IGFBP7-transfectants revealed two bands in response to IGFBP7 staining, a 38 kD band seen also in cell lysates, and a weaker, smaller 29 kD band. N-terminal sequencing revealed that both bands are IGFBP7 gene products [85]. The 38 kD band corresponded to the full length protein minus the signal sequence, whereas the smaller 29 kD band was cleaved after amino acid lys^{97}, suggesting cleavage by the enzyme matriptase [39,85](fig 2, 3). IGFBP7 overexpression in MDA-MB-468 cells reduced cell growth and migration compared to parental MDA-MB-468 cells. Similarly, conditioned medium from IGFBP7 overexpressing breast cancer cell lines also lowered the growth of MDA-MB-468 cells. In order to examine the mechanism of IGFBP7-mediated growth inhibition, the effect of IGFBP7 overexpression on the MAP kinase pathway was analyzed. IGFBP7 overexpression inhibited the phosphorylation of MEK-1/2 and ERK-1/2 compared to parental MDA-MB-468 cells [85](fig. 5). These results are consistent with those observed in melanoma studies, whereby IGFBP7 is thought to act through autocrine and paracrine pathways to inhibit BRAF-MEK-ERK signaling resulting in induction of senescence or apoptosis [75].

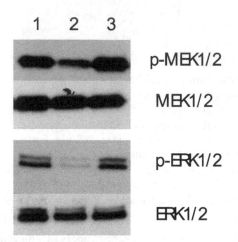

Fig. 5. Effect of IGFBP7 overexpression on the MAP kinase signaling pathway. Western blotting using equal amounts of protein from total cell lysates from MDA-MB-468 (lane 1), MDA-MB-468/IGFBP7 (lane 2), and empty vector control (lane 3) cells were examined by western blotting with antibodies to pERK-1/2,ERK-1/2, pMEK-1/2, and MEK-1/2.

The effects of IGFBP7 mediated growth inhibition were also examined *in vivo*. Parental MDA-MB-468 breast cancer cells and the IGFBP7-overexpressing variant were injected into NOD/SCID or NSG mice. Examination of tumor growth revealed a significant inhibition of tumor growth from the IGFBP7 overexpressing MDA-MB-468 cells (fig 6). Tumors were considerably smaller in the presence of IGFBP7. Immunohistochemistry and qRT-PCR of revealed the expression IGFBP7 in tumors derived from IGFBP7 overexpressing cells, confirming continual production of IGFBP7 *in vivo* during the duration of the experiment, which suggested that IGFBP7 was responsible for tumor growth suppression [85].

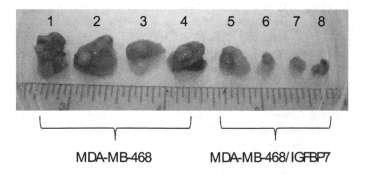

Fig. 6. Effect of IGFBP7 overexpression on breast tumor formation in vivo. 5×10^6 MDA-MB-468 cells or MDA-MB-468/IGFBP7 cells were injected into NSG or NOD/SCID mice. After 36 days, tumors were removed and analyzed.

Melanoma

IGFBP7 was shown to be a tumor suppressor in melanoma studies, in that loss of IGFBP7 expression was critical step in melanoma development [75]. Activating BRAF mutations are found at a high frequency in melanomas (50-70%)[88]. In normal melanocytes, IGFBP7 is expressed at low levels. Following expression of the activating BRAFV600E mutation in melanocytic nevi, IGFBP7 is upregulated and induces senescence [75]. Melanoma cell lines harboring the activating BRAFV600E mutation, did not express IGFBP7, due to epigenetic silencing through promoter methylation of IGFBP7 [75,89]. Upon exposure to IGFBP7, BRAFV600E-positive melanoma cells underwent apoptosis. BRAFV600E expression in melanoma cells results in hyperactivation of the BRAF-MEK-ERK pathway. IGFBP7 treatment blocked cellular proliferation in part through inhibition of this pathway. Specifically, the phosphorylation of MEK by BRAF was prevented by upregulation of the RAF inhibitory protein (RKIP) by IGFBP7 through autocrine/paracrine pathways [75]. The apoptotic pathway induced by IGFBP7 involved the upregulation of BNIP3L, a proapoptotic BCL2 family protein. Furthermore, systemically administered IGFBP7 markedly suppressed the growth of BRAF-positive melanomas in xenografted mice, also through induction of apoptosis [75]. Epigenetic silencing of IGFBP7 is even more pronounced in human metastatic samples [89]. In a mouse model of metastatic melanoma, where mice were injected via tail vein with the highly metastatic BRAFV600E-positive malignant melanoma cells A375M-F*luc*, IGFBP7 systemic administration suppressed tumor growth and increased survival [89]. Another group demonstrated that intratumoral injection of IGFBP7 in the form of the plasmid, pcDNA3.1-IGFBP7, promoted stable expression of IGFBP7, and suppressed the growth of the murine malignant melanoma cell line, B16-F10, by inducing apoptosis. Caspase 3 levels were increased and VEGF levels were decreased in the pcDNA3.1-IGFBP7 treated group [90].

Colorectal cancer

In the normal colon, IGFBP7 expression varies from the basal compartment to the surface epithelium. Epithelial cells at the surface contain very strong IGFBP7 expression, whereas IGFBP7 staining was much weaker at the crypt base, which indicates that IGFBP7 expression is stronger in the differentiating areas of the colonic epithelium. Interestingly, IGFBP7 expression is actually increased in colorectal cancer. In colon carcinoma, IGFBP7 expression is strongest in the well differentiated colorectal adenocarcinoma, while weakly expressed in poorly differentiated colorectal adenocarcinoma [91]. IGFBP7 expression was correlated with differentiation, low grade tumor, and better prognosis. Cell differentiation and apoptosis are considered a result of normal colonocyte terminal differentiation in vivo. Introduction of IGFBP7 into colon cancer cells induced a more differentiated morphology. Upregulation of several colonic epithelial cell differentiation markers, such as AKP and CEA occurred with reintroduction of IGFBP7 [91]. This study identified IGFBP7 as a potential key marker associated with colon cancer differentiation.

The inhibition of IGFBP7 expression in colon cancer cell lines was shown to be due to aberrant DNA hypermethylation of the CpG island in exon 1 of IGFBP7, specifically in the promoter region [92]. Reactivation of IGFBP7 by 5-aza-dC treatment inhibited colon cancer cell proliferation in a dose dependent manner [93]. Demethylation restored p53-induced IGFBP7 expression[94]. Epigenetic inactivation of IGFBP7 appears to play a key role in tumorigenesis of CRCs with CpG island methylator phenotype (CIMP) by enabling escape from p53-induced senescence [94]. Cell cycle was arrested, as cells accumulated in G2/M phase. 5-aza-dC treatment also increased the percentage of cells undergoing apoptosis. Cell migration and invasion were also reduced after treatment with 5-aza-dC [93]. The authors argue that demethylation increased the expression of tumor suppressor proteins, specifically IGFBP7, which was involved in the 5-aza-dC induced growth inhibitory effects.

A more direct effect of IGFBP7 as a tumor suppressor in colon cancer was shown in a subsequent study. Colorectal carcinoma cells, RKO and CW2, transfected with pcDNA3.1-IGFBP7 showed reduced proliferation. Cells were arrested in G1 phase of cell cycle (15% increased compared to control cells). The expression of E-cadherin and β-catenin were reduced in IGFBP7-transduced CW2 cells. Migration was not affected. A senescence like phenotype was induced, as judged by increased SA-β-Gal activity, together with increased p53 and reduced pRB expression [95]. Cellular senescence is a barrier to cancer, preventing cells from unlimited proliferation [96,97]. This study suggested that IGFBP7 is an important molecule that triggers senescence through two important pathways, the p53-dependent pathway and the p16/p21-pRB pathway [95].

IGFBP7 was also shown to inhibit colon cancer tumor growth. Overexpression of IGFBP7 in the human colon cancer cell line, DLD-1, reduced its tumorgenicity *in vivo* [98]. Anchorage independent growth was also reduced. IGFBP7 expression increased cell adhesion of DLD-1 cells to laminin-5 and fibronectin [98]. In a separate study, two human CRC cell lines, one with an activating BRAF mutation (HT29) and the second with an activating KRAS mutation (SW-620), when xenografted into nude mice, were significantly growth inhibited upon systemic IGFBP7 treatment [89].

Proteomics was used to identify proteins associated with IGFBP7 in CRC. Six proteins were downregulated upon IGFBP7 reintroduction in colon cancer RKO cells, one of which was heat shock protein (HSP) 60 [99]. The authors focused on HSP60, as a key protein involved in IGFBP7-mediated growth inhibition, since it is overexpressed in CRC tissue and involved in proliferation and inhibition of apoptosis. They argue that one mechanism by which IGFBP7 overexpression inhibits growth of CRC cells, is through downregulation of HSP60.

Prostate cancer

IGFBP7 expression is found in primary cultures of prostate epithelial cells, and within the conditioned media from these cells. Peripheral nerves and stromal components associated with prostate tissue were strongly positive for IGFBP7 [100]. IGFBP7 protein and mRNA expression was up-regulated by IGF-I, TGF-β, and retinoic acid in the nontumorigenic prostate epithelial line, P69, derived by immortalization of human primary prostate epithelial cells with simian virus-40 T antigen. IGFBP7 was undetectable by northern blot from malignant prostate lines such as LNCap, DU145, and PC-3 cells, and M12 cells (the tumorigeneic and metastatic subclone of P69) [101,100]. There was a significant loss of detectable IGFBP7 mRNA in metastatic prostate tissue [28]. Re-expression of IGFBP7 in the human prostate cancer cell line, M12, results in an increase in cell doubling time, a decrease in colony formation in soft agar, a marked change in epithelial morphology along with an increased sensitivity to apoptosis, and finally decreased tumor formation and size *in vivo* [102]. In order to identify genes upregulated by IGFBP7 expression in prostate epithelial cells, a cDNA array analysis of IGFBP7-overexpressing M12 was performed, identifying SOX9, a transcription factor associated with differentiation [103]. The overexpression of

SOX9 in M12 cells seemed to recapitulate the effects seen with overexpression of IGFBP7 alone, suggesting that SOX9 is at least partly responsible for the growth inhibitory effect of IGFBP7 on prostate cancer cells. Another group used similar techniques and identified another transcription factor, manganese superoxide dismutase (SOD-2), which they argue was at least in part responsible for the growth inhibitory effects of IGFBP7 in prostate cancer cells [104]. Whether these transcription factors were indeed part of the anti-proliferative mechanism of IGFBP7, or merely a consequence of IGFBP7 overexpression in M12 cells remains to be determined.

Thyroid cancer

In accordance with prostate, colon and breast cancer, IGFBP7 expression is also significantly downregulated in thyroid cancer tissue samples compared to normal thyroid tissue [105]. IGFBP7 is epigenetically silenced by promoter hypermethylation in PTC-derived NIM1 thyroid tumor cell line. NIM1, along with most other thyroid cancer cell lines, carries the BRAFV600E mutation. Restoration of IGFBP7 in NIM1 cells by cDNA transfection resulted in growth inhibition, reduced colony formation in soft agar, and decreased migration capability in wound healing assay. Furthermore, tumor growth was inhibited upon injection in nude mice [105]. Examination of the mechanism governing IGFBP7 mediated growth inhibition revealed that IGFBP7-expressing NIM1 cells were impaired in cell cycle progression, manifesting cell cycle arrest in G1. The G1 arrest was associated with a strong decline in phospho-ERK levels, and an upregulation of p53 and p21 tumor suppressors. IGFBP7 expression alone resulted in increased apoptosis, as judged by increased cleaved PARP, which was even more pronounced upon exposure to the TRAIL, a proapoptotic agent effective in NIM1 cells [105]. These results suggest that IGFBP7 is a tumor suppressor in thyroid carcinogenesis.

Hepatocellular carcinoma (HCC)

A strong antitumor activity against HCC has been demonstrated for interferon (IFN)-based combination therapy (IFN-α/ 5-FU therapy) [106-116]. However continuous exposure to IFN-α can result in IFN-resistant HCC cells. IGFBP7 was identified by microarray analysis as one of the most significantly downregulated genes in IFN resistant clones. Parental PLC/PRF/5 cells transfected with short hairpin RNA for IGFBP7 showed IFN-α resistance. IGFBP7 transfection into IFN-resistant HCC cells restored IFN sensitivity [106]. These results suggested that IGFBP7 could be a novel marker to predict clinical outcome to IFN-α/5-FU therapy.

A recent report studied PLC/PRF/5 cells treated with shRNA directed towards IGFBP7. They found that in the absence of IGFBP7 expression, the cells grew more rapidly, phospho-ERK was significantly increased, and apoptosis was decreased, as compared to the parental IGFBP7 expressing cells [117]. They found that apoptosis was decreased as a result of decreased expression of proapoptotic proteins, *SMARCB1* and *BNIP3L* by qRT-PCR. Furthermore, upon suppression of IGFBP7 expression, cell cycle progression was increased, concomittently with increased cyclin D1 and cyclin E, and decreased p27. IGFBP7 reexpression in an HCC line that had very low IGFBP7 levels resulted in growth inhibition and decreased invasive ability. IGFBP7 downregulation was also significantly associated with tumor progression and postoperative poor prognosis in resected human HCC samples [117]. These studies identify IGFBP7 as a tumor suppressor and also an independent significant prognostic factor in HCC.

Lung cancer

Expression of IGFBP7 in lung cancer cell lines using RT-PCR revealed decreased expression of IGFBP7 compared to controls, and 42 out of 90 patients with primary lung tumors exhibited negative staining of IGFBP7 by immunohistochemical analysis [118]. There was a significant correlation between DNA methylation of exon/intron 1 region and IGFBP7 downregulation. When a p53 expression vector was transfected into lung cancer cell lines, it could only induce expression of IGFBP7 in the unmethylated cell line, but not in the methylated cell lines, suggesting that IGFBP7 might be regulated by p53 in lung cancer cell lines.

Squamous cell carcinoma of the head and neck (SCCHN)

A study found that a single nucleotide polymorphism (G to A) in the IGFBP7 promoter region was significantly associated with a reduced risk of SCCHN, when analyzed in a hospital-based case-control study of 1065 SCCHN patients and 1112 cancer-free control subjects. Upon analyzing reporter gene constructs, the G to A allelic change at -418 of the IGFBP7 promoter had increased promoter and DNA binding activity, suggesting increased IGFBP7 protein expression [119].

Although IGFBP7 has been shown to function as a tumor suppressor in a wide variety of cancers, a few studies suggest that IGFBP7 has an opposite effect, ie. promoting cancer growth. These cancers include the blood cancer, leukemia, and the brain cancer, glioblastoma.

Glioblastoma

IGFBP7 is a selective biomarker of glioblastoma (GBM) vessels, strongly expressed in tumor endothelial cells and vascular basement membrane [120]. IGFBP7 was strongly expressed in GBM specimens but not nontumor brain tissue. Moreover, statistical analysis showed that expression of IGFBP7 correlated inversely with overall GBM survival rates. Inhibition of IGFBP7 expression using siRNA transfection in a glioma cell line inhibited cell growth [121]. Addition of IGFBP7 to cell culture medium stimulated cell proliferation. IGFBP7 also promoted glioma cell migration, through downregulation of AKT phosphorylation and enhanced ERK1/2 activation [121]. IGFBP7 expression in brain endothelial cells was found to be upregulated by secreted factors from GBM cells through TGF-β1/ALK5/Smad2 signaling pathway, which has been implicated in angiogenesis [122].

Acute leukemia

Overexpression of the human gene BAALC (brain and acute leukemia, cytoplasmic), was shown to be associated with inferior outcome and chemotherapy resistance in adult patients with cytogenetically-normal acute myeloid leukemia (CN-AML), T cell-acute lymphoblastic leukemia (T-ALL) and B-precursor acute lymphoblastic leukemia (B-ALL)[123,124,125,126,127]. IGFBP7 was strongly correlated with BAALC-expression, implicating IGFBP7 in acute leukemia [128]. Aberrant expression of IGFBP7 in adult leukemia was correlated with chemotherapy resistance and inferior survival. Addition of IGFBP7 to leukemic cell lines inhibited cell growth without induction of apoptosis or senescence, suggesting a role of IGFBP7 in contributing to drug resistance through reduced sensitivity to cytostatic drugs [128]. Aberrantly increased levels of IGFBP7 were found in

CSF from children with acute lymphoblastic leukemia, implicating IGFBP7 with a more aggressive subtype of ALL [129]. IGFBP7 was also aberrantly overexpressed in the majority of AML at diagnosis and upon relapse, but not at remission stage [130]. Thus, IGFBP7 was shown to play a positive contributing role in the interaction between leukemia cells and the microenvironment, which may promote the leukemic cells' adhesion, invasion, and migration.

While the data observed in studies of leukemia and glioblastoma portray IGFBP7 in a negative role with respect to cancer, the vast majority of data from studies of solid tumors are in disagreement with these conclusions. It is possible that cell signaling pathways that result in senescence or apoptosis due to IGFBP7 are not present or functional in hematopoietic or glioma cells.

4. Conclusions and perspectives

IGFBP7 has been shown to have tumor suppressive function in breast and other cancers. When examining the summarized data in Table 1, a common thread appears. Overexpression of IGFBP7 leads to inhibition of growth both *in vitro* and *in vivo*, increased expression of apoptotic markers (caspases, cleaved PARP), senescence associated proteins (*i.e.* p21, p27, p53), and decreased expression of proteins associated with proliferation (p-ERK). IGFBP7 appears to affect signaling through the MAP kinase pathway in many tumor models, including breast cancer. OIS may be a mechanism of tumor suppression by IGFBP7. The breast cancer cell lines used in our study, MDA-MB-468 cells, have a mutated PTEN, disregulating the PI3K pathway [131]. OIS can be triggered not only by the activation of oncogenes but also by the loss of tumor suppressor genes, such as PTEN. By upregulating proteins that counteract proliferation, such as cyclin dependent kinase inhibitors, ie. p21, which we have shown to occur upon IGFBP7 addition to breast cancer cells, the combined effect can lead to OIS [132]. Our model for the role of IGFBP7 in breast cancer inhibition depicts the entrance of IGFBP7 full length or cleaved IGFBP7 (through matriptase) into the cell, where signals are propagated to the nucleus, leading to the upregulation of expression of cyclin dependent kinase inhibitors, such as p21 and p27 (fig 7). This together with an already hyperstimulated MAP kinase pathway due to oncogenic mutations such as RAS, leads to MAP kinase pathway inhibition, growth arrest, and senescence, as suggested by the conflicting signal model of senescence[132].

The strong link to breast cancer outcome suggests that IGFBP7 may not only be a good prognostic indicator for malignant disease progression, but also a useful surrogate marker for monitoring therapeutic responses in the treatment of breast cancers. Senescence has been shown to be a method of halting tumor growth by many standard chemotherapeutic drugs [133]. Preliminary results indicate that senescence may be one mechanism by which IGFBP7 inhibits breast cancer cell growth in our system. Inhibition of breast cancer growth in vivo and in vitro together with induction of senescence indicates that IGFBP7 could be further developed as a potential drug to treat breast cancers. The fact that IGFBP7 has growth inhibitory effects when expressed in triple negative breast cancer cells, *i.e.* MDA-MB-468, provides an exciting opportunity to bring to the clinic a potential drug for hard to treat breast tumors.

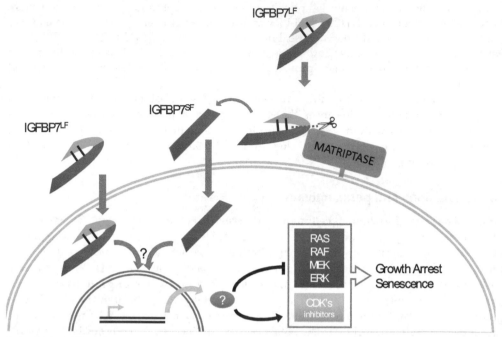

Fig. 7. Model for IGFBP7-mediated inhibition of breast cancer cell growth. IGFBP7 full length (FL) is cleaved by cell surface matriptase to short form (SF). Both forms enter breast cancer cells through an as yet unknown receptor, followed by signal propagation to the nucleus, which leads to upregulation of expression of cyclin dependent kinase (CDK) inhibitors, such as p21 and p27. This ultimately leads to growth arrest and senescence.

5. Acknowledgements

This work was supported by a CIHR grant, #MOP-97996 to Arun Seth. We thank Pearl Lam for her contribution to some of the microarray work and Stephanie Bacopulos for help with graphics.

6. References

[1] Chaves, J. and Saif, M. W. (2011) IGF system in cancer: from bench to clinic. Anticancer Drugs 22:206-212.

[2] Stewart, C. E. and Rotwein, P. (1996) Growth, differentiation, and survival: multiple physiological functions for insulin-like growth factors. Physiol Rev 76:1005-1026.

[3] Roberts, C. T., Jr., Brown, A. L., Graham, D. E., Seelig, S., Berry, S., Gabbay, K. H., and Rechler, M. M. (1986) Growth hormone regulates the abundance of insulin-like growth factor I RNA in adult rat liver. J Biol Chem 261:10025-10028.

[4] Steele-Perkins, G., Turner, J., Edman, J. C., Hari, J., Pierce, S. B., Stover, C., Rutter, W. J., and Roth, R. A. (1988) Expression and characterization of a functional human insulin-like growth factor I receptor. J Biol Chem 263:11486-11492.

[5] Soos, M. A., Whittaker, J., Lammers, R., Ullrich, A., and Siddle, K. (1990) Receptors for insulin and insulin-like growth factor-I can form hybrid dimers. Characterisation of hybrid receptors in transfected cells. Biochem J 270:383-390.

[6] Siddle, K., Urso, B., Niesler, C. A., Cope, D. L., Molina, L., Surinya, K. H., and Soos, M. A. (2001) Specificity in ligand binding and intracellular signalling by insulin and insulin-like growth factor receptors. Biochem Soc Trans 29:513-525.

[7] Braulke, T. (1999) Type-2 IGF receptor: a multi-ligand binding protein. Horm Metab Res 31:242-246.

[8] Mosthaf, L., Grako, K., Dull, T. J., Coussens, L., Ullrich, A., and McClain, D. A. (1990) Functionally distinct insulin receptors generated by tissue-specific alternative splicing. EMBO J 9:2409-2413.

[9] Yamaguchi, Y., Flier, J. S., Benecke, H., Ransil, B. J., and Moller, D. E. (1993) Ligand-binding properties of the two isoforms of the human insulin receptor. Endocrinology 132:1132-1138.

[10] Yamaguchi, Y., Flier, J. S., Yokota, A., Benecke, H., Backer, J. M., and Moller, D. E. (1991) Functional properties of two naturally occurring isoforms of the human insulin receptor in Chinese hamster ovary cells. Endocrinology 129:2058-2066.

[11] Denley, A., Wallace, J. C., Cosgrove, L. J., and Forbes, B. E. (2003) The insulin receptor isoform exon 11- (IR-A) in cancer and other diseases: a review. Horm Metab Res 35:778-785.

[12] Sciacca, L., Prisco, M., Wu, A., Belfiore, A., Vigneri, R., and Baserga, R. (2003) Signaling differences from the A and B isoforms of the insulin receptor (IR) in 32D cells in the presence or absence of IR substrate-1. Endocrinology 144:2650-2658.

[13] Frasca, F., Pandini, G., Scalia, P., Sciacca, L., Mineo, R., Costantino, A., Goldfine, I. D., Belfiore, A., and Vigneri, R. (1999) Insulin receptor isoform A, a newly recognized, high-affinity insulin-like growth factor II receptor in fetal and cancer cells. Mol Cell Biol 19:3278-3288.

[14] Blanquart, C., Achi, J., and Issad, T. (2008) Characterization of IRA/IRB hybrid insulin receptors using bioluminescence resonance energy transfer. Biochem Pharmacol 76:873-883.

[15] Soos, M. A., Field, C. E., and Siddle, K. (1993) Purified hybrid insulin/insulin-like growth factor-I receptors bind insulin-like growth factor-I, but not insulin, with high affinity. Biochem J 290 (Pt 2):419-426.

[16] Kim, H. S., Nagalla, S. R., Oh, Y., Wilson, E., Roberts, C. T., Jr., and Rosenfeld, R. G. (1997) Identification of a family of low-affinity insulin-like growth factor binding proteins (IGFBPs): characterization of connective tissue growth factor as a member of the IGFBP superfamily. Proc Natl Acad Sci U S A 94:12981-12986.

[17] Grimberg, A. and Cohen, P. (2000) Role of insulin-like growth factors and their binding proteins in growth control and carcinogenesis. J Cell Physiol 183:1-9.

[18] Jones, J. I. and Clemmons, D. R. (1995) Insulin-like growth factors and their binding proteins: biological actions. Endocr Rev 16:3-34.

[19] Hwa, V., Oh, Y., and Rosenfeld, R. G. (1999) The insulin-like growth factor-binding protein (IGFBP) superfamily. Endocr Rev 20:761-787.

[20] Zhu, W., Shiojima, I., Ito, Y., Li, Z., Ikeda, H., Yoshida, M., Naito, A. T., Nishi, J., Ueno, H., Umezawa, A., Minamino, T., Nagai, T., Kikuchi, A., Asashima, M., and Komuro, I. (2008) IGFBP-4 is an inhibitor of canonical Wnt signalling required for cardiogenesis. Nature 454:345-349.

[21] Perks, C. M., Newcomb, P. V., Norman, M. R., and Holly, J. M. (1999) Effect of insulin-like growth factor binding protein-1 on integrin signalling and the induction of apoptosis in human breast cancer cells. J Mol Endocrinol 22:141-150.

[22] Fu, P., Thompson, J. A., and Bach, L. A. (2007) Promotion of cancer cell migration: an insulin-like growth factor (IGF)-independent action of IGF-binding protein-6. J Biol Chem 282:22298-22306.

[23] Kiepe, D., Van Der Pas, A., Ciarmatori, S., Standker, L., Schutt, B., Hoeflich, A., Hugel, U., Oh, J., and Tonshoff, B. (2008) Defined carboxy-terminal fragments of insulin-like growth factor (IGF) binding protein-2 exert similar mitogenic activity on cultured rat growth plate chondrocytes as IGF-I. Endocrinology 149:4901-4911.

[24] Mihelic, M. and Turk, D. (2007) Two decades of thyroglobulin type-1 domain research. Biol Chem 388:1123-1130.

[25] Neumann, G. M., Marinaro, J. A., and Bach, L. A. (1998) Identification of O-glycosylation sites and partial characterization of carbohydrate structure and disulfide linkages of human insulin-like growth factor binding protein 6. Biochemistry 37:6572-6585.

[26] Forbes, B. E., Turner, D., Hodge, S. J., McNeil, K. A., Forsberg, G., and Wallace, J. C. (1998) Localization of an insulin-like growth factor (IGF) binding site of bovine IGF binding protein-2 using disulfide mapping and deletion mutation analysis of the C-terminal domain. J Biol Chem 273:4647-4652.

[27] Hwa, V., Oh, Y., and Rosenfeld, R. G. (1999) Insulin-like growth factor binding proteins: a proposed superfamily. Acta Paediatr Suppl 88:37-45.

[28] Hwa, V., Tomasini-Sprenger, C., Bermejo, A. L., Rosenfeld, R. G., and Plymate, S. R. (1998) Characterization of insulin-like growth factor-binding protein-related protein-1 in prostate cells. J Clin Endocrinol Metab 83:4355-4362.

[29] Akaogi, K., Sato, J., Okabe, Y., Sakamoto, Y., Yasumitsu, H., and Miyazaki, K. (1996) Synergistic growth stimulation of mouse fibroblasts by tumor-derived adhesion factor with insulin-like growth factors and insulin. Cell Growth Differ 7:1671-1677.

[30] Oh, Y., Nagalla, S. R., Yamanaka, Y., Kim, H. S., Wilson, E., and Rosenfeld, R. G. (1996) Synthesis and characterization of insulin-like growth factor-binding protein (IGFBP)-7. Recombinant human mac25 protein specifically binds IGF-I and -II. J Biol Chem 271:30322-30325.

[31] Martinerie, C., Viegas-Pequignot, E., Guenard, I., Dutrillaux, B., Nguyen, V. C., Bernheim, A., and Perbal, B. (1992) Physical mapping of human loci homologous to the chicken nov proto-oncogene. Oncogene 7:2529-2534.

[32] O'Brien, T. P., Yang, G. P., Sanders, L., and Lau, L. F. (1990) Expression of cyr61, a growth factor-inducible immediate-early gene. Mol Cell Biol 10:3569-3577.

[33] Pennica, D., Swanson, T. A., Welsh, J. W., Roy, M. A., Lawrence, D. A., Lee, J., Brush, J., Taneyhill, L. A., Deuel, B., Lew, M., Watanabe, C., Cohen, R. L., Melhem, M. F., Finley, G. G., Quirke, P., Goddard, A. D., Hillan, K. J., Gurney, A. L., Botstein, D., and Levine, A. J. (1998) WISP genes are members of the connective tissue growth factor family that are up-regulated in wnt-1-transformed cells and aberrantly expressed in human colon tumors. Proc Natl Acad Sci U S A 95:14717-14722.

[34] Swisshelm, K., Ryan, K., Tsuchiya, K., and Sager, R. (1995) Enhanced expression of an insulin growth factor-like binding protein (mac25) in senescent human mammary epithelial cells and induced expression with retinoic acid. Proc Natl Acad Sci U S A 92:4472-4476.

[35] Kato, M. V., Sato, H., Tsukada, T., Ikawa, Y., Aizawa, S., and Nagayoshi, M. (1996) A follistatin-like gene, mac25, may act as a growth suppressor of osteosarcoma cells. Oncogene 12:1361-1364.

[36] Murphy, M., Pykett, M. J., Harnish, P., Zang, K. D., and George, D. L. (1993) Identification and characterization of genes differentially expressed in meningiomas. Cell Growth Differ 4:715-722.

[37] Sato, J., Hasegawa, S., Akaogi, K., Yasumitsu, H., Yamada, S., Sugahara, K., and Miyazaki, K. (1999) Identification of cell-binding site of angiomodulin (AGM/TAF/Mac25) that interacts with heparan sulfates on cell surface

[38] Bartelt, D. C., Shapanka, R., and Greene, L. J. (1977) The primary structure of the human pancreatic secretory trypsin inhibitor. Amino acid sequence of the reduced S-aminoethylated protein. Arch Biochem Biophys 179:189-199.

[39] Ahmed, S., Jin, X., Yagi, M., Yasuda, C., Sato, Y., Higashi, S., Lin, C. Y., Dickson, R. B., and Miyazaki, K. (2006) Identification of membrane-bound serine proteinase matriptase as processing enzyme of insulin-like growth factor binding protein-related protein-1 (IGFBP-rP1/angiomodulin/mac25). FEBS J 273:615-627.

[40] Ahmed, S., Yamamoto, K., Sato, Y., Ogawa, T., Herrmann, A., Higashi, S., and Miyazaki, K. (2003) Proteolytic processing of IGFBP-related protein-1 (TAF/angiomodulin/mac25) modulates its biological activity. Biochem Biophys Res Commun 310:612-618.

[41] Akaogi, K., Okabe, Y., Funahashi, K., Yoshitake, Y., Nishikawa, K., Yasumitsu, H., Umeda, M., and Miyazaki, K. (1994) Cell adhesion activity of a 30-kDa major secreted protein from human bladder carcinoma cells. Biochem Biophys Res Commun 198:1046-1053.

[42] Yamauchi, T., Umeda, F., Masakado, M., Isaji, M., Mizushima, S., and Nawata, H. (1994) Purification and molecular cloning of prostacyclin-stimulating factor from serum-free conditioned medium of human diploid fibroblast cells. Biochem J 303 (Pt 2):591-598.

[43] Inoguchi, T., Umeda, F., Ono, H., Kunisaki, M., Watanabe, J., and Nawata, H. (1989) Abnormality in prostacyclin-stimulatory activity in sera from diabetics. Metabolism 38:837-842.

[44] Inoguchi, T., Umeda, F., Watanabe, J., and Ibayashi, H. (1986) Reduced serum-stimulatory activity on prostacyclin production by cultured aortic endothelial cells in diabetes mellitus. Haemostasis 16:447-452.

[45] Burger, A. M., Zhang, X., Li, H., Ostrowski, J. L., Beatty, B., Venanzoni, M., Papas, T., and Seth, A. (1998) Down-regulation of T1A12/mac25, a novel insulin-like growth factor binding protein related gene, is associated with disease progression in breast carcinomas. Oncogene 16:2459-2467.

[46] Firth, S. M. and Baxter, R. C. (2002) Cellular actions of the insulin-like growth factor binding proteins. Endocr Rev 23:824-854.

[47] Yamanaka, Y., Wilson, E. M., Rosenfeld, R. G., and Oh, Y. (1997) Inhibition of insulin receptor activation by insulin-like growth factor binding proteins. J Biol Chem 272:30729-30734.

[48] Kato, M. V. (2000) A secreted tumor-suppressor, mac25, with activin-binding activity. Mol Med 6:126-135.

[49] Jeruss, J. S., Sturgis, C. D., Rademaker, A. W., and Woodruff, T. K. (2003) Down-regulation of activin, activin receptors, and Smads in high-grade breast cancer. Cancer Res 63:3783-3790.

[50] Nagakubo, D., Murai, T., Tanaka, T., Usui, T., Matsumoto, M., Sekiguchi, K., and Miyasaka, M. (2003) A high endothelial venule secretory protein, mac25/angiomodulin, interacts with multiple high endothelial venule-associated molecules including chemokines. J Immunol 171:553-561.

[51] Wilson, E. M., Oh, Y., and Rosenfeld, R. G. (1997) Generation and characterization of an IGFBP-7 antibody: identification of 31kD IGFBP-7 in human biological fluids and Hs578T human breast cancer conditioned media. J Clin Endocrinol Metab 82:1301-1303.

[52] Degeorges, A., Wang, F., Frierson, H. F., Jr., Seth, A., and Sikes, R. A. (2000) Distribution of IGFBP-rP1 in normal human tissues. J Histochem Cytochem 48:747-754.

[53] Dominguez, F., Avila, S., Cervero, A., Martin, J., Pellicer, A., Castrillo, J. L., and Simon, C. (2003) A combined approach for gene discovery identifies insulin-like growth factor-binding protein-related protein 1 as a new gene implicated in human endometrial receptivity. J Clin Endocrinol Metab 88:1849-1857.

[54] HAYFLICK, L. and MOORHEAD, P. S. (1961) The serial cultivation of human diploid cell strains. Exp Cell Res 25:585-621.

[55] Steinert, S., Shay, J. W., and Wright, W. E. (2000) Transient expression of human telomerase extends the life span of normal human fibroblasts. Biochem Biophys Res Commun 273:1095-1098.

[56] Campisi, J. and d'Adda di, Fagagna F. (2007) Cellular senescence: when bad things happen to good cells. Nat Rev Mol Cell Biol 8:729-740.

[57] Newbold, R. F. and Overell, R. W. (1983) Fibroblast immortality is a prerequisite for transformation by EJ c-Ha-ras oncogene. Nature 304:648-651.

[58] Serrano, M., Lin, A. W., McCurrach, M. E., Beach, D., and Lowe, S. W. (1997) Oncogenic ras provokes premature cell senescence associated with accumulation of p53 and p16INK4a. Cell 88:593-602.

[59] Wei, S., Wei, S., and Sedivy, J. M. (1999) Expression of catalytically active telomerase does not prevent premature senescence caused by overexpression of oncogenic Ha-Ras in normal human fibroblasts. Cancer Res 59:1539-1543.

[60] Lowe, S. W., Cepero, E., and Evan, G. (2004) Intrinsic tumour suppression. Nature 432:307-315.

[61] Courtois-Cox, S., Genther Williams, S. M., Reczek, E. E., Johnson, B. W., McGillicuddy, L. T., Johannessen, C. M., Hollstein, P. E., MacCollin, M., and Cichowski, K. (2006) A negative feedback signaling network underlies oncogene-induced senescence. Cancer Cell 10:459-472.

[62] Michaloglou, C., Vredeveld, L. C., Soengas, M. S., Denoyelle, C., Kuilman, T., van der Horst, C. M., Majoor, D. M., Shay, J. W., Mooi, W. J., and Peeper, D. S. (2005) BRAFE600-associated senescence-like cell cycle arrest of human naevi. Nature 436:720-724.

[63] Chen, Z., Trotman, L. C., Shaffer, D., Lin, H. K., Dotan, Z. A., Niki, M., Koutcher, J. A., Scher, H. I., Ludwig, T., Gerald, W., Cordon-Cardo, C., and Pandolfi, P. P. (2005) Crucial role of p53-dependent cellular senescence in suppression of Pten-deficient tumorigenesis. Nature 436:725-730.

[64] Dimri, G. P., Lee, X., Basile, G., Acosta, M., Scott, G., Roskelley, C., Medrano, E. E., Linskens, M., Rubelj, I., Pereira-Smith, O., and . (1995) A biomarker that identifies senescent human cells in culture and in aging skin in vivo. Proc Natl Acad Sci U S A 92:9363-9367.

[65] Campisi, J. (2005) Senescent cells, tumor suppression, and organismal aging: good citizens, bad neighbors. Cell 120:513-522.

[66] Beausejour, C. M., Krtolica, A., Galimi, F., Narita, M., Lowe, S. W., Yaswen, P., and Campisi, J. (2003) Reversal of human cellular senescence: roles of the p53 and p16 pathways. EMBO J 22:4212-4222.

[67] Dirac, A. M. and Bernards, R. (2003) Reversal of senescence in mouse fibroblasts through lentiviral suppression of p53. J Biol Chem 278:11731-11734.

[68] Sage, J., Miller, A. L., Perez-Mancera, P. A., Wysocki, J. M., and Jacks, T. (2003) Acute mutation of retinoblastoma gene function is sufficient for cell cycle re-entry. Nature 424:223-228.

[69] Bennett, D. C. (2003) Human melanocyte senescence and melanoma susceptibility genes. Oncogene 22:3063-3069.

[70] Chin, L., Merlino, G., and DePinho, R. A. (1998) Malignant melanoma: modern black plague and genetic black box. Genes Dev 12:3467-3481.

[71] Sparrow, L. E., Eldon, M. J., English, D. R., and Heenan, P. J. (1998) p16 and p21WAF1 protein expression in melanocytic tumors by immunohistochemistry. Am J Dermatopathol 20:255-261.

[72] Wang, Y. L., Uhara, H., Yamazaki, Y., Nikaido, T., and Saida, T. (1996) Immunohistochemical detection of CDK4 and p16INK4 proteins in cutaneous malignant melanoma. Br J Dermatol 134:269-275.

[73] Pollock, P. M., Harper, U. L., Hansen, K. S., Yudt, L. M., Stark, M., Robbins, C. M., Moses, T. Y., Hostetter, G., Wagner, U., Kakareka, J., Salem, G., Pohida, T., Heenan, P., Duray, P., Kallioniemi, O., Hayward, N. K., Trent, J. M., and Meltzer, P. S. (2003) High frequency of BRAF mutations in nevi. Nat Genet 33:19-20.

[74] Kuilman, T., Michaloglou, C., Vredeveld, L. C., Douma, S., van, Doorn R., Desmet, C. J., Aarden, L. A., Mooi, W. J., and Peeper, D. S. (2008) Oncogene-induced senescence relayed by an interleukin-dependent inflammatory network. Cell 133:1019-1031.

[75] Wajapeyee, N., Serra, R. W., Zhu, X., Mahalingam, M., and Green, M. R. (2-8-2008) Oncogenic BRAF induces senescence and apoptosis through pathways mediated by the secreted protein IGFBP7. Cell 132:363-374.

[76] Acosta, J. C., O'Loghlen, A., Banito, A., Guijarro, M. V., Augert, A., Raguz, S., Fumagalli, M., Da, Costa M., Brown, C., Popov, N., Takatsu, Y., Melamed, J., d'Adda di, Fagagna F., Bernard, D., Hernando, E., and Gil, J. (2008) Chemokine signaling via the CXCR2 receptor reinforces senescence. Cell 133:1006-1018.

[77] Kortlever, R. M., Higgins, P. J., and Bernards, R. (2006) Plasminogen activator inhibitor-1 is a critical downstream target of p53 in the induction of replicative senescence. Nat Cell Biol 8:877-884.

[78] Coppe, J. P., Patil, C. K., Rodier, F., Sun, Y., Munoz, D. P., Goldstein, J., Nelson, P. S., Desprez, P. Y., and Campisi, J. (2008) Senescence-associated secretory phenotypes reveal cell-nonautonomous functions of oncogenic RAS and the p53 tumor suppressor. PLoS Biol 6:2853-2868.

[79] Kuilman, T. and Peeper, D. S. (2009) Senescence-messaging secretome: SMS-ing cellular stress. Nat Rev Cancer 9:81-94.

[80] Burger, A. M., Leyland-Jones, B., Banerjee, K., Spyropoulos, D. D., and Seth, A. K. (2005) Essential roles of IGFBP-3 and IGFBP-rP1 in breast cancer. Eur J Cancer 41:1515-1527.

[81] Burger, A. M., Zhang, X., and Seth, A. (1998) Detection of novel genes that are up-regulated (Di12) or down-regulated (T1A12) with disease progression in breast cancer. Eur J Cancer Prev 7 Suppl 1:S29-S35.

[82] Komatsu, S., Okazaki, Y., Tateno, M., Kawai, J., Konno, H., Kusakabe, M., Yoshiki, A., Muramatsu, M., Held, W. A., and Hayashizaki, Y. (2000) Methylation and downregulated expression of mac25/insulin-like growth factor binding protein-7 is associated with liver tumorigenesis in SV40T/t antigen transgenic mice, screened by restriction landmark genomic scanning for methylation (RLGS-M). Biochem Biophys Res Commun 267:109-117.

[83] Smith, P., Nicholson, L. J., Syed, N., Payne, A., Hiller, L., Garrone, O., Occelli, M., Gasco, M., and Crook, T. (2007) Epigenetic inactivation implies independent functions for insulin-like growth factor binding protein (IGFBP)-related protein 1 and the related IGFBPL1 in inhibiting breast cancer phenotypes. Clin Cancer Res 13:4061-4068.

[84] Landberg, G., Ostlund, H., Nielsen, N. H., Roos, G., Emdin, S., Burger, A. M., and Seth, A. (2001) Downregulation of the potential suppressor gene IGFBP-rP1 in human breast cancer is associated with inactivation of the retinoblastoma protein, cyclin E overexpression and increased proliferation in estrogen receptor negative tumors. Oncogene 20:3497-3505.

[85] Amemiya, Y., Yang, W., Benatar, T., Nofech-Mozes, S., Yee, A., Kahn, H., Holloway, C., and Seth, A. (2010) Insulin like growth factor binding protein-7 reduces growth of human breast cancer cells and xenografted tumors. Breast Cancer Res Treat

[86] Wilson, H. M., Birnbaum, R. S., Poot, M., Quinn, L. S., and Swisshelm, K. (2002) Insulin-like growth factor binding protein-related protein 1 inhibits proliferation of MCF-7 breast cancer cells via a senescence-like mechanism. Cell Growth Differ 13:205-213.

[87] Cailleau, R., Olive, M., and Cruciger, Q. V. (1978) Long-term human breast carcinoma cell lines of metastatic origin: preliminary characterization. In Vitro 14:911-915.

[88] Davies, H., Bignell, G. R., Cox, C., Stephens, P., Edkins, S., Clegg, S., Teague, J., Woffendin, H., Garnett, M. J., Bottomley, W., Davis, N., Dicks, E., Ewing, R., Floyd, Y., Gray, K., Hall, S., Hawes, R., Hughes, J., Kosmidou, V., Menzies, A., Mould, C., Parker, A., Stevens, C., Watt, S., Hooper, S., Wilson, R., Jayatilake, H., Gusterson, B. A., Cooper, C., Shipley, J., Hargrave, D., Pritchard-Jones, K., Maitland, N., Chenevix-Trench, G., Riggins, G. J., Bigner, D. D., Palmieri, G., Cossu, A., Flanagan, A., Nicholson, A., Ho, J. W., Leung, S. Y., Yuen, S. T., Weber, B. L., Seigler, H. F., Darrow, T. L., Paterson, H., Marais, R., Marshall, C. J., Wooster, R., Stratton, M. R., and Futreal, P. A. (2002) Mutations of the BRAF gene in human cancer. Nature 417:949-954.

[89] Wajapeyee, N., Kapoor, V., Mahalingam, M., and Green, M. R. (2009) Efficacy of IGFBP7 for treatment of metastatic melanoma and other cancers in mouse models and human cell lines. Mol Cancer Ther 8:3009-3014.

[90] Chen, R. Y., Chen, H. X., Jian, P., Xu, L., Li, J., Fan, Y. M., and Tu, Y. T. (2010) Intratumoral injection of pEGFC1-IGFBP7 inhibits malignant melanoma growth in C57BL/6J mice by inducing apoptosis and down-regulating VEGF expression. Oncol Rep 23:981-988.

[91] Ruan, W., Xu, E., Xu, F., Ma, Y., Deng, H., Huang, Q., Lv, B., Hu, H., Lin, J., Cui, J., Di, M., Dong, J., and Lai, M. (2007) IGFBP7 plays a potential tumor suppressor role in colorectal carcinogenesis. Cancer Biol Ther 6:354-359.

[92] Lin, J., Lai, M., Huang, Q., Ma, Y., Cui, J., and Ruan, W. (2007) Methylation patterns of IGFBP7 in colon cancer cell lines are associated with levels of gene expression. J Pathol 212:83-90.

[93] Lin, J., Lai, M., Huang, Q., Ruan, W., Ma, Y., and Cui, J. (2008) Reactivation of IGFBP7 by DNA demethylation inhibits human colon cancer cell growth in vitro. Cancer Biol Ther 7:1896-1900.

[94] Suzuki, H., Igarashi, S., Nojima, M., Maruyama, R., Yamamoto, E., Kai, M., Akashi, H., Watanabe, Y., Yamamoto, H., Sasaki, Y., Itoh, F., Imai, K., Sugai, T., Shen, L., Issa, J. P., Shinomura, Y., Tokino, T., and Toyota, M. (2009) IGFBP7 is a p53 Responsive Gene Specifically Silenced in Colorectal Cancer with CpG Island Methylator Phenotype. Carcinogenesis

[95] Ma, Y., Lu, B., Ruan, W., Wang, H., Lin, J., Hu, H., Deng, H., Huang, Q., and Lai, M. (2008) Tumor suppressor gene insulin-like growth factor binding protein-related protein 1 (IGFBP-rP1) induces senescence-like growth arrest in colorectal cancer cells. Exp Mol Pathol 85:141-145.

[96] Braig, M., Lee, S., Loddenkemper, C., Rudolph, C., Peters, A. H., Schlegelberger, B., Stein, H., Dorken, B., Jenuwein, T., and Schmitt, C. A. (2005) Oncogene-induced senescence as an initial barrier in lymphoma development. Nature 436:660-665.

[97] Collado, M., Gil, J., Efeyan, A., Guerra, C., Schuhmacher, A. J., Barradas, M., Benguria, A., Zaballos, A., Flores, J. M., Barbacid, M., Beach, D., and Serrano, M. (2005) Tumour biology: senescence in premalignant tumours. Nature 436:642-

[98] Sato, Y., Chen, Z., and Miyazaki, K. (2007) Strong suppression of tumor growth by insulin-like growth factor-binding protein-related protein 1/tumor-derived cell adhesion factor/mac25. Cancer Sci 98:1055-1063.

[99] Ruan, W., Wang, Y., Ma, Y., Xing, X., Lin, J., Cui, J., and Lai, M. (2010) HSP60, a protein downregulated by IGFBP7 in colorectal carcinoma. J Exp Clin Cancer Res 29:41-

[100] Degeorges, A., Wang, F., Frierson, H. F., Jr., Seth, A., Chung, L. W., and Sikes, R. A. (1999) Human prostate cancer expresses the low affinity insulin-like growth factor binding protein IGFBP-rP1. Cancer Res 59:2787-2790.

[101] Lopez-Bermejo, A., Buckway, C. K., Devi, G. R., Hwa, V., Plymate, S. R., Oh, Y., and Rosenfeld, R. G. (2000) Characterization of insulin-like growth factor-binding protein-related proteins (IGFBP-rPs) 1, 2, and 3 in human prostate epithelial cells: potential roles for IGFBP-rP1 and 2 in senescence of the prostatic epithelium. Endocrinology 141:4072-4080.

[102] Sprenger, C. C., Damon, S. E., Hwa, V., Rosenfeld, R. G., and Plymate, S. R. (1999) Insulin-like growth factor binding protein-related protein 1 (IGFBP-rP1) is a potential tumor suppressor protein for prostate cancer. Cancer Res 59:2370-2375.

[103] Drivdahl, R., Haugk, K. H., Sprenger, C. C., Nelson, P. S., Tennant, M. K., and Plymate, S. R. (2004) Suppression of growth and tumorigenicity in the prostate tumor cell line M12 by overexpression of the transcription factor SOX9. Oncogene 23:4584-4593.

[104] Plymate, S. R., Haugk, K. H., Sprenger, C. C., Nelson, P. S., Tennant, M. K., Zhang, Y., Oberley, L. W., Zhong, W., Drivdahl, R., and Oberley, T. D. (2003) Increased manganese superoxide dismutase (SOD-2) is part of the mechanism for prostate

tumor suppression by Mac25/insulin-like growth factor binding-protein-related protein-1. Oncogene 22:1024-1034.

[105] Vizioli, M. G., Sensi, M., Miranda, C., Cleris, L., Formelli, F., Anania, M. C., Pierotti, M. A., and Greco, A. (2010) IGFBP7: an oncosuppressor gene in thyroid carcinogenesis. Oncogene 29:3835-3844.

[106] Tomimaru, Y., Eguchi, H., Wada, H., Noda, T., Murakami, M., Kobayashi, S., Marubashi, S., Takeda, Y., Tanemura, M., Umeshita, K., Doki, Y., Mori, M., and Nagano, H. (2010) Insulin-like growth factor-binding protein 7 alters the sensitivity to interferon-based anticancer therapy in hepatocellular carcinoma cells. Br J Cancer 102:1483-1490.

[107] Eguchi, H., Nagano, H., Yamamoto, H., Miyamoto, A., Kondo, M., Dono, K., Nakamori, S., Umeshita, K., Sakon, M., and Monden, M. (2000) Augmentation of antitumor activity of 5-fluorouracil by interferon alpha is associated with up-regulation of p27Kip1 in human hepatocellular carcinoma cells. Clin Cancer Res 6:2881-2890.

[108] Kondo, M., Nagano, H., Sakon, M., Yamamoto, H., Morimoto, O., Arai, I., Miyamoto, A., Eguchi, H., Dono, K., Nakamori, S., Umeshita, K., Wakasa, K., Ohmoto, Y., and Monden, M. (2000) Expression of interferon alpha/beta receptor in human hepatocellular carcinoma. Int J Oncol 17:83-88.

[109] Kondo, M., Nagano, H., Wada, H., Damdinsuren, B., Yamamoto, H., Hiraoka, N., Eguchi, H., Miyamoto, A., Yamamoto, T., Ota, H., Nakamura, M., Marubashi, S., Dono, K., Umeshita, K., Nakamori, S., Sakon, M., and Monden, M. (2005) Combination of IFN-alpha and 5-fluorouracil induces apoptosis through IFN-alpha/beta receptor in human hepatocellular carcinoma cells. Clin Cancer Res 11:1277-1286.

[110] Wada, H., Nagano, H., Yamamoto, H., Arai, I., Ota, H., Nakamura, M., Damdinsuren, B., Noda, T., Marubashi, S., Miyamoto, A., Takeda, Y., Umeshita, K., Doki, Y., Dono, K., Nakamori, S., Sakon, M., and Monden, M. (2007) Combination therapy of interferon-alpha and 5-fluorouracil inhibits tumor angiogenesis in human hepatocellular carcinoma cells by regulating vascular endothelial growth factor and angiopoietins. Oncol Rep 18:801-809.

[111] Sakon, M., Nagano, H., Dono, K., Nakamori, S., Umeshita, K., Yamada, A., Kawata, S., Imai, Y., Iijima, S., and Monden, M. (2002) Combined intraarterial 5-fluorouracil and subcutaneous interferon-alpha therapy for advanced hepatocellular carcinoma with tumor thrombi in the major portal branches. Cancer 94:435-442.

[112] Yamamoto, T., Nagano, H., Sakon, M., Wada, H., Eguchi, H., Kondo, M., Damdinsuren, B., Ota, H., Nakamura, M., Wada, H., Marubashi, S., Miyamoto, A., Dono, K., Umeshita, K., Nakamori, S., Yagita, H., and Monden, M. (2004) Partial contribution of tumor necrosis factor-related apoptosis-inducing ligand (TRAIL)/TRAIL receptor pathway to antitumor effects of interferon-alpha/5-fluorouracil against Hepatocellular Carcinoma. Clin Cancer Res 10:7884-7895.

[113] Ota, H., Nagano, H., Sakon, M., Eguchi, H., Kondo, M., Yamamoto, T., Nakamura, M., Damdinsuren, B., Wada, H., Marubashi, S., Miyamoto, A., Dono, K., Umeshita, K., Nakamori, S., Wakasa, K., and Monden, M. (2005) Treatment of hepatocellular carcinoma with major portal vein thrombosis by combined therapy with subcutaneous interferon-alpha and intra-arterial 5-fluorouracil; role of type 1 interferon receptor expression. Br J Cancer 93:557-564.

[114] Nakamura, M., Nagano, H., Sakon, M., Yamamoto, T., Ota, H., Wada, H., Damdinsuren, B., Noda, T., Marubashi, S., Miyamoto, A., Takeda, Y., Umeshita, K., Nakamori, S., Dono, K., and Monden, M. (2007) Role of the Fas/FasL pathway in combination therapy with interferon-alpha and fluorouracil against hepatocellular carcinoma in vitro. J Hepatol 46:77-88.

[115] Damdinsuren, B., Nagano, H., and Monden, M. (2007) Combined intra-arterial 5-fluorouracil and subcutaneous interferon-alpha therapy for highly advanced hepatocellular carcinoma. Hepatol Res 37 Suppl 2:S238-S250.

[116] Nagano, H., Sakon, M., Eguchi, H., Kondo, M., Yamamoto, T., Ota, H., Nakamura, M., Wada, H., Damdinsuren, B., Marubashi, S., Miyamoto, A., Takeda, Y., Dono, K., Umeshit, K., Nakamori, S., and Monden, M. (2007) Hepatic resection followed by IFN-alpha and 5-FU for advanced hepatocellular carcinoma with tumor thrombus in the major portal branch. Hepatogastroenterology 54:172-179.

[117] Tomimaru, Y., Eguchi, H., Wada, H., Kobayashi, S., Marubashi, S., Tanemura, M., Umeshita, K., Kim, T., Wakasa, K., Doki, Y., Mori, M., and Nagano, H. (2011) IGFBP7 downregulation is associated with tumor progression and clinical outcome in hepatocellular carcinoma. Int J Cancer

[118] Chen, Y., Pacyna-Gengelbach, M., Ye, F., Knosel, T., Lund, P., Deutschmann, N., Schluns, K., Kotb, W. F., Sers, C., Yasumoto, H., Usui, T., and Petersen, I. (2007) Insulin-like growth factor binding protein-related protein 1 (IGFBP-rP1) has potential tumour-suppressive activity in human lung cancer. J Pathol 211:431-438.

[119] Huang, Y. J., Niu, J., Liu, Z., Wang, L. E., Sturgis, E. M., and Wei, Q. (2010) The functional IGFBP7 promoter -418G>A polymorphism and risk of head and neck cancer. Mutat Res 702:32 39.

[120] Pen, A., Moreno, M. J., Martin, J., and Stanimirovic, D. B. (2007) Molecular markers of extracellular matrix remodeling in glioblastoma vessels: microarray study of laser-captured glioblastoma vessels. Glia 55:559-572.

[121] Jiang, W., Xiang, C., Cazacu, S., Brodie, C., and Mikkelsen, T. (2008) Insulin-like growth factor binding protein 7 mediates glioma cell growth and migration. Neoplasia 10:1335-1342.

[122] Pen, A., Moreno, M. J., Durocher, Y., Deb-Rinker, P., and Stanimirovic, D. B. (2008) Glioblastoma-secreted factors induce IGFBP7 and angiogenesis by modulating Smad-2-dependent TGF-beta signaling. Oncogene 27:6834-6844.

[123] Tanner, S. M., Austin, J. L., Leone, G., Rush, L. J., Plass, C., Heinonen, K., Mrozek, K., Sill, H., Knuutila, S., Kolitz, J. E., Archer, K. J., Caligiuri, M. A., Bloomfield, C. D., and de La, Chapelle A. (2001) BAALC, the human member of a novel mammalian neuroectoderm gene lineage, is implicated in hematopoiesis and acute leukemia. Proc Natl Acad Sci U S A 98:13901-13906.

[124] Baldus, C. D., Tanner, S. M., Ruppert, A. S., Whitman, S. P., Archer, K. J., Marcucci, G., Caligiuri, M. A., Carroll, A. J., Vardiman, J. W., Powell, B. L., Allen, S. L., Moore, J. O., Larson, R. A., Kolitz, J. E., de la Chapelle, A., and Bloomfield, C. D. (2003) BAALC expression predicts clinical outcome of de novo acute myeloid leukemia patients with normal cytogenetics: a Cancer and Leukemia Group B Study. Blood 102:1613-1618.

[125] Bienz, M., Ludwig, M., Leibundgut, E. O., Mueller, B. U., Ratschiller, D., Solenthaler, M., Fey, M. F., and Pabst, T. (2005) Risk assessment in patients with acute myeloid leukemia and a normal karyotype. Clin Cancer Res 11:1416-1424.

[126] Baldus, C. D., Martus, P., Burmeister, T., Schwartz, S., Gokbuget, N., Bloomfield, C. D., Hoelzer, D., Thiel, E., and Hofmann, W. K. (2007) Low ERG and BAALC expression identifies a new subgroup of adult acute T-lymphoblastic leukemia with a highly favorable outcome. J Clin Oncol 25:3739-3745.

[127] Langer, C., Radmacher, M. D., Ruppert, A. S., Whitman, S. P., Paschka, P., Mrozek, K., Baldus, C. D., Vukosavljevic, T., Liu, C. G., Ross, M. E., Powell, B. L., de la Chapelle, A., Kolitz, J. E., Larson, R. A., Marcucci, G., and Bloomfield, C. D. (2008) High BAALC expression associates with other molecular prognostic markers, poor outcome, and a distinct gene-expression signature in cytogenetically normal patients younger than 60 years with acute myeloid leukemia: a Cancer and Leukemia Group B (CALGB) study. Blood 111:5371-5379.

[128] Heesch, S., Schlee, C., Neumann, M., Stroux, A., Kuhnl, A., Schwartz, S., Haferlach, T., Goekbuget, N., Hoelzer, D., Thiel, E., Hofmann, W. K., and Baldus, C. D. (2010) BAALC-associated gene expression profiles define IGFBP7 as a novel molecular marker in acute leukemia. Leukemia 24:1429-1436.

[129] How, H. K., Yeoh, A., Quah, T. C., Oh, Y., Rosenfeld, R. G., and Lee, K. O. (1999) Insulin-like growth factor binding proteins (IGFBPs) and IGFBP-related protein 1-levels in cerebrospinal fluid of children with acute lymphoblastic leukemia. J Clin Endocrinol Metab 84:1283-1287.

[130] Hu, S., Chen, R., Man, X., Feng, X., Cen, J., Gu, W., He, H., Li, J., Chai, Y., and Chen, Z. (2011) Function and Expression of Insulin-Like Growth Factor-Binding Protein 7 (IGFBP7) Gene in Childhood Acute Myeloid Leukemia. Pediatr Hematol Oncol

[131] Hollestelle, A., Elstrodt, F., Nagel, J. H., Kallemeijn, W. W., and Schutte, M. (2007) Phosphatidylinositol-3-OH kinase or RAS pathway mutations in human breast cancer cell lines. Mol Cancer Res 5:195-201.

[132] Blagosklonny, M. V. (2003) Cell senescence and hypermitogenic arrest. EMBO Rep 4:358-362.

[133] Schmitt, C. A. (2007) Cellular senescence and cancer treatment. Biochim Biophys Acta 1775:5-20.

[134] Clausen, T., Kaiser, M., Huber, R., and Ehrmann, M. (2011) HTRA proteases: regulated proteolysis in protein quality control. Nat.Rev.Mol.Cell Biol. 12:152-162.

[135] Shibata, Y., Tsukazaki, T., Hirata, K., Xin, C., and Yamaguchi, A. (2004) Role of a new member of IGFBP superfamily, IGFBP-rP10, in proliferation and differentiation of osteoblastic cells. Biochem.Biophys.Res.Commun. 325:1194-1200.

3

In Vitro Breast Cancer Models as Useful Tools in Therapeutics?

Emilie Bana and Denyse Bagrel
Université Paul Verlaine – Metz
Laboratoire d'Ingénierie Moléculaire et Biochimie Pharmacologique
France

1. Introduction

The increased use of animals in fundamental and applied research due to the remarkable drug development in the 20th century has been an important matter of concern for people at large, but also for the scientific community. This led Russel and Burch to examine the decisions which could meliorate this situation, and they proposed, in 1959, the principle of the 3Rs (Reduce, Refine, and Replace) nowadays largely admitted as an ethical and incontrovertible principle (Russell & Bursch 1959). Alternatives to animal experiments (Scheme 1) then knew a fantastic boom with the permanent objective of a high scientific quality in order to prevent, treat and cure human illness.

Reaching the equilibrium between *in vitro* and *in vivo* models, observing the 3Rs rules, is very difficult. Effectively, *in vitro* systems allow an excellent control of all parameters of the experiments, and then, good quantifications. More the models are simple, more they are easy to handle, but more they also are dedifferentiated and keep away from the *in vivo* situation.

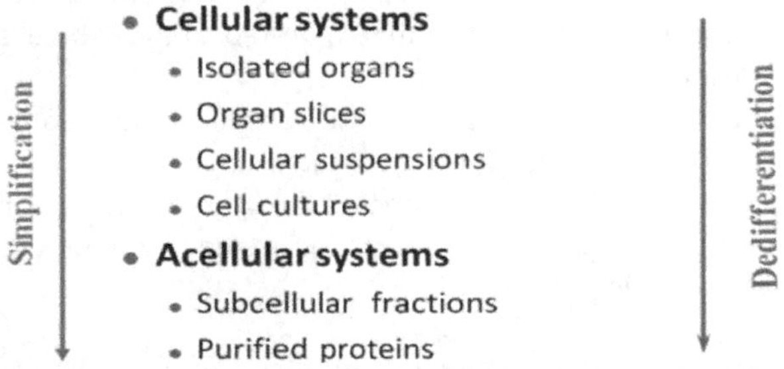

- **Cellular systems**
  - Isolated organs
  - Organ slices
  - Cellular suspensions
  - Cell cultures
- **Acellular systems**
  - Subcellular fractions
  - Purified proteins

Simplification (left vertical axis) — *Dedifferentiation* (right vertical axis)

Scheme 1. *In vitro* systems as alternatives to the use of animals.

Within the framework of this book, the question becomes now: how the 3Rs could be the best way to phase out animal experiments when considering breast cancer? We try to bring some response elements in this chapter, emphasising the *in vitro* models the most useful and the most frequently used. But we also show that no model is perfect and sufficient by itself, and that pure *in vitro* models also need assistance of *in vivo* ones.

2. Models for investigation on breast cancer

2.1 Established breast cancer cell lines
2.1.1 The different cell lines and their main properties

Significant amounts of data on breast cancer have been collected over the past 40 years, thanks to the use of established cell lines. The first breast cancer cell lines (BCCL) have been established in the sixties-seventies and very few new cell lines have been developed since. Only a hundred of BCCL are currently available and three of them have been extensively studied and represent now nearly 80% of the 35 000 publications mentioning breast cancer cell lines (Lacroix & Leclercq 2004).

Most of the cell lines were created from cells derived from metastasis or from pleural effusion. Pleural effusions contain large amounts of well isolated tumour cells and few contaminating cells such as fibroblasts, thus making their recovery and growing easier than those of cells directly derived from primary tumours or metastasis. Moreover, metastatic cells are highly dedifferentiated cells, which allow their cultivation more successfully than the primary tumour cells.

The three more used BCCL (MCF-7, MDA-MB-231 and T47D) are issued from pleural effusion of an invasive ductal carcinoma (Soule *et al.* 1973; Cailleau *et al.* 1974; Keydar *et al.* 1979), and they mainly differ by their oestrogen receptor (ER) and progesterone receptor (PgR) status: MCF-7 and T47D are ER+ PgR+ while MDA-MB-231 is ER- PgR-. Among these three cell lines, MCF-7 was the most often used during the last ten years: it has been cited in 53% of all the scientific papers mentioning BCCL, while MDA-MB-231 and T47D were respectively cited in about 18% and 7% of these articles (calculation made on the basis of a Medline-based survey in March 2011).

The use of these lines has many technical advantages.

- The complete control of environmental conditions and standardised culture conditions ensures the reproducibility of results between experiments and laboratories.
- Maintaining cells in culture is much less costly than working on animal models. Besides the fact that some animal models are expensive by themselves, the care of animals and the staff necessary to a good work in an animal house are the main drain of resources. Conversely, the medium and the staff time required to growth cells are cheaper, thus allowing the widespread use of BCCL.
- Cryopreservation enables long-term conservation of the same strain and can theoretically permit the use of these cell lines indefinitely.

These advantages have allowed to gather essential data for the study of breast cancer in the last 40 years, making these cell lines reference models in the field with the establishment of a complete genetic and proteinic profile.

2.1.2 The main drawbacks of these models
-    Stability/instability

In practice, these strains, although cryopreserved, undergo dedifferentiation resulting from multiple subcultures, and leading to the lost of special characteristics. Moreover, differences in the culturing practices (medium composition, time between subcultures, subculturing technique, etc.), can explain some divergences observed for a same strain in different laboratories.

- Simplicity

The relevance of cellular models is controversial since their over-simplicity implies difficulties in extrapolating results from the cell line to the tumour in humans and thus raises the question of their representativeness.

Indeed, cell lines are homogeneous, theoretically consisting only of a single cell type (pure and clonal) due to the way they are established:

- The dislocation of tumours is followed by isolation of cells, in order to obtain the most stable culture during subcultures.
- The culture conditions eliminate some types of cells present in the original tumour, unable to grow on a synthetic surface, or whose rate of development is much lower than the one of the surviving cells.
- Cells in culture do not undergo the influence of nervous and hormonal regulatory systems active *in vivo*.

These particularities reduce the similarity with the primary tumour.

- Limited representativeness

The hundred of available cell lines do not cover all of the tumour features found in patients. Furthermore, the proportions of some characteristics are sometimes reversed, such as the ER and PgR status which is very different in cell lines, compared to that found in the patient population (Lacroix & Leclercq 2004). These dissimilarities can be explained by the fact that most lines are derived from pleural effusion and metastases containing cells which are already different from the original tumour and thus, more or less representative of this tumour. Indeed, the ER/PgR status sometimes differs between the metastasis and the original tumour from the same patient. Based on these observations, several teams have worked on the development of cell lines derived from a primary tumour (Amadori *et al.* 1993; Gazdar *et al.* 1998; Shen *et al.* 2009), which are much more representative of the *in vivo* cancerous tissues that lines derived from metastases, but which suffer from the same problems related to their relative homogeneity and instability in a long term use. Moreover, the establishment of cell lines from primary tumours remains a difficult achievement, failures mainly being the result of contamination by the stroma surrounding the tumour.

- Confusion with some cell lines

Besides these previous drawbacks, many criticisms have been made against BCCL because some of them have been proven not being from breast cancer origin. Indeed, some lines were contaminated by other cell types during their first years of use, then spread to other laboratories, and used on a large scale without further verifications of their true origin. Several cell lines were denounced as false, whereas it was not the case (Fogh *et al.* 1977; Nelson-Rees & Flandermeyer 1977). These contaminations have been subjects of controversial for a long time. However, studies have shown with certitude that two cell lines were not from their supposed origin.

The MCF-7-ADRr cell line was developed in 1986 by Batist. It is derived from the lineage of human mammary adenocarcinoma MCF-7 and was rendered resistant to adriamycin treatment after exposition to increased concentrations of this drug. The obtained resistant cell line was also resistant to other agents such as actinomycin D, vinblastine and vincristine. However in 1998, the lineage between MCF-7 and MCF-7-ADRr became controversial, as shown by DNA fingerprinting studies and genetic comparison, so that the true origin of the cell line was undetermined and the cell line was renamed NCI/ADR-RES. Liscovitch and Ravid, in 2007, have collected data showing that NCI/ADR-RES were carcinoma ovarian cells (Liscovitch & Ravid 2007), and experiments of Affymetrix SNP array analysis at the Sanger Institute (Cancer Genome Project) and of karyotyping, helped to put in evidence an indisputable resemblance of NCI/ADR-RES with the OVCAR-8 human ovarian carcinoma cell line. The most likely scenario is that the stock of MCF-7 cells from the National Cancer Institute used in 1986 for the development of the lineage, was contaminated with OVCAR-8 cells before the first generation of MCF-7-ADR-r. OVCAR-8 cells are naturally resistant to adriamycin, and the *in vitro* selection probably eliminated the MCF-7 cells and allowed the survival of OVCAR-8 cells (Liscovitch & Ravid 2007). It can be noted that MCF-7-ADRr are no longer distributed by the international cell bank ATCC.

The second misidentification concerns the MDA-MB-435 cell line established by Cailleau and colleagues in 1978. This cell line has been controversial in 2000, further to the results of DNA microarray analysis which suggested that these cells might be of melanocyte origin (Ross & Perou 2001). Some other results, obtained by microsatellite comparison analysis, karyotyping and comparative genomic hybridisation experiments (Rae *et al.* 2007), confirmed that MDA-MB-435 cells are in fact M14 melanoma cells.

However, these two cell lines, MCF-7-ADRr and MDA-MB-235, are still used as breast cancer cell lines for some studies and are used for publications in international journals, while it has been proven that they are not from breast cancer origin (Lacroix 2008). The verification of the origin of a cell line is essential, and a way of ensuring that the cell lines are really from a well-defined origin is to make a short tandem repeat (STR) profiling. This method is used to confirm the identity of a cell line by comparison to a known profile and a periodic re-authentication of cell lines is advisable. Moreover, banks of cell lines such as ATCC guarantee the exact origin of their cells. Several authors suggested to prove the authenticity of the cell lines used for each publications (Burdall *et al.* 2003; Lacroix 2008).

2.1.3 Non cancerous immortalised cells as controls

It should be noticed that the study of mammary tumours also involves the use of non cancerous cells which were immortalised. These cell lines were derived from healthy breast tissue, but only few models, obtained by different methods, are available.

- The immortalisation could be the consequence of a particular composition of the growth medium. This is the case for the non-tumourigenic epithelial cell lines MCF-10A (adherent cells) and MCF-10F (floating cells) which were established from the same sample in the nineties (Soule *et al.* 1990). These cell lines were produced by a long-term culture in a special medium containing a low concentration of Ca^{2+} and no serum addition, which resulted in the apparition of immortalised cells with normal features of mammalian epithelial cells.

- Two other cell lines were derived from a mammoplastic surgery. These cells named MCF-12A and MCF-12F became spontaneously immortal after unexpected exposition to high temperatures (45°C during 72 hours, Pauley *et al.* 1991).

- Another cell line, hTERT-HME1 was obtained from the HME1 cells (Human Mammary Epithelial) which were immortalised by infection with the retrovirus pBabepuro+hTER. The immortality feature results from the exogenous expression of the telomerase gene coming from the viral infection (Van der Haegen & Shay 1993; Gollahon & Shay 1996).

- Under chemical pressure, normal cells in culture can also be immortalised. This is the case for some cell lines as 184A1 and 184B5 which were obtained by exposition to benzo[a]pyrène, a chemical carcinogen, leading to clonal events which are the origin of these immortal cell lines (Stampfer 1989).

The use of these "non cancerous" cell lines is important to give a comparison point to results obtained with cancerous cell lines. However, there are drawbacks and controversy to their use, the major one concerning the way they were obtained. Indeed, if they are still non-tumourigenic, they suffer of genetic modifications which lead them to become immortal. They are looking like normal cells, but they are not.

2.1.4 Breast cell lines and metabolism of therapeutic drugs
- Drug metabolism

The metabolic equipment of a cell can explain its sensitivity/resistance to drugs. Indeed, any xenobiotic molecule (therapeutic drugs included) undergoes the same metabolic fate in the cells. Briefly, enzymes of Phase I (essentially cytochromes P450 (CYP) dependent enzymes) ensure a bioactivation of the molecules while enzymes of Phase II conjugate the metabolites issued from Phase I to endogenous molecules (glucuronic acid, glutathione, sulfates...) in order to make them more water-soluble and to facilitate their elimination. Finally, transporters of Phase III are responsible for exporting these last products out of the cells. Each human organ is equipped with these enzymes, but their expression pattern differs quantitatively and qualitatively. The liver is the most efficient organ in metabolising processes, even if we know that some enzymes are more specifically expressed in non hepatic tissues.

When considering the usefulness of breast cell lines as *in vitro* tools to predict sensitivity or resistance to a molecule, it is easy to perform, in first line, simple cytotoxicity tests. However, in order to explain the reasons of these cells behavior, or to predict the metabolism of a new compound, the knowledge of the metabolic equipment of the cells is necessary. As it is impossible, and not very interesting, to decline the results of the literature concerning breast cell lines and assays with the numerous chemical molecules which have been, precisely or not precisely, tested, we chose two examples of therapeutic drugs, used in breast cancer, that need to be bioactivated by CYP before exerting their deleterious effects in the cells: oxazaphosphorines and ellipticine.

- Metabolism of oxazaphosphorines

The oxazaphosphorines generally used in pharmacology (*i.e.* cyclophosphamide (CPA), ifosfamide (IFO), and trofosfamide) represent an important group of chemotherapeutic agents. However, their use is limited by severe toxic side effects. New oxazaphosphorines derivatives have been developed in order to improve selectivity and to reduce toxicity but they won't be studied here, due to their bioactivation process which is different from that of previous molecules (Zhang *et al.* 2005).

Both CPA and IFO, the most widely used as alkylating agents, are prodrugs whose metabolism involves different cytochromes P450 (CYPs) catalysing 4-hydroxylations leading to acrolein and nitrogen mustards capable of reacting with DNA molecules leading to cell apoptosis and/or necrosis. Another pathway consists in an N-dealkylation whose last product is the toxic chloroacetaldehyde (Figure 1) (Rooseboom *et al.* 2004; Zhang *et al.* 2005). All these metabolites are highly reactive metabolites responsible for urotoxicity, neurotoxicity and nephrotoxicity. As all the mechanisms underlying these toxicities are not elucidated, Mesna (Sodium 2-mercaptoethanesulfonate) is often used to limit these side effects (Giraud *et al.* 2010).

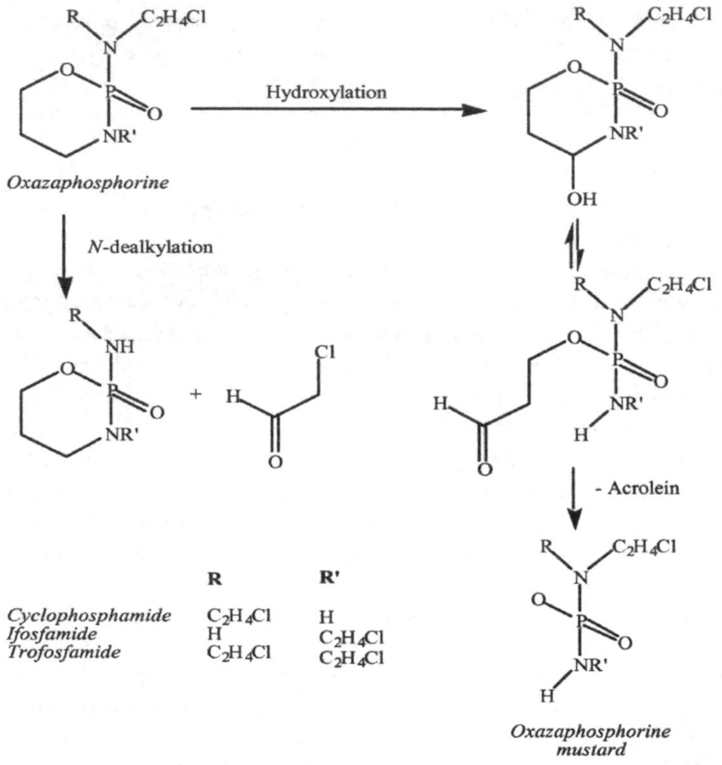

Fig. 1. **First phase of metabolism of the oxazaphosphorines by CYPs:** hydroxylation leads to oxazaphosphorine mustards, and N-dealkylation results in chloracetaldehyde formation. From Rooseboom *et al.* 2004 with permission from ASPET.

As already mentioned, several CYPs are involved in these drug metabolism: CYP2B6 (Wang & Tompkins 2008; Mo *et al.* 2009; Bray *et al.* 2010), CYP3A4 (Kivisto *et al.* 1995), but also CYP2A6 (Di *et al.* 2009), CYP2C9, CYP2C19, CYP3A5 (Bray *et al.* 2010) and probably others. Figure 2 below, extracted from Wang & Tompkins 2008, shows the expression of the different human hepatic CYP and their contribution to metabolize clinically-used drugs. No analog study was performed in breast tissue, and *a fortiori* in breast cancer cell lines. However, the literature reports the presence of CYP3A4 (the CYP enzyme the most involved in drug metabolism) in MCF-7, T47D and MDA-MB-231 (Nagaoka *et al.* 2006; Chen *et al.* 2009; Mitra *et al.* 2011), of CYP2B6 in MCF-7 and T47D (Lo *et al.* 2010) whereas this information is not available for MDA-MB-231. While CYP2D6 and splicing variants similar to those found in breast cancer tissues were shown expressed in MCF-7 (Huang *et al.* 1997), no information about this CYP, to our knowledge, was related for T47D and MDA-MB-231.

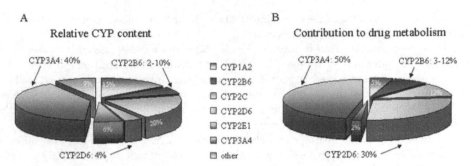

Fig. 2. Hepatic CYP expression (A) and their contribution to metabolism of clinically-used drugs (B). From Wang & Tompkins 2008, permission granted by Bentham Science Publishers Ltd.

- Metabolism of ellipticine

Another example is given by ellipticine. This alkaloid compound found in several plants (Ochrosia, Aspidoserma subincanum, Bleekeria vitiensis) is a topoisomerase poison often used in ovarian and breast cancer treatment. It is also a prodrug whose efficiency depends on CYP activation. 13-hydroxy- and 12-hydroxy-ellipticine, responsible for the formation of DNA adducts, are generated by CYP1A1/2, CYP3A4 and CYP2C9.

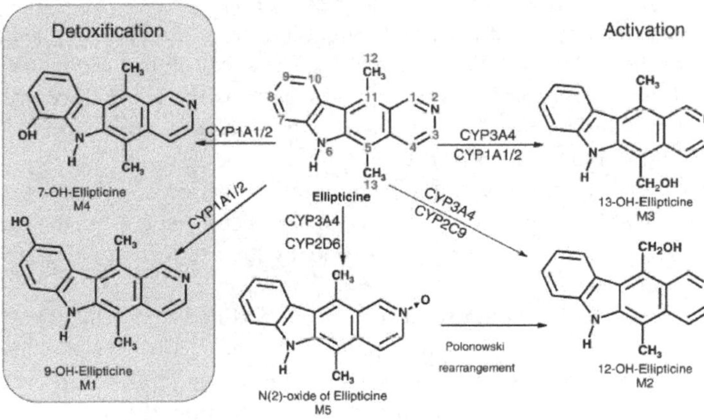

Fig. 3. Main pathways of ellipticine metabolism. Reprinted from Stiborova *et al.* 2011, ©2011, with permission from Elsevier.

Members of the CYP1 family are usually expressed in extrahepatic tissues and it is not strange to find CYP1A1 in MCF-7 (Androutsopoulos *et al.* 2009; Stiborova *et al.* 2011), in MDA-MB-231 and T47D (Macpherson & Matthews 2010). We already mentioned the presence of CYP3A4 in the three cell lines, but no precise information is available for CYP2C9.

This slight overview shows that the three main breast cancer cell lines are able to give interesting information about drugs that have to be bioactivated before exerting their deleterious effects in cancer cells. However, we must keep in mind that polymorphic variants of the genes coding these enzymes, or splicing variants, may influence the pharmacology of any drugs. Very few information about that are available in patients, but no study was performed in breast cancer cells.

BCCL have been created to study tumour development and related mechanisms and to test molecules potentially active. They are inevitable models for many studies. However, their extensive use in all areas of research on breast cancer remains sometimes controversial due to the over simplicity of the model, the instability of the strain, the existence of "false cell lines" and the failures of representativeness of the tumour. Thus, it clearly appears that these models are not sufficient to answer all the questions on breast cancer, and it is essential to turn to complementary models. Consequently, new models were introduced in the late 70s. They were used to a lesser extent than cell lines for a long time, but they tend to be more used now.

2.2 Improving representativeness of the model: Direct culture of tumour fragment

There are several methods to circumvent the problem of representativeness of BCCL, e.g. the direct culture of tumour fragments. The first attempts in this direction were made in the late 60s from tumours of 1mm^3 volume (Matoska & Stricker 1967). However, these cultures were proven difficult due to the high thickness of the samples, preventing the diffusion of nutrients and oxygen to the center of the sample, and thus, avoiding a long-term cultivation *in vitro*. This method has been modified over time, and with the use of microtome, problems associated with diffusion of nutrients have been resolved. The samples are now constituted of extremely thin slices of about 150 to 200 µM thick (Nissen *et al.* 1983).

This type of model was used to study the different inter-tumoural cell interactions and also to test the sensitivity to drugs (Milani *et al.* 2010). The slice tumour model associated with the development of microscopic analysis methods, such as the triple-fluorescence viability assay developed by Van Der Kuip, allowed the study of the cytotoxic effect of Taxol on this breast cancer model (Van Der Kuip *et al.* 2006).

Another example of drug study is the evaluation of the action of cytokines and cytotoxic drugs on animal (MMTV-Neu mice) breast cancer slices, especially the monitoring of apoptosis increase and DNA damage after treatment with interferon-gamma or doxorubicin (Parajuli & Doppler 2009).

The last noticeable example is the use of a tropism-modified oncolytic adenovirus, and a wild-type adenovirus on these slices to treat breast cancer. The results showed that the modified oncolytic adenovirus can infect and replicate in breast cancer tissue slices, suggesting the great potential of this model for evaluating the potential of oncolytic adenovirus constructs (Pennington *et al.* 2010).

This list is not exhaustive and the literature shows that a lot of results were obtained by the slice culturing method, more particularly on the study of drugs effects like tamoxifen or paclitaxel (Conde *et al.* 2008; Sonnenberg *et al.* 2008; Rajendran *et al.* 2011).

Although used since the late 70's, the slice technique evolved over time and was adapted to technological innovations. We may especially underline the use of silicon sensor chips wearing electrodes and sensors as a carrier of culture slice. The samples are deposited on the chip and data concerning the tumour-slice are analysed continuously during its cultivation and during its contact with drugs; measurements are made in real-time by the readout of ionic-sensitive field effect transistors and an oxygen electrode. This model was used to study the effects of Taxol on 200 slices of breast cancer, which revealed a dose-dependent decrease of the metabolic activity showed by the measurement of a decrease in the acidification of the medium (Mestres *et al.* 2006).

This technique has advantages and drawbacks. The direct culture of tumour fragment has the major advantage of preserving tissue architecture and all the cell populations constituting the human tumour. This method is thus a valuable technique which permits to take into account the whole tumour environment *in vivo*, allowing the investigation of the role of 3-dimensional structures and stromal interactions in tumour. It also allows to study the response of a particular tumour type to environmental stimulations, drugs, and cytokines under well-defined and reproducible conditions.

However, the culture of tumour samples presents limitations that do not allow its widespread use. Obtaining tumour samples is submitted to ethical constraints relative to the use of patient samples for research. In addition, it must be performed under ideal conditions. Thus, the samples have to be prepared very quickly after their excision, which means that the research laboratory should have particular facilities to have a direct access to fresh tissues. Moreover, the samples excised by the surgeon are becoming smaller and smaller, due to early diagnoses, and the major part of the samples is kept for diagnosis. Then, if some sample is still available for research, priority is given to research on biomarkers of the tumour in order to give personalised therapies, and, only after, it is disposable for fundamental research. Additionally to the availability restrictions, the same sample cannot be used for many tests because of the limitations of growth of this tissue *in vitro*. Repetition of assays and comparative measurements are thus more difficult with this model.

The use of samples from animal models with mammary tumour partially resolves the problem of availability of samples, but it also raises questions on the representativeness of the samples with human breast tumours. High improvements for providing human tissues of good quality will be brought by the emergence of biobanks.

2.3 Circumventing the lack of diversity: Co-culturing of cell lines

The co-culturing represents another way to circumvent the lack of cell diversity found in cell lines and to allow understanding of the tumoural proliferation mechanisms and inter-cellular interactions within a tumour. It is an indispensable tool to elucidate the regulation of the tumour by epithelial and stromal components surrounding it.

This model can be used by different ways: co-culturing of two cell types with a direct contact or co-culturing with a separating porous membrane between both cell types. The first method implicates to be able to differentiate the two cell types by microscopy. For that the use of fluorescent markers is a valuable tool (see Figure 4 for an example of co-culture of MDA-MB-231 with hASCs (adipose stem cells) respectively stained by the lipophilic tracers DiI (dialkylindocarbocyanines) and DiO (dialkyloxacarbocyanines), Pinilla *et al.* 2009).

The second method allows a relative isolation of the two cell types, the porosity of the membrane separating them allowing the exchange of substances. The two techniques give complementary information on the behavior of cells studied, especially the crucial role of the inter-cellular communication (Cappelletti *et al.* 1991).

In example, we could cite the co-culture of MDA-MB-231 and MCF-7, which has highlighted the importance of the heterogeneity of tumours for their growth and the role of oestrogen receptors. In this study, the co-culture of MCF-7 and MDA-MB-231 (respectively ER+ and

ER-) in a membrane separation system, was characterised by an increase of the MCF-7 cells growth rate in comparison with monocultures. This suggests that complex interactions between heterogenous cells population in tumour could explain the variability in tumour progression between different patients and the failure in response to endocrine treatment for some patients with ER+ tumours.

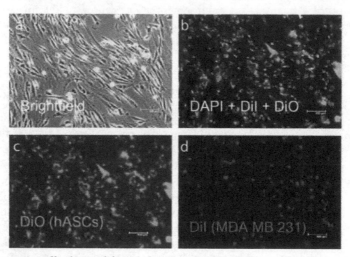

Fig. 4. Human stem cells derived from adipose tissue (hASCs) and breast cancer cells (MDA-MB-231) cultured in a monolayer co-culture system. (a) Direct microscopic observation of the co-culture of MDA-MB-231 and hASCs cells. (b) Overlay of DiO (hASCs), DiI (MDA-MB-231) and DAPI (nucleus) stainings. (c) DiO staining of hASCs derived stem cells (green). (d) DiI staining of MDA-MB-231 breast cancer cells (red). Reprinted from Pinilla *et al.* 2009, ©2009, with permission from Elsevier.

Another example concerns the direct co-culturing of MCF-10A, a non-cancerous breast cell line, with the cancerous one MCF-7. An exposure to hormonal treatment with 17β-estradiol was able to inhibit the proliferation of MCF-7 cells in this co-culture, whereas this phenomenon was not observed in a monoculture of MCF-7. This highlighted the complex interactions between ER+ MCF-7 and ER- MCF-10A cells which may reflect physiologically relevant mechanisms of the paracrine regulation of cell proliferation (Spink *et al.* 2006).
The co-culture of MCF-7 with fibroblasts derived from normal biopsies or from cancer biopsies also allowed to highlight the crucial role of fibroblasts in breast tumours. The results of two studies, one in direct co-culturing (Samoszuk *et al.* 2005) the second in membrane separated system (Dong-Le Bourhis *et al.* 1997), showed that MCF-7 growth rate was inhibited by fibroblasts issued from non cancerous tissues, but not by fibroblasts issued from tumourous tissues or serum-activated fibroblasts which enhanced MCF-7 growth rate. This suggests that fibroblasts could release some tumour growth inhibiting or activating factors.
The role of tumour-associated macrophages in the proliferation of tumour cells was also studied by co-culturing macrophages with MCF-7 cells in a membrane separated system. This co-culture lead to a significant increase of MCF-7 invasiveness *in vitro* (Hagemann *et al.* 2004).

These repeatable techniques have permitted to highlight the regulation of mammary tumours by the surrounding stroma and the complex interactions between the cell subtypes of the tumour.

2.4 A model with a tumour-like structure and cell diversity: 3-D culture

Another particular model allows cells to grow in 3-dimensions, generally with a matrix support (Yuhas *et al.* 1978). This type of culture permits an *in vitro* depiction of tumour tissue more accurate than classical 2-dimensional cultures in monolayers, as this last model does not correctly imitate the architecture and cellular gradients of oxygen and nutrients that are found in poorly vascularised regions of the tumour.

Only few cell lines are spontaneously able to establish spheroid architectures under certain culture conditions, but most of the systems require the use of synthetic or non-synthetic matrix. Systems are most often made of agar matrices or collagen support (Kim *et al.* 2004b). The Figure 5 show the growth of a MCF-7 spheroid growth in a hydrogel agarose matrix system (Fritsch *et al.* 2010).

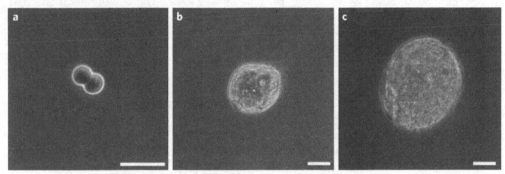

Fig. 5. Growth of a MCF-7 tumour spheroid in agarose hydrogel. The pictures represent the spheroid at 2 days old (a), 11 days old (b) and 27 days old (c) (the scale bar represent 50 µm). Reprinted by permission from Macmillan Publishers Ltd: Nature Physics, Fritsch *et al.* 2010, ©2010. http://www.nature.com/nphys.

Co-culturing of multiple cell types on these 3-dimensional systems is often used to study the relationship between cells, while simulating the tumour architecture with the most fidelity. These systems generally implicate the cultivation of tumour cells with other cell types like stromal, endothelial, fibroblasts and immune-competent cells. Moreover, this type of model, structurally like-looking the tumour, can be used quite indefinitely because it relies on the use of immortalised cells lines. This allows circumventing the problem of the lack of samples which is the major drawback of the tumour fragment culturing.

More advanced systems have been derived from this principle; one can cite the microfluidic-based 3-dimensional culturing (Bauer *et al.* 2010) that allows to grow multicellular tumour spheroid on a microchannel support, in order to analyze complex and heterotypic cellular interactions between breast cancer cells and fibroblast from the surrounding stroma. It has many advantages compared to the standard 3D culture: the culture volume and the number of needed cells are smaller than in standard support, the molecules are only distributed by diffusion mechanisms and the model is adapted to high throughput screenings.

2.5 Xenografts: An intermediary model between cell lines and *in vivo* models

We previously saw that some *in vitro* models tend to provide essential information on the inter-cellular interactions, by taking more or less into account the 3-dimensional structure of the tumour, but none of them benefit from the nervous and hormonal regulations found in the living organism.

There are particular models which can do perfectly the junction between *in vitro* and *in vivo* models, the xenografts. They are obtained by injecting cancer cells, usually derived from established cell lines, into a living organism. They are called xenografts because the injected cells are of human origin but are introduced into an animal organism, usually an immunodeficient rodent. The injection can be orthotopic (in breast gland) or heterotopic (localised in another part of the body, usually subcutaneously).

The xenograft model has the advantage of using cells from human tumour cell lines for which a significant amount of data was collected *in vitro*, and to study their behavior *in vivo*. There are several models available for research on breast cancer, principally using immunodeficient mice. The model nude is by far the most commonly used (Kim *et al.* 2004a). It is characterised by an absence of a functional thymus and active T cells (Kindred 1971). The second common model is the SCID mouse (severe combined immunodeficiency). These mice have a deficit in VDJ recombinases that allow the binding of specific and non-specific parts of immunoglobulin and T cell receptor (Bosma & Carroll 1991). See Figure 6 illustrating the two common models of mice used for breast cancer xenografts: nude and SCID.

A   B

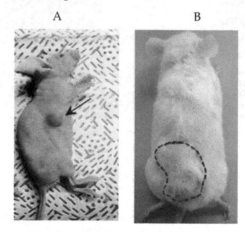

Fig. 6. **Nude (A) and SCID (B) mice models** xenografted respectively with MCF-7 and MDA-MB-231 breast cancer cell lines. (A) was taken from Nizamutdinova *et al.* 2008, by permission of Oxford University Press, and (B) was taken from Wang et al. 2010, with permission from ASBMB journals.

The injected breast cancer cells mostly come from established cell lines like MCF-7, MDA-MB-231, T-47-D or ZR-75-1. The first experiments of cell transplantations were made in the 80s, and opened onto success in the establishment of malignant tumours in nude mice (Ozzello & Sordat 1980; Kim *et al.* 2004a). Since then, a lot of models have been developed for investigation of new treatments, therapeutic targets and establishment of new cancer detection method by medical imaging.

This technique is widely used to test the effect of new antitumourous compounds or therapeutic methods, for example to test new virotherapies. Thus, a benign virus

Coxsackievirus 21 (CVA21) was intravenously injected in SCID mice xenografted with MDA-MB-231 breast cancer cells. CVA21 virus targets the receptors ICAM-1 and DAF that are overexpressed in breast cancer cells. In this experiment a rapid lysis focused on cancer cells was observed in all mice, making this virus a good candidate for use in systemic therapy (Skelding *et al.* 2009). See Figure 7 illustrating the effect of the virus on xenografted mice, visualised by bioluminescent analysis.

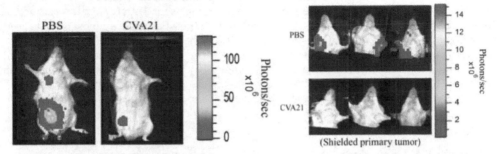

Fig. 7. **Observation of the oncolytic activity of CVA21 virus in SCID mouse xenografted with MDA-MB-231-luc**. The breast cancer cells were xenografted into the mammary fat pad, mice were then treated with PBS or CVA21. Metastases were detected 3 weeks post-cell injection. The mice on the pictures are representative for bioluminescent observation at day 42 post treatment. From Skelding *et al.* 2009, with kind permission from Springer Science and Business Media B.V.

In the investigation of new treatments, the vitamin D3 receptors constitute good targets as they are present in over 80% of mammary tumours and they are negative growth regulator of both oestrogen-dependent and independent breast cancer cells *in vitro*. In a study published in 1998 it was shown that EB1089, a vitamin D3 analog, was able to highly reduce the growth of tumour in nude mice xenografted with MCF-7 cells (tumours were 4-fold smaller than those in untreated mice). This reduction was resulting from an enhancement of apoptosis and reducing proliferation of tumour epithelial cells, suggesting the great potential of vitamin D3 analogs such as EB1089 against human breast cancer (VanWeelden *et al.* 1998).

This model can also be used to explore new potential targets for anticancer therapies. A good example is the targeting of receptor ERβ. In an experiment, standard T47D ERα+ ERβ- and modified T47D ERα+ ERβ+ (T47D stably transfected with a plasmid allowing the expression of the receptor ERβ), were xenografted in SCID mice. 17β-estradiol was then injected into mice. The treatment triggered an acceleration of tumour growth in mice xenografted with the native T47D strain, and conversely a regression of tumours T47D ERβ+. These results emphasize the antagonistic role of ERβ receptors that appear to play an antitumourigenic role, and offered prospects for the development of ER-selective inhibitors. (Hartman *et al.* 2006).

The targets cited above are non exhaustive. Many other therapeutic targets are tested with xenografts models, as it is the case of the VEGF pathway implicated in tumour angiogenesis (Le *et al.* 2008), or of cell cycle regulating proteins such as CDK kinases (Fry *et al.* 2004).

The use of established cell lines for producing xenografts raises several questions about their relevance. The murine model presents considerable differences with the human body, concerning the biochemical and physiological regulation. Moreover, the stroma that will grow surround the tumour will be of murine origin and it will result in a chimeric tumour which biology may significantly differ from human one (Kim *et al.* 2004a). Furthermore, in humans, the immune system plays an important role in the fight against tumour, whereas in xenografts models the immune system is totally absent.

The xenograft model has some limitations but is the most accomplished of all models because it takes into account the complexity of the organism.

Besides the xenografts, there are also murine models which can develop tumours spontaneously or under the influence of inducing compounds (Russo & Russo 1996). Although the achievement of these models is easy, their use is largely debated because of their relevance to the clinical situation. Indeed, murine breast cancers are most often caused by viral infections and are not hormone dependent, whereas a considerable proportion of human cancers are oestrogen dependent. To date there is no evidence suggesting a viral induction of breast cancer in humans. The biology of spontaneous rodent tumours differs from the human ones. The size, the oncogenic targets or the degree of maturation and differentiation of cells differ between the two species, making them hardly comparable.

3. Conclusion

In this chapter, we described the main models used in breast cancer research in order to obtain results of high scientific quality. In summary, we can say that BCCL models allow repeatable experiments with simple material and methods. They are inevitable models for basic studies and mechanistic explorations, but their use is still controversial owing to their approximate representativeness of breast tumours in human and to the existence of misidentified cell lines.

Cultures of cancerous tissues preserve the tumour architecture and the cell diversity of a tumour but this model suffers of limited reproducibility and cannot be easily maintained for a long time. Co-culture systems offer an alternative with reproducible long term culture systems, and offer the possibility to study the relations between different types of cells in tumour, but this model suffers from the same controversies as BCCL as it mainly relies on their use.

3-dimensional systems allow the mimicking of the tumour architecture and microenvironment, but very few cell lines are able to form spheroids under specific conditions.

Considering the advantages and drawbacks of these models, the xenografts appear to be good alternative models as they enable to take into account the tumour structure, its microenvironment, the role of the metabolism and they preserve the cell diversity of the tumour. But as other models, they also have drawbacks principally due to the metabolic and physiological differences existing between human and rodents, and to the fact that the role of the immune system against tumour is not taken into account with the immunodeficient rodent models used for xenografts.

Application of the 3Rs principle leaded to the development of all these models, but we showed that none of them is sufficient by itself and able to perfectly mimic breast cancer in human. However it clearly appears that all these models are essential to accumulate data and information to fight breast cancer.

4. Acknowledgements

The "Ligue contre le Cancer" (54, 55, 57 and 88 Departmental committees) is acknowledged for its financial support. E.B is recipient of an AFR grant of the National Research Fund, Luxembourg.

5. References

Amadori, D., Bertoni, L., Flamigni, A., Savini, S., De Giovanni, C., Casanova, S., De Paola, F., Amadori, A., Giulotto, E. and Zoli, W. (1993). Establishment and characterization of a new cell line from primary human breast carcinoma. *Breast Cancer Res Treat*, Vol. 28, No.3: 251-260.

Androutsopoulos, V. P., Li, N. and Arroo, R. R. (2009). The methoxylated flavones eupatorin and cirsiliol induce CYP1 enzyme expression in MCF7 cells. *J Nat Prod*, Vol. 72, No.8: 1390-1394.

Bauer, M., Su, G., Beebe, D. J. and Friedl, A. (2010). 3D microchannel co-culture: method and biological validation. *Integr Biol (Camb)*, Vol. 2, No.7-8: 371-378.

Bosma, M. J. and Carroll, A. M. (1991). The SCID mouse mutant: definition, characterization, and potential uses. *Annu Rev Immunol*, Vol. 9: 323-350.

Bray, J., Sludden, J., Griffin, M. J., Cole, M., Verrill, M., Jamieson, D. and Boddy, A. V. (2010). Influence of pharmacogenetics on response and toxicity in breast cancer patients treated with doxorubicin and cyclophosphamide. *Br J Cancer*, Vol. 102, No.6: 1003-1009.

Burdall, S. E., Hanby, A. M., Lansdown, M. R. and Speirs, V. (2003). Breast cancer cell lines: friend or foe? *Breast Cancer Research*, Vol. 5, No.2: 89-95.

Cailleau, R., Young, R., Olive, M. and Reeves, W. J., Jr. (1974). Breast tumor cell lines from pleural effusions. *J Natl Cancer Inst*, Vol. 53, No.3: 661-674.

Cappelletti, V., Ruedl, C., Granata, G., Coradini, D., Del Bino, G. and Di Fronzo, G. (1991). Interaction between hormone-dependent and hormone-independent human breast cancer cells. *Eur J Cancer*, Vol. 27, No.9: 1154-1157.

Chen, Y., Tang, Y., Chen, S. and Nie, D. (2009). Regulation of drug resistance by human pregnane X receptor in breast cancer. *Cancer Biol Ther*, Vol. 8, No.13: 1265-1272.

Conde, S. J., Luvizotto, R. A., Sibio, M. T., Katayama, M. L., Brentani, M. M. and Nogueira, C. R. (2008). Tamoxifen inhibits transforming growth factor-alpha gene expression in human breast carcinoma samples treated with triiodothyronine. *J Endocrinol Invest*, Vol. 31, No.12: 1047-1051.

Di, Y. M., Chow, V. D., Yang, L. P. and Zhou, S. F. (2009). Structure, function, regulation and polymorphism of human cytochrome P450 2A6. *Curr Drug Metab*, Vol. 10, No.7: 754-780.

Dong-Le Bourhis, X., Berthois, Y., Millot, G., Degeorges, A., Sylvi, M., Martin, P. M. and Calvo, F. (1997). Effect of stromal and epithelial cells derived from normal and tumorous breast tissue on the proliferation of human breast cancer cell lines in co-culture. *Int J Cancer*, Vol. 71, No.1: 42-48.

Fogh, J., Wright, W. C. and Loveless, J. D. (1977). Absence of HeLa cell contamination in 169 cell lines derived from human tumors. *J Natl Cancer Inst*, Vol. 58, No.2: 209-214.

Fritsch, A., Höckel, M., Kiessling, T., Nnetu, K. D., Wetzel, F., Zink, M. and Käs, J. A. (2010). Are biomechanical changes necessary for tumour progression? *Nature Physics*, Vol. 6: 730-732.

Fry, D. W., Harvey, P. J., Keller, P. R., Elliott, W. L., Meade, M., Trachet, E., Albassam, M., Zheng, X., Leopold, W. R., Pryer, N. K. and Toogood, P. L. (2004). Specific inhibition of cyclin-dependent kinase 4/6 by PD 0332991 and associated antitumor activity in human tumor xenografts. *Mol Cancer Ther*, Vol. 3, No.11: 1427-1438.

Gazdar, A. F., Kurvari, V., Virmani, A., Gollahon, L., Sakaguchi, M., Westerfield, M., Kodagoda, D., Stasny, V., Cunningham, H. T., Wistuba, II, Tomlinson, G., Tonk, V., Ashfaq, R., Leitch, A. M., Minna, J. D. and Shay, J. W. (1998). Characterization of paired tumor and non-tumor cell lines established from patients with breast cancer. *Int J Cancer*, Vol. 78, No.6: 766-774.

Giraud, B., Hebert, G., Deroussent, A., Veal, G. J., Vassal, G. and Paci, A. (2010). Oxazaphosphorines: new therapeutic strategies for an old class of drugs. *Expert Opin Drug Metab Toxicol*, Vol. 6, No.8: 919-938.

Gollahon, L. S. and Shay, J. W. (1996). Immortalization of human mammary epithelial cells transfected with mutant p53 (273his). *Oncogene*, Vol. 12, No.4: 715-725.

Hagemann, T., Robinson, S. C., Schulz, M., Trumper, L., Balkwill, F. R. and Binder, C. (2004). Enhanced invasiveness of breast cancer cell lines upon co-cultivation with macrophages is due to TNF-alpha dependent up-regulation of matrix metalloproteases. *Carcinogenesis*, Vol. 25, No.8: 1543-1549.

Hartman, J., Lindberg, K., Morani, A., Inzunza, J., Strom, A. and Gustafsson, J. A. (2006). Estrogen receptor beta inhibits angiogenesis and growth of T47D breast cancer xenografts. *Cancer Res*, Vol. 66, No.23: 11207-11213.

Huang, Z., Fasco, M. J. and Kaminsky, L. S. (1997). Alternative splicing of CYP2D mRNA in human breast tissue. *Arch Biochem Biophys*, Vol. 343, No.1: 101-108.

Keydar, I., Chen, L., Karby, S., Weiss, F. R., Delarea, J., Radu, M., Chaitcik, S. and Brenner, H. J. (1979). Establishment and characterization of a cell line of human breast carcinoma origin. *Eur J Cancer*, Vol. 15, No.5: 659-670.

Kim, J. B., O'Hare, M. J. and Stein, R. (2004a). Models of breast cancer: is merging human and animal models the future? *Breast Cancer Res*, Vol. 6, No.1: 22-30.

Kim, J. B., Stein, R. and O'Hare, M. J. (2004b). Three-dimensional *in vitro* tissue culture models of breast cancer-- a review. *Breast Cancer Res Treat*, Vol. 85, No.3: 281-291.

Kindred, B. (1971). Antibody response in genetically thymus-less nude mice injected with normal thymus cells. *J Immunol*, Vol. 107, No.5: 1291-1295.

Kivisto, K. T., Kroemer, H. K. and Eichelbaum, M. (1995). The role of human cytochrome P450 enzymes in the metabolism of anticancer agents: implications for drug interactions. *Br J Clin Pharmacol*, Vol. 40, No.6: 523-530.

Lacroix, M. (2008). Persistent use of "false" cell lines. *Int J Cancer*, Vol. 122, No.1: 1-4.

Lacroix, M. and Leclercq, G. (2004). Relevance of breast cancer cell lines as models for breast tumours: an update. *Breast Cancer Res Treat*, Vol. 83, No.3: 249-289.

Le, X. F., Mao, W., Lu, C., Thornton, A., Heymach, J. V., Sood, A. K. and Bast, R. C., Jr. (2008). Specific blockade of VEGF and HER2 pathways results in greater growth inhibition of breast cancer xenografts that overexpress HER2. *Cell Cycle*, Vol. 7, No.23: 3747-3758.

Liscovitch, M. and Ravid, D. (2007). A case study in misidentification of cancer cell lines: MCF-7/AdrR cells (re-designated NCI/ADR-RES) are derived from OVCAR-8 human ovarian carcinoma cells. *Cancer Lett*, Vol. 245, No.1-2: 350-352.

Lo, R., Burgoon, L., Macpherson, L., Ahmed, S. and Matthews, J. (2010). Estrogen receptor-dependent regulation of CYP2B6 in human breast cancer cells. *Biochim Biophys Acta*, Vol. 1799, No.5-6: 469-479.

Macpherson, L. and Matthews, J. (2010). Inhibition of aryl hydrocarbon receptor-dependent transcription by resveratrol or kaempferol is independent of estrogen receptor alpha expression in human breast cancer cells. *Cancer Lett*, Vol. 299, No.2: 119-129.

Matoska, J. and Stricker, F. (1967). Following human tumours in primary organ culture. *Neoplasma*, Vol. 14, No.5: 507-519.

Mestres, P., Morguet, A., Schmidt, W., Kob, A. and Thedinga, E. (2006). A new method to assess drug sensitivity on breast tumor acute slices preparation. *Ann N Y Acad Sci*, Vol. 1091: 460-469.

Milani, C., Welsh, J., Katayama, M. L., Lyra, E. C., Maciel, M. S., Brentani, M. M. and Folgueira, M. A. (2010). Human breast tumor slices: a model for identification of vitamin D regulated genes in the tumor microenvironment. *J Steroid Biochem Mol Biol*, Vol. 121, No.1-2: 151-155.

Mitra, R., Guo, Z., Milani, M., Mesaros, C., Rodriguez, M., Nguyen, J., Luo, X., Clarke, D., Lamba, J., Schuetz, E., Donner, D. B., Puli, N., Falck, J. R., Capdevila, J., Gupta, K., Blair, I. A. and Potter, D. A. (2011). CYP3A4 mediates growth of ER+ breast cancer cells, in part, by nuclear translocation of phospho-Stat3 through biosynthesis of ({+/-})-14,15-EET. *J Biol Chem*, Vol.:

Mo, S. L., Liu, Y. H., Duan, W., Wei, M. Q., Kanwar, J. R. and Zhou, S. F. (2009). Substrate specificity, regulation, and polymorphism of human cytochrome P450 2B6. *Curr Drug Metab*, Vol. 10, No.7: 730-753.

Nagaoka, R., Iwasaki, T., Rokutanda, N., Takeshita, A., Koibuchi, Y., Horiguchi, J., Shimokawa, N., Iino, Y., Morishita, Y. and Koibuchi, N. (2006). Tamoxifen activates CYP3A4 and MDR1 genes through steroid and xenobiotic receptor in breast cancer cells. *Endocrine*, Vol. 30, No.3: 261-268.

Nelson-Rees, W. A. and Flandermeyer, R. R. (1977). Inter- and intraspecies contamination of human breast tumor cell lines HBC and BrCa5 and other cell cultures. *Science*, Vol. 195, No.4284: 1343-1344.

Nissen, E., Tanneberger, S., Weiss, H. and Bender, E. (1983). [*In vitro* cultivation of vital tissue slices: a new variation of organ culture technics]. *Biomed Biochim Acta*, Vol. 42, No.7-8: 907-916.

Nizamutdinova, I. T., Lee, G. W., Lee, J. S., Cho, M. K., Son, K. H., Jeon, S. J., Kang, S. S., Kim, Y. S., Lee, J. H., Seo, H. G., Chang, K. C. and Kim, H. J. (2008). Tanshinone I suppresses growth and invasion of human breast cancer cells, MDA-MB-231, through regulation of adhesion molecules. *Carcinogenesis*, Vol. 29, No.10: 1885-1892.

Ozzello, L. and Sordat, M. (1980). Behavior of tumors produced by transplantation of human mammary cell lines in athymic nude mice. *Eur J Cancer*, Vol. 16, No.4: 553-559.

Parajuli, N. and Doppler, W. (2009). Precision-cut slice cultures of tumors from MMTV-neu mice for the study of the ex vivo response to cytokines and cytotoxic drugs. *In Vitro Cell Dev Biol Anim*, Vol. 45, No.8: 442-450.

Pauley, R. J., Paine, T. J., Herbert, D. and Soule, D. N. (1991). Immortal Human Mammary Epithelial Cell Sublines. *United States Patent*, Patent n°. 5206165,

Pennington, K., Chu, Q. D., Curiel, D. T., Li, B. D. and Mathis, J. M. (2010). The utility of a tissue slice model system to determine breast cancer infectivity by oncolytic adenoviruses. *J Surg Res*, Vol. 163, No.2: 270-275.

Pinilla, S., Alt, E., Abdul Khalek, F. J., Jotzu, C., Muehlberg, F., Beckmann, C. and Song, Y. H. (2009). Tissue resident stem cells produce CCL5 under the influence of cancer cells and thereby promote breast cancer cell invasion. *Cancer Lett*, Vol. 284, No.1: 80-85.

Rae, J. M., Creighton, C. J., Meck, J. M., Haddad, B. R. and Johnson, M. D. (2007). MDA-MB-435 cells are derived from M14 melanoma cells--a loss for breast cancer, but a boon for melanoma research. *Breast Cancer Res Treat*, Vol. 104, No.1: 13-19.

Rajendran, S., O'Hanlon, D., Morrissey, D., O'Donovan, T., O'Sullivan, G. C. and Tangney, M. (2011). Preclinical evaluation of gene delivery methods for the treatment of loco-regional disease in breast cancer. *Exp Biol Med (Maywood)*, Vol. 236, No.4: 423-434.

Rooseboom, M., Commandeur, J. N. and Vermeulen, N. P. (2004). Enzyme-catalyzed activation of anticancer prodrugs. *Pharmacol Rev*, Vol. 56, No.1: 53-102.

Ross, D. T. and Perou, C. M. (2001). A comparison of gene expression signatures from breast tumors and breast tissue derived cell lines. *Dis Markers*, Vol. 17, No.2: 99-109.

Russell, W. M. S. and Bursch, R. L. (1959). The Principles of Humane Experimental Technique. London, Methuen, 978-0900767784.

Russo, I. H. and Russo, J. (1996). Mammary gland neoplasia in long-term rodent studies. *Environ Health Perspect,* Vol. 104, No.9: 938-967.

Shen, C., Gu, M., Liang, D., Miao, L., Hu, L., Zheng, C. and Chen, J. (2009). Establishment and characterization of three new human breast cancer cell lines derived from Chinese breast cancer tissues. *Cancer Cell Int,* Vol. 9: 2.

Skelding, K. A., Barry, R. D. and Shafren, D. R. (2009). Systemic targeting of metastatic human breast tumor xenografts by Coxsackievirus A21. *Breast Cancer Res Treat,* Vol. 113, No.1: 21-30.

Sonnenberg, M., van der Kuip, H., Haubeis, S., Fritz, P., Schroth, W., Friedel, G., Simon, W., Murdter, T. E. and Aulitzky, W. E. (2008). Highly variable response to cytotoxic chemotherapy in carcinoma-associated fibroblasts (CAFs) from lung and breast. *BMC Cancer,* Vol. 8: 364.

Soule, H. D., Maloney, T. M., Wolman, S. R., Peterson, W. D., Jr., Brenz, R., McGrath, C. M., Russo, J., Pauley, R. J., Jones, R. F. and Brooks, S. C. (1990). Isolation and characterization of a spontaneously immortalized human breast epithelial cell line, MCF-10. *Cancer Res,* Vol. 50, No.18: 6075-6086.

Soule, H. D., Vazguez, J., Long, A., Albert, S. and Brennan, M. (1973). A human cell line from a pleural effusion derived from a breast carcinoma. *J Natl Cancer Inst,* Vol. 51, No.5: 1409-1416.

Spink, B. C., Cole, R. W., Katz, B. H., Gierthy, J. F., Bradley, L. M. and Spink, D. C. (2006). Inhibition of MCF-7 breast cancer cell proliferation by MCF-10A breast epithelial cells in coculture. *Cell Biol Int,* Vol. 30, No.3: 227-238.

Stampfer, M. R. (1989). Continuous human cell lines and method of making same. *United States Patent,* Patent n°. 4808532,

Stiborova, M., Rupertova, M. and Frei, E. (2011). Cytochrome P450- and peroxidase-mediated oxidation of anticancer alkaloid ellipticine dictates its anti-tumor efficiency. *Biochim Biophys Acta,* Vol. 1814, No.1: 175-185.

Van der Haegen, B. A. and Shay, J. W. (1993). Immortalization of human mammary epithelial cells by SV40 large T-antigen involves a two step mechanism. *In Vitro Cell Dev Biol,* Vol. 29A, No.3 Pt 1: 180-182.

Van Der Kuip, H., Murdter, T. E., Sonnenberg, M., McClellan, M., Gutzeit, S., Gerteis, A., Simon, W., Fritz, P. and Aulitzky, W. E. (2006). Short term culture of breast cancer tissues to study the activity of the anticancer drug taxol in an intact tumor environment. *BMC Cancer,* Vol. 6: 86.

VanWeelden, K., Flanagan, L., Binderup, L., Tenniswood, M. and Welsh, J. (1998). Apoptotic regression of MCF-7 xenografts in nude mice treated with the vitamin D3 analog, EB1089. *Endocrinology,* Vol. 139, No.4: 2102-2110.

Wang, H. and Tompkins, L. M. (2008). CYP2B6: new insights into a historically overlooked cytochrome P450 isozyme. *Curr Drug Metab,* Vol. 9, No.7: 598-610.

Wang, Z., Bryan, J., Franz, C., Havlioglu, N. and Sandell, L. J. (2010). Type IIB procollagen NH(2)-propeptide induces death of tumor cells via interaction with integrins alpha(V)beta(3) and alpha(V)beta(5). *J Biol Chem,* Vol. 285, No.27: 20806-20817.

Yuhas, J. M., Tarleton, A. E. and Molzen, K. B. (1978). Multicellular tumor spheroid formation by breast cancer cells isolated from different sites. *Cancer Res,* Vol. 38, No.8: 2486-2491.

Zhang, J., Tian, Q., Yung Chan, S., Chuen Li, S., Zhou, S., Duan, W. and Zhu, Y. Z. (2005). Metabolism and transport of oxazaphosphorines and the clinical implications. *Drug Metab Rev,* Vol. 37, No.4: 611-703.

4

Breast Cancer: Classification Based on Molecular Etiology Influencing Prognosis and Prediction

Siddik Sarkar[1] and Mahitosh Mandal[1]

[1]*School of Medical Science and Technology, Indian Institute of Technology Kharagpur*
Kharagpur, West Bengal
India

1. Introduction

Cancer is a group of diseases that leads to uncontrolled cell division and eventually forms a lump or mass called a tumor. They are classified and named after the part of the body where the tumor originates. Breast cancer begins in breast tissue, which is made up of glands for milk production, called lobules, and the ducts that connect lobules to the nipple. The remainder of the breast is made up of fatty, connective, and lymphatic tissue. On the basis of origin, it is of two types (i) ductal and (ii) lobular. Ductal carcinoma constitutes 80-90% and lobular carcinoma constitutes 10-20% breast cancer cases.

Breast cancer is one of the most frequently diagnosed cancers in women worldwide, comprising 16% of all female cancers cases. It is estimated that this disease will affect one in eight females in America during their lifetime. It is estimated that occurrence of female breast cancer is 28% of cancers from all sites in U.S.A, and the relative risk of ever developing breast cancer is 0.125 (1 in 8) (American Cancer Society, 2009). Although breast cancer is thought to be a disease of the developed world, a majority (69%) of all breast cancer deaths occurs in developing countries (WHO Global Burden of Disease, 2004) and relative survival is poor in underdeveloped and developing countries (Coleman et al., 2008). The relative risk of developing breast cancer in the lifetime of women in the developed and developing countries is 0.048 (1 in 21) and 0.018 (1 in 56) respectively. In India, breast cancer is the leading cancer among women (Fig. 1) and the relative risk is 0.033 (1 in 30) (NCRP, 2008).

2. Risk factors of breast cancer

Every woman is at risk for developing breast cancer. Several relatively strong risk factors for breast cancer that affect large proportion of the general population have been known for some time. However, the vast majority of breast cancer cases occur in women who have no identifiable risk factors other than their gender and age (Kelsey & Gammon, 1990). The other established risk factors are previous family history, age at first full-term pregnancy, early menarche, late menopause, genetic and breast tissue density. These factors are not easily modifiable and classified under unmodified factors. However, other factors associated with increased breast cancer risk are postmenopausal obesity, hormone replacement therapy (HRT), alcohol consumption, and physical inactivity, no breast feeding are modifiable and classified under modified factors. The relative risk of various factors responsible for breast cancer are shown in Table 1 (Hulka & Moorman, 2001).

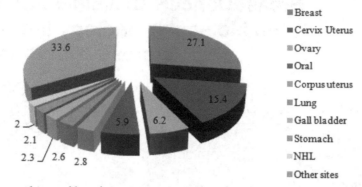

Fig. 1. Demographic profiles of cancer cases in Indian females. Based on 2004-2005 data for Bangalore, Barshi, Bhopal, Chennai, Delhi, Mumbai, Ahmedabad and 2005 data for Kolkata.

3. Classification of breast cancer

3.1.1 Histopathological classification

Each breast has 15 to 25 sections called lobes, formed by groups of lobules, the milk glands. Each lobule is composed of grape-like clusters of acini (also called alveoli), the hollow sacs that make and hold breast milk. The lobes and lobules are connected by thin tubes, called ducts that deliver milk to nipple (Fig. 2). The pink or the brown pigmented region surrounding the nipple is called areola. Connective and fatty tissue fills the remaining space in between the lobes and ducts. The most common type of breast cancer is ductal cancer. It is found in the cells of the ducts. Cancer that starts in lobes or lobules is called lobular cancer. It is more often found in both breasts than other types of breast cancer. Rarely breast cancer

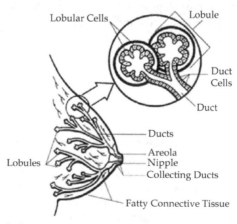

Fig. 2. Anatomy of female breast.

can begin in the connective tissue that's made up of muscles, fat and blood vessels. Cancer that begins in the connective tissue is called sarcoma. It accounts for less than 5% of all soft tissue sarcomas and less than 1% of breast cancer (Moore and Kinne, 1996). Phyllodes tumor and angiosarcoma are two common forms of sarcoma. Cancers are also classified as non invasive (in situ) and invasive (infiltrating). The term in situ means "in its original place" and refers to cancer that has not spread past the area where it initially developed. Invasive breast cancer has a tendency to spread (invade) to other tissues of the breast and/or other regions of the body. A less common type of breast cancer is inflammatory breast cancer characterized by general inflammation (red and swollen) of the breast (Fig. 3). The different types of invasive cancers, their frequency and percentage survival is shown in Table 1.2.

Relative Risk	Factor
>4.0	Female
	Age (65+ vs. <65 years, although risk increases across all ages until age 80)
	Certain inherited genetic mutations for breast cancer (BRCA1 and/or BRCA2)
	Two or more first-degree relatives with breast cancer diagnosed at an early age
	Personal history of breast cancer
	High breast tissue density or 75% dense
2.1-4.0	Biopsy-confirmed atypical hyperplasia
	One first-degree relative with breast cancer
	High-dose radiation to chest
	High bone density (postmenopausal)
1.1-2.0 Factors that affect circulating hormones	Late age at first full-term pregnancy (>30 years)
	Early menarche (<12 years)
	Late menopause (>55 years)
	No full-term pregnancies
	No breast feeding
	Recent oral contraceptive use
	Recent and long-term use of HRT
	Obesity (postmenopausal)
	Personal history of endometrial or ovarian cancer
1.1 -2.0 Other factors	Alcohol consumption
	Height (tall)
	High socioeconomic status

Hulka BS, and Moorman PG 2001. Maturitas 2008; 38:103-113
© 2001 Elsevier Science Ireland Ltd.

Table 1. Factors that increase the Relative Risk for Breast Cancer.

Invasive ductal carcinoma is the most common breast cancer and it accounts more than 75% of breast cancer cases. Most are invasive ductal carcinoma (IDC) not otherwise specified (IDC NOS), and remaining IDC includes Inflammatory breast cancer, medullary carcinoma, metaplastic, apocrine and tubular carcinoma. Medullary carcinoma accounts <5% of breast cancers diagnosed, and takes its name from its color, which is close to the color of brain tissue, or medulla. It is an invasive breast cancer that forms a distinct boundary between tumor tissue and normal tissue. Metaplastic breast cancer is a form of invasive ductal cancer, meaning that it forms in the milk ducts and then moves into other tissues of the breast. Metaplastic breast carcinomas constitute a heterogeneous group of neoplasms, accounting for less than 1% of all invasive mammary carcinomas (Reis-Filho et al., 2005), such as squamous (skin) or osseous (bone) cells. The other groups of invasive breast cancers are invasive lobular carcinoma, adenoid cystic carcinoma, micropapillary carcinoma, mucinous carcinoma (formed by the mucus-producing cancer cells), etc as shown in Fig. 3.

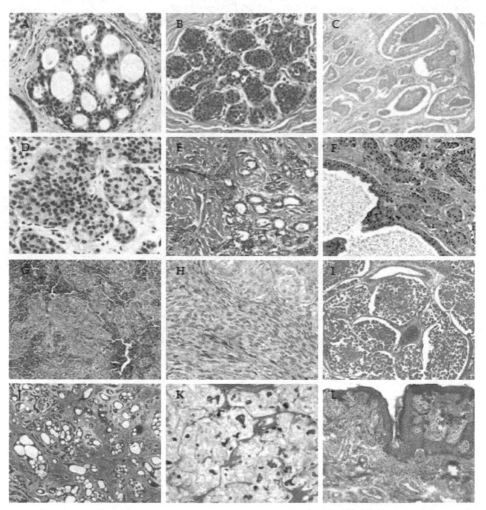

Fig. 3. Histology of breast carcinoma. Breast carcinoma is classified into Ductal (A), Lobular carcinoma (B) and Inflammatory carcinoma. (C). It can be further classified into non-invasive (A-B) and invasive carcinoma (C-L). Invasive cancer includes Inflammatory (C), Invasive lobular (D), tubular (E) apocrine (F), medullary, (G) metaplastic (H), micropapillary, (I) adenoid cystic (J), mucunous carcinoma (K), and paget disease (L).

Histopathological type of invasive breast carcinoma	Frequency (%)	10-year OS (%)
Invasive ductal carcinoma not otherwise specified (IDC NOS)	50-60	35-50
Inflammatory carcinoma	1-6	30-40
Apocrine carcinoma	1-4	Like IDC NOS
Medullary carcinoma	5-7	50-90
Metaplastic carcinoma	<5	Unknown
Micropapillary carcinoma	1-2	Unknown
Tubular carcinoma	1-2	90-100
Invasive lobular carcinoma	5-15	35-50
Adenoid cystic carcinoma	0.1	85-100
Mucinous carcinoma	<3	85-95
Neuroendocrine carcinoma	2-5	Unknown
Mammary Paget disease	1-4	40-50

Table 2. Frequency and outcome of histological types of invasive breast cancer.

3.1.2 Molecular classification

Breast cancer is a clinically heterogeneous disease. Histologically similar tumors may have different prognosis and may respond to therapy differently. It is believed that these differences in clinical behavior are due to molecular differences between histologically similar tumors. DNA microarray technology, Immuno-histochemistry (IHC), Fluorescent in situ hybridization (FISH), and quantitative reverse transcription polymerase chain reaction (RT-PCR) are ideally suitable techniques to reveal molecular differences among the same or different groups of histopathological specimens. Each of these molecular techniques has the potential for proper prognosis and prediction of human cancers, including breast. IHC was developed more than 30 years back and it is used for classification of breast cancer into ER positive and ER negative tumors. FISH was developed 20 years back and is used to classify breast tumors into HER-2 amplified or non amplified categories. Breast cancer cells generally overexpress estrogen receptor (ER)/ progesterone receptor (PR), and human epidermal growth factor-2 (HER-2) receptor for breast tumor formation and progression. Thus, breast cancer can be classified into three sub-groups (i) ER/PR positive (ii) ER negative or HER-2 positive and triple negative (ER, PR and HER-2 negative) on the basis of receptor status. The classification of breast cancer on the basis of ER status improves the prognosis and clinical outcome of ER+ tumors as ER+ cancer cells depend on estrogen for their growth, and the treatment of patients with anti-estrogen agents (e.g. tamoxifen) will inhibit the effect of estrogen and thus improves the treatment outcome. Generally, HER-2+ had a worse prognosis, however HER-2+ cancer cells respond to drugs such as the monoclonal antibody, trastuzumab, (in combination with conventional chemotherapy) and this has improved the prognosis and pathological complete response significantly (Chang et al., 2010). Triple-negative breast cancer is a high risk breast cancer that lacks the benefit of specific therapy that targets these proteins. It can be categorized in basal subtypes (Rakha et al., 2007). It is found in 10-20% of breast cancer cases and mostly diagnosed in younger women with BRCA1 and BRCA2 mutations (Dent et al., 2007; Dawood et al., 2009). The rate of recurrence is very high, and it reaches its peak within first 3 years and then declines after that. Patients with triple negative breast cancer are most likely to die within 5 years than patients with other breast cancers. All deaths due to breast cancer in patients' with triple-negative cancer occurred within 10 years of diagnosis.

A novel molecular classification of breast cancer based on gene expression profiles segregates breast cancer into four types (i) luminal, (ii) basal, (iii) HER-2 and (iv) normal type (Perou et al., 2000; Sotiriou et al., 2003; Tamimi et al., 2008) (Fig. 4).

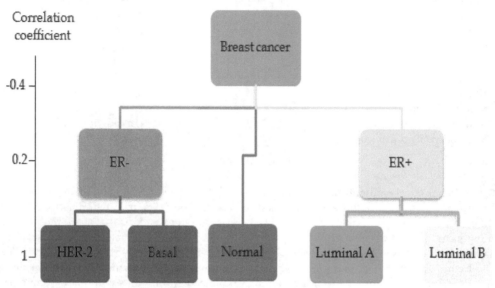

Fig. 4. Dendrogram of breast cancer. The tumors were separated into two main groups mainly associated with ER status as analyzed by hierarchical cluster analysis generated by using gene profile data. The dendrogram is further branched into smaller subgroups within the ER+ and ER- classes based on their basal and luminal characteristics: HER-2 subgroup, dark red; basal-like 1 subgroup, pink; luminal-like A subgroup, green; luminal-like B subgroup, yellow; and normal-like breast subgroup, blue.

Luminal express keratin 8/18, ER, GATA binding protein, X-box binding protein 1, annexin XXXI, cytochrome P450 and basal type express keratin 5, keratin 17, integrin β4, matrix metalloprotease 14, laminin α3, basonuclin and mutated *TP53* gene. Luminal type is further classified into luminal A and luminal B. Luminal B expresses HER-2 along with ER where as luminal A doesn't express HER-2. HER-2 subtype express ERB-2/HER-2, growth factor receptor bound protein 7, TNF receptor-associated factor IV, GRB 7. Normal–breast-like group showed the highest expression of many genes known to be expressed by adipose tissue and other non-epithelial cell types. These tumors also showed strong expression of basal epithelial genes and low expression of luminal epithelial genes. It expresses CD36 antigen collagen type I, glycerol 3 phosphate dehydrogenase I, lipoprotein lipase A, alcohol dehydrogenase 2 (Sorlie et al., 2001). The molecular subclasses show difference in clinical outcome as per as overall survival (OS) and relapse free survival (RFS) is concerned as shown in Table 1.3. There was a significant difference in overall survival between the subtypes with basal and HER-2 is as associated with worse outcome and shortest survival time.

Molecular types of breast carcinoma	Frequency (%)	5-year OS+ (%)	5-year RFS* (%)	10-year OS (%)	10-year RFS (%)
Luminal A	50-60	85-95	80-90	75-85	75-85
Luminal B	5-10	70-80	65-75	55-65	54-64
Basal	10-20	63-73	60-70	57-67	45-55
ERB-2	10-20	55-65	15-20	45-55	15-30
Normal-like	10-15	84-94	80-90	75-85	72-82

Table 3. Breast cancer outcomes in molecular types of breast cancer.RFS: The percentage of people without any further symptoms of breast cancer during the interval elapsed between the date of breast surgery and the date of diagnosed further episode of breast cancer, whether the breast cancer was classified as a recurrence or second primary, and whatever the histology. OS: The percentage of people survived during the interval elapsed between the date of breast surgery and the date of breast cancer-related or un-related death (documented from hospital records).

4. Clinical outcomes of breast cancer in association with clinical, histopathological and molecular classification

Breast cancers can be classified by different schemata. Classification aspects include clinical (age, tumor, node), histopathological (grade, ER and HER-2 status, ductal, lobular, invasive) and molecular (normal-like, luminal, basal, HER-2) values. Every aspect influences treatment response and prognosis as shown in Table 2 and Table 3. The true prognostic or predictive value of the various molecular classes is unknown because there is a strong correlation between molecular class and conventional histopathologic variables (ER status, grade). For example, in one study, all luminal-type cancers were ER-positive and 63% of these were also low or intermediate grade, in contrast to 95% of basal-like cancers that were ER-negative, 91% of which were high grade (Pusztai et al., 2003). These associations partly explain the different clinical outcome observed in different molecular classes. Rouzier et al. studied the pathological outcomes of different molecular subclasses of breast cancer patients. They obtained tumor tissue biopsies from 82 patients with newly diagnosed breast cancer before they were given a commonly used chemotherapy (Taxol/5-fluorouracil, doxorubicin, and cyclophosphamide). Patients with basal-like and erbb-2+ subgroups were found to have the highest rates (45% each) of a pathological complete response (CR), while only 6% of luminal tumors had a complete response. Among the normal-like cancers, no response was seen (Rouzier et al., 2005). None of the 61 genes associated with pathologic CR in the basal-like group were associated with pathologic CR in the HER-2+ group, which suggest that the mechanisms of chemotherapy sensitivity may vary across the subtypes. As molecular classification was not independently associated with pathologic CR, the predictive accuracy of the logistic regression models including (a) clinical + pathologic variables, (b) clinical variables + molecular classification, and (c) clinical + pathologic variables + molecular class (Fig. 5) was measured by constructing Receiver Operating Characteristics curve.

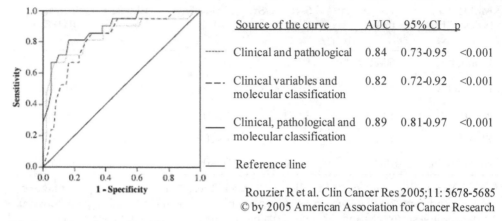

Source of the curve	AUC	95% CI	p
------ Clinical and pathological	0.84	0.73-0.95	<0.001
— —· Clinical variables and molecular classification	0.82	0.72-0.92	<0.001
——— Clinical, pathological and molecular classification	0.89	0.81-0.97	<0.001
——— Reference line			

Rouzier R et al. Clin Cancer Res 2005;11: 5678-5685
© by 2005 American Association for Cancer Research

Fig. 5. Receiver Operating Characteristic curves for logistic regression models. Three different prediction models were compared including clinical plus histopathologic variables (model 1), clinical variables plus molecular classification (model 2), and clinical plus histopathologic plus molecularclassification (model 3). All three models were similarly done.

The three models yielded similar area under curve (AUC). This indicates that the molecular class alone can replace histopathological characteristics (estrogen receptor, HER-2 status, or grade) for prediction of pathologic CR but provides little additional information when these characteristics are included. The basal-like and HER-2 tumors were predominantly high nuclear grade and the basal-like tumors were almost all estrogen receptor negative and 80% of HER-2 molecular class expresses HER-2. These characteristics are known to be associated with higher likelihood of pathologic CR to preoperative chemotherapy (Rouzier et al., 2002; Abrial et al., 2005; Gennari et al., 2008). Because of this association, incorporation of molecular class into a logistic regression–based predictor of response didn't improve the prediction accuracy compared with using routine clinical and pathologic variables only. Therefore, it is likely that more focused gene signature–based predictors will need to be developed through supervised outcome prediction methods that are differentially expressed between cases of pathologic CR and residual disease.

5. Screening and detection of breast cancer

Screening uses test/techniques to check people who might have that disease (breast cancer) and to allow it to be treated at an early stage when a cure is more likely. Breast cancer screening is done by mammography (low dose x-ray technique to visualize the internal structure of the breast). On average, mammography will detect about 80-90% of the breast cancers in women without symptoms. Testing is somewhat more accurate in postmenopausal than in premenopausal women (Michaelson et al., 2002). It can reduce breast cancer mortality by 20-30% in women over 50 yrs old in high-income countries when the screening coverage is over 70% (IARC, 2008). MRI, or magnetic resonance imaging, is a technology that uses magnets and radio waves to produce detailed cross-sectional images of the inside of the body. MRI does not use x-rays, so it does not involve any radiation exposure. Breast MRI is not recommended as a routine screening tool for all women as MRI screening results in more false positives results. However, it is recommended for screening women who are at high risk for breast cancer, usually due to a strong family history and/or a mutation in genes such as BRCA1 or BRCA2. It is also used for gathering more information about the suspicious area found on mammogram and ultrasound and also used for monitoring recurrence after treatment. Positron emission tomography (PET) scan creates computerized images of chemical changes that take place in the tissue. PET scans may play a role in determining whether a breast mass is cancerous. However, PET scans are more accurate in detecting larger and more aggressive tumors than they are in locating tumors that are smaller than 8 mm and/or less aggressive. They may also detect cancer when other imaging techniques show normal results. PET scans may be helpful in evaluating and staging recurrent disease. Clinical breast examination (CBE) is recommended for average risk asymptomatic in the age group of 20-30 to observe any changes in shape, texture, and location of lumps (situated in skin or deeper tissues). The breasts should also be inspected for skin changes (e.g., dimpling, redness) and asymmetry. The area under both arms will also be examined. CBE is also an opportunity for a woman and her health care provider to discuss changes in her breasts, early detection testing, and factors in the woman's history that might make her more likely to develop. All women should become familiar with both the appearance and feel of their breasts to detect any changes and report them promptly to their physician. A woman who chooses to perform breast self-exams (BSE) should receive instructions and have her technique reviewed by a health care professional who performs clinical examinations. Finding and reporting breast changes early offers women the best opportunity for improving breast cancer treatment and reducing breast cancer deaths. Mammotome® is a vacuum assisted breast biopsy that uses image guidance such as stereotactic x-ray, ultrasound, MRI and/or molecular imaging to perform breast biopsies. Mammotome offers a full array of tissue markers to mark the biopsy site for follow-up observations. There have been no reports of serious complications resulting from the Mammotome breast biopsy system. Ductal lavage is another screening and investigational technique for collecting samples of cells from breast ducts for analysis under a microscope. A saline (salt water) solution is introduced into a milk duct through a catheter (a thin, flexible tube) that is inserted into the opening of the duct on the surface of the nipple. Fluid, which contains cells from the duct, is withdrawn through the catheter. The cells are checked under a microscope to identify changes that may indicate cancer or changes that may increase the risk for breast cancer. The procedure is used to identify precancerous cells, called atypical cells. Ductal lavage is currently performed only on women who have multiple breast cancer risk factors to detect breast cancer before it starts. Ductal lavage appears to have low sensitivity and high specificity for breast cancer detection, possibly because cancer-containing ducts fail to yield fluid or have benign or mildly atypical cytology (Khan et al., 2004).

6. Breast cancer treatment

Breast cancer treatment depends on stage, age, hormonal and receptor status. Most women with breast cancer will undergo some type of surgery. Surgery is often combined with other treatments such as radiation therapy, chemotherapy, hormone therapy, and targeted therapy.

6.1 Surgery

Most patients with breast cancer have surgery to remove the tumor mass from the breast. The types of breast cancer surgery differ in the amount of tissue that is removed with the tumor, depending on the tumor's characteristics, whether it has spread (metastasized), and patient's personal feelings. Some of the lymph nodes under the arm are usually taken out and looked under a microscope to see if they contain cancer cells. Breast-conserving surgery or lumpectomy is done to remove the cancer cells but not the breast itself. Lumpectomy is almost always followed by about 5 to 7 weeks of radiation therapy. A woman who chooses lumpectomy and radiation will have the same expected long-term survival as if she had chosen mastectomy (Fisher et al., 2002). Simple or total mastectomy includes removal of the entire breast. Modified radical mastectomy includes removal of the entire breast and lymph nodes under the arm, but does not include removal of the underlying chest wall muscle, as with a radical mastectomy. Both lumpectomy and mastectomy are often accompanied by removal of regional lymph nodes from the axilla, or armpit, to determine the involvement of lymph nodes and spreading of the disease. Axillary lymph node metastasis is the most important prognostic factor for the disease-free and overall survival. Patients with multiple unfavorable risk factors such as positive axillary lymph nodes, high nuclear grade, young age and large tumor showed poorer local control and disease-free survival than patients without any risk factors, and so more aggressive treatment is required for these patients. Adjuvant radio-, chemo-, or targeted therapy has improved the prognosis of patients with higher risk factors (Lee & Chan, 1984; Kim et al., 2005).

6.2 Radiation therapy

Radiation therapy is a cancer treatment that uses high-energy x-rays or other types of radiation to destroy cancer cells remaining in the breast, chest wall, or underarm area after surgery, or to reduce the size of a tumor before surgery (Early Breast Cancer Trialists' Collaborative Group, 2000). There are two types of radiation therapy. External radiation therapy uses a machine outside the body to send radiation toward the cancer. Internal radiation therapy uses a radioactive substance sealed in needles, seeds, wires, or catheters that are placed directly into or near the cancer. The way the radiation therapy is given depends on the type and stage of the cancer being treated. Using traditional clinical and pathological factors, patients can be classified into subgroups by the risk of loco-regional recurrence. In the high-risk groups the absolute benefit of irradiation is larger. However, the patients are over-treated in every subgroup. Substantial proportion of the patients remains free of loco-regional recurrence even in the absence of irradiation, and some patients develop loco-regional recurrence despite postoperative irradiation. Molecular subtypes on the basis of receptors may provide sufficient information to allow accurate individual risk assessment to identify patients who might benefit from receiving post mastectomy radiotherapy (PMRT). A significantly improved overall survival after PMRT was seen only among patients of luminal subtypes. No significant overall survival improvement after PMRT was found among patients with basal and ERB2 subtypes (Fig. 6). There was also smaller improvements in loco-regional recurrence of breast cancer in basal and ERB2 subtypes as compared to luminal A and luminal B (Kyndi et al., 2008). Hence, the improvement in survival resulting from the use of irradiation is more related to the prevention of local recurrences. Post-irradiation local recurrence increases the risk of mortality, but with good prognostic factors (<4 positive nodes, tumor size <2 cm, Grade 1 malignancy, ER- and PR-positive, HER-2-negative) the 10-year survival is 80-90% (Fodor, 2009).

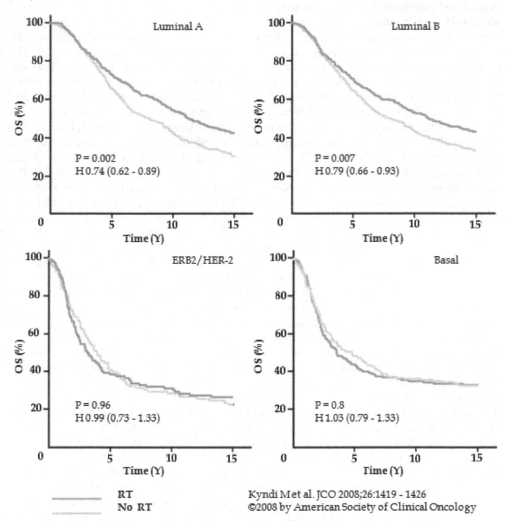

Fig. 6. Overall survival (OS)% of different molecular subtypes of breast cancer patients after receiving post mastectomy radiation therapy (RT). P values and 95% CI of Hazard (H) ratios are shown.

6.3 Chemotherapy and molecular targeted-therapy

Chemotherapeutic drugs are applied in neoadjuvant settingsto shrink the size of tumor that has metastasized and also in adjuvant settings to delay the further growth and spread of the tumor. It is found that combinations of drugs are more effective than just one drug alone for breast cancer treatment. The most common drugs recommended to be used in combination in early breast cancer are cyclophosphamide, methotrexate, 5-fluorouracil (CMF combinations), doxorubicin (Adriamycin), epirubicin, paclitaxel (Taxol), and docetaxol (Taxotere). Although the benefit and clinical outcome of chemotherapy is dependent on clinical and histopathological parameters, but there are a percentage of cases that behave in an unexpected manner, even if the clinical and pathological parameters indicate the opposite (Gonzalez-Angulo et al., 2007). The introduction of hormonal receptor status to the classical clinical parameters improved the clinical outcome (Goldhirsch et al., 2003). The chemotherapeutic drugs are designed to target the specific molecular markers (molecular targeted therapy) overexpressed in cancer tissues. The presence of ER is correlated with a better prognosis, predicting response to hormonal therapies such as tamoxifen and aromatase inhibitors. But still 15-20% of breast cancer patients with ER+ have recurrent disease. It's the luminal B subgroup of previously classified ER+ tumor that is irresponsive to tamoxifen treatment as they co-express EGFRs and shows poor relapse-free survival (RFS) and over-all survival (OS). Thus over-simplified classification based on ER status required additional molecular makers for sub-classification for optimal treatment. The molecular portraits based on gene profiling divides breast carcinomas into luminal (A and B), basal, HER-2 and normal like. Basal and HER-2 types normally overexpress EGFR and HER-2 respectively. EGFR and HER-2 is overexpressed in 17-30% and 20-30% respectively in breast cancer. Both EGFR and HER-2 is associated with poor prognosis and worse clinical outcome. Basal like subtypes are more aggressive and less responsive to conventional chemotherapy and expected to benefit from EGFR-targeted therapies. Tyrosine kinase inhibitors (TKI) (ZD1839, ZD6474) in combined with anthracyclines (doxorubicin, epirubicin) or taxanes based regimens will improve the clinical outcome of the basal subtypes. HER-2 might serve as a marker for tissue HER-2 status, especially for the prediction of benefit from trastuzumab and/or chemotherapy regimens (anthracyclines) (Sandri et al., 2004). Although the molecular profile of the tumor is a major determinant of disease progression and response to treatment, other factors including chemo- sensitvity or resistivity may be of considerable importance. It is found that for 100 node-negative, premenopausal women receiving chemotherapy according to standard criteria, at 5 years 3 are cured by chemotherapy, 83.50 would have been alive without chemotherapy and 13.50 die despite chemotherapy. With application of molecular profiling to predict the outcome (for the same 100 people), the number treated would be reduced to 39.05 (allowing for a false-positive rate equivalent to that seen in the van 't Veer study (van 't Veer et al., 2002), resulting in an increase in the proportion cured (from 3 out of 100 to 3 out of 39 or 8%). If it were possible to predict chemo-responsiveness, it is possible that the number receiving chemotherapy would reduce further from 39.05 to 29.20 (allowing for a false-positive rate equivalent to that seen in the van't Veer study). In this scenario, the proportion cured by chemotherapy would be 3 out of 29.20 (10.16%) (>3-fold increase in survival rate using chemotherapy), and the number of women treated has been reduced by 70.80%. Thus it is found that molecular profiling will enhance the survival benefit of chemotherapeutic regimens, which will be further improved applying the knowledge of chemo-responsiveness as shown in Fig. 7. If accurate determination of chemo-sensitivity were achieved by observing the set of genes responsible for treatment response, the overall number receiving cytotoxic treatment unnecessarily would decrease, and the overall survival benefit derived, per person treated, increase accordingly, as shown in Fig. 7. However, the absolute survival benefit of patients diagnosed with breast cancer would be unaffected and would be improved with more molecular subtypes along with the development of specific agents targeting particular biomarkers (molecular targeted therapy).

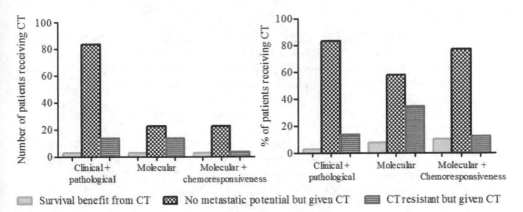

Cleator S and Ashworth A. Br J Cancer 2004; 90:1120 – 1124
©2004 by CancerResearch UK

Fig. 7. Model for the effect of molecular profiling on breast cancer. The data shows numbers of premenopausal women with node negative breast cancer receiving chemotherapy (CT), and associated benefit at 5 years. 100 node-negative, premenopausal women receiving chemotherapy according to standard criteria, at 5 years showed survival benefit, no benefit and breast cancer specific death. The two bar graph represents absolute survival benefit and % survival benefit of breast cancer patients receiving chemotherapy. Note that in neither figure has consideration been given to the false-negative rate inherent in molecular profiling. It has been assumed that all deaths occurring were breast cancer related.

7. Conclusion

Adjuvant chemo- and radiotherapy improves survival of patients but it is being increasingly recognized that the benefit is not equal for all patients of breast cancer. Molecular characteristics of the cancer affect sensitivity to chemo- and radiotherapy. In general, ER- (Basal and HER-2) is more sensitive to chemotherapy than ER+ (Luminal A and Luminal B) breast cancer where as ER+ is more sensitive to radiotherapy than ER- breast cancer. The prognostic predictions made by traditional histopathological based models and molecular based models are discordant in about 30% of the cases (van de Vijver et al., 2002), suggesting that one of these methods may be superior to the other or at least that the information they capture is complementary. Corollary to this, it is found that when both the type of classifications are combined (histopathological and molecular), it yield better prognostic values as observed in Fig. 6. It is currently unknown whether genomic tests based on molecular signatures yield a more accurate risk prediction than conventional models. A better prognostic test based on molecular classification with the knowledge of chemo-responsiveness could lead to a reduction in overtreatment of low-risk individuals who are falsely assigned to high-risk category by clinical variables. Such a test could also lead to better overall survival by correctly identifying high-risk individuals who might currently miss out on systemic therapy. Even if molecular classification do not prove to be better than clinical models in prognosis and prediction outcome of breast cancer, inclusion of their results, as additional variables, in current models could improve prognostic predictions.

8. References

Abrial, C., Van Praagh, I., Delva, R., Leduc, B., Fleury, J., Gamelin, E., Sillet-Bach, I., Penault-Llorca, F., Amat, S., & Chollet, P. (2005). Pathological and clinical response of a primary chemotherapy regimen combining vinorelbine, epirubicin, and paclitaxel as neoadjuvant treatment in patients with operable breast cancer. *Oncologist*, Vol.10, pp.242-49.

American Cancer Society. (2010). Breast Cancer Facts and Figures 2009-10: *American Cancer Society*, Inc., Atlanta

Chang, H. R., Glaspy, J., Allison M. A., Kass, F. C., Elashoff, R., Chung, D. U., & Gornbein, J. (2010). Differential response of triple-negative breast cancer to a docetaxel and carboplatin-based neoadjuvant treatment. *Cancer*, Vol.116, pp.4227-32.

Coleman, M. P., Quaresma, M., Berrino, F., Lutz, J. M., De Angelis, R., Capocaccia, R., Baili, P., Rachet, B., Gatta, G., Hakulinen, T., Micheli, A., Sant, M., Weir, H. K., Elwood, J. M., Tsukuma, H., Koifman, S., E Silva, G. A, Francisci, S., Santaquilani, M., Verdecchia, A., Storm, H. H., & Young, J. L. (2008). Cancer survival in five continents: a worldwide population-based study (CONCORD). *Lancet Oncol*, Vol.9, pp.730-56.

Dawood, S., Broglio, K., Kau, S. W., Green, M. C., Giordano, S. H., Meric-Bernstam, F., Buchholz, T. A., Albarracin, C., Yang, W. T., Hennessy, B. T., Hortobagyi, G. N., & Gonzalez-Angulo, A. M. (2009). Triple receptor-negative breast cancer: the effect of race on response to primary systemic treatment and survival outcomes. *J Clin Oncol*, Vol.27, pp.220-26.

Dent, R., Trudeau, M., Pritchard, K. I., Hanna, W. M., Kahn, H. K., Sawka, C. A., Lickley, L. A., Rawlinson, E., Sun, P., & Narod, S. A. (2007). Triple-negative breast cancer: clinical features and patterns of recurrence. *Clin Cancer Res*, Vol.13, pp.4429-34.

Early Breast Cancer Trialists' Collaborative Group. (2000). Favourable and unfavourable effects on long-term survival of radiotherapy for early breast cancer: an overview of the randomised trials. Early Breast Cancer Trialists' Collaborative Group. *Lancet*, Vol.355, pp.1757-70.

Fisher, B., Anderson, S., Bryant, J., Margolese, R. G., Deutsch, M., Fisher, E. R., Jeong, J. H., & Wolmark, N. (2002). Twenty-year follow-up of a randomized trial comparing total mastectomy, lumpectomy, and lumpectomy plus irradiation for the treatment of invasive breast cancer. *N Engl J Med*, Vol.347, pp.1233-41.

Fodor, J. (2009). [Evidence-based radiotherapy in the treatment of early-stage invasive breast cancer: traditional clinical features and biomarkers]. *Magy Onkol*, Vol.53, pp.7-14.

Gennari. A., Sormani, M. P., Pronzato, P., Puntoni, M., Colozza, M., Pfeffer, U., & Bruzzi, P. (2008). HER2 status and efficacy of adjuvant anthracyclines in early breast cancer: a pooled analysis of randomized trials. *J Natl Cancer Inst*, Vol.100, pp.14-20.

Goldhirsch, A., Wood, W. C., Gelber, R. D., Coates, A. S., Thurlimann, B., & Senn, H. J. (2003). Meeting highlights: updated international expert consensus on the primary therapy of early breast cancer. *J Clin Oncol*, Vol.21, pp.3357-65.

Gonzalez-Angulo, A. M., Morales-Vasquez, F., & Hortobagyi, G. N. (2007). Overview of resistance to systemic therapy in patients with breast cancer. *Adv Exp Med Biol*, Vol.608, pp.1-22.

Hulka, B. S., & Moorman, P. G. (2001). Breast cancer: hormones and other risk factors. *Maturitas*, 38:103-113; discussion 103-6.

Kelsey, J. L., & Gammon, M. D. (1990). Epidemiology of breast cancer. *Epidemiol Rev*, Vol. 12, pp.228-40.

Khan, S. A., Wiley, E. L., Rodriguez, N., Baird, C., Ramakrishnan, R., Nayar, R., Bryk, M., Bethke, K. B., Staradub, V. L., Wolfman, J., Rademaker, A., Ljung, B. M., & Morrow, M. (2004). Ductal lavage findings in women with known breast cancer undergoing mastectomy. *J Natl Cancer Inst*, Vol. 96, pp.1510-17.

Kim, K. J., Huh, S. J., Yang, J. H., Park, W., Nam, S. J., Kim, J. H., Lee, J. H., Kang, S. S., Lee, J. E., Kang, M. K., Park, Y. J., & Nam, H. R. (2005). Treatment results and prognostic factors of early breast cancer treated with a breast conserving operation and radiotherapy. *Jpn J Clin Oncol*, Vol. 35, pp.126-33.

Kyndi, M., Sorensen, F. B., Knudsen, H., Overgaard, M., Nielsen, H. M., & Overgaard, J. (2008). Estrogen receptor, progesterone receptor, HER-2, and response to postmastectomy radiotherapy in high-risk breast cancer: the Danish Breast Cancer Cooperative Group. *J Clin Oncol*, Vol.26, pp.1419-26.

Lee, Y. T., & Chan, L. S. (1984). Surgical treatment of carcinoma of the breast: IV. Prognosis according to extent of involvement of the axillary lymph nodes. *J Surg Oncol*, Vol. 27, pp.35-41.

Michaelson, J., Satija, S., Moore, R., Weber, G., Halpern, E., Garland, A., Puri, D., & Kopans, D. B. (2002). The pattern of breast cancer screening utilization and its consequences. *Cancer*, Vol. 94, pp.37-43.

Moore, M. P., & Kinne, D. W. (1996). Breast sarcoma. *Surg Clin North Am*, Vol.76, pp.383-92.

Perou, C. M., Sorlie, T., Eisen, M. B., van de Rijn, M., Jeffrey, S. S., Rees, C. A., Pollack, J. R., Ross, D. T., Johnsen, H., Akslen, L. A., Fluge, O., Pergamenschikov, A., Williams, C., Zhu, S. X., Lonning, P. E., Borresen-Dale, A. L., Brown, P. O., & Botstein, D. (2000). Molecular portraits of human breast tumours. *Nature*, Vol.406, pp.747-52.

Pusztai, L., Ayers, M., Stec, J., Clark, E., Hess, K., Stivers, D., Damokosh, A., Sneige, N., Buchholz, T. A., Esteva, F. J., Arun, B., Cristofanilli, M., Booser, D., Rosales, M., Valero, V., Adams, C., Hortobagyi, G. N., & Symmans, W. F. (2003). Gene expression profiles obtained from fine-needle aspirations of breast cancer reliably identify routine prognostic markers and reveal large-scale molecular differences between estrogen-negative and estrogen-positive tumors. *Clin Cancer Res*, Vol. 9, pp.2406-15.

Rakha, E. A., El-Sayed, M. E., Green, A. R., Lee, A. H., Robertson, J. F., & Ellis, I. O. (2007). Prognostic markers in triple-negative breast cancer. *Cancer*, Vol. 109, pp.25-32.

Reis-Filho, J. S., Milanezi, F., Carvalho, S., Simpson, P. T., Steele, D., Savage, K., Lambros, M. B., Pereira, E. M., Nesland, J. M., Lakhani, S. R., & Schmitt, F. C. (2005). Metaplastic breast carcinomas exhibit EGFR, but not HER2, gene amplification and overexpression: immunohistochemical and chromogenic in situ hybridization analysis. *Breast Cancer Res*, Vol. 7, pp.R1028-35.

Rouzier, R., Extra, J. M., Klijanienko, J., Falcou, M. C., Asselain, B., Vincent-Salomon, A., Vielh, P., & Bourstyn, E. (2002). Incidence and prognostic significance of complete axillary downstaging after primary chemotherapy in breast cancer patients with T1 to T3 tumors and cytologically proven axillary metastatic lymph nodes. *J Clin Oncol*, Vol. 20, pp.1304-10.

Rouzier, R., Perou, C. M., Symmans, W. F., Ibrahim, N., Cristofanilli, M., Anderson, K., Hess, K. R., Stec, J., Ayers, M., Wagner, P., Morandi, P., Fan, C., Rabiul, I., Ross, J.

S., Hortobagyi, G. N., & Pusztai, L. (2005). Breast cancer molecular subtypes respond differently to preoperative chemotherapy. *Clin Cancer Res*, Vol. 11:5678-85.

Sandri, M. T., Johansson, H., Colleoni, M., Zorzino, L., Passerini, R., Orlando, L., & Viale, G. (2004). Serum levels of HER2 ECD can determine the response rate to low dose oral cyclophosphamide and methotrexate in patients with advanced stage breast carcinoma. *Anticancer Res*, Vol. 24, pp.1261-66.

Sorlie, T., Perou, C. M., Tibshirani, R., Aas, T., Geisler, S., Johnsen, H., Hastie, T., Eisen, M. B., van de Rijn, M., Jeffrey, S. S., Thorsen, T., Quist, H., Matese, J. C., Brown, P. O., Botstein, D., Eystein Lonning, P., & Borresen-Dale, A. L. (2001). Gene expression patterns of breast carcinomas distinguish tumor subclasses with clinical implications. *Proc Natl Acad Sci U S A*, Vol. 98, pp.10869-74.

Sotiriou, C., Neo, S. Y., McShane, L. M., Korn, E. L., Long, P. M., Jazaeri, A., Martiat, P., Fox, S. B., Harris, A. L., & Liu, E. T. (2003). Breast cancer classification and prognosis based on gene expression profiles from a population-based study. *Proc Natl Acad Sci U S A*, Vol. 100, pp.10393-98.

Tamimi, R. M., Baer, H. J., Marotti, J., Galan, M., Galaburda, L., Fu, Y., Deitz, A. C., Connolly, J. L., Schnitt, S. J., Colditz, G. A., & Collins, L. C. (2008). Comparison of molecular phenotypes of ductal carcinoma in situ and invasive breast cancer. *Breast Cancer Res*, Vol. 10, pp.R67.

van 't Veer, L. J., Dai, H., van de Vijver, M. J., He, Y. D., Hart, A. A., Mao, M., Peterse, H. L., van der Kooy, K., Marton, M. J., Witteveen, A. T., Schreiber, G. J., Kerkhoven, R. M., Roberts, C., Linsley, P. S., Bernards, R., & Friend, S. H. (2002). Gene expression profiling predicts clinical outcome of breast cancer. *Nature*, Vol. 415, pp.530-36.

van de Vijver, M. J., He, Y. D., van't Veer, L. J., Dai, H., Hart, A. A., Voskuil, D. W., Schreiber, G. J., Peterse, J. L., Roberts, C., Marton, M. J., Parrish, M., Atsma, D., Witteveen, A., Glas, A., Delahaye, L., van der Velde, T., Bartelink, H., Rodenhuis, S., Rutgers, E. T., Friend, S. H., & Bernards, R. (2002). A gene-expression signature as a predictor of survival in breast cancer. *N Engl J Med*, Vol. 347, pp.1999-2009.

5

Breast Cancer from Molecular Point of View: Pathogenesis and Biomarkers

Seyed Nasser Ostad and Maliheh Parsa

Faculty of Pharmacy, Tehran University of Medical Sciences, Tehran,
Iran

1. Introduction

1.1 Breast cancer and risk factors

Breast cancer is the most common female cancer, the second most common cause of cancer death in women, and the main cause of death in women ages 40 to 59 (1). It has been reported that mortality rate from breast cancer has been significantly greater in women whose cancer was first diagnosed during pregnancy compared with those who had never been pregnant (2). Nowadays, many women all over the world faced the challenge of living with breast cancer. The lifetime probability of developing breast cancer is one in six overall (3). High prevalence of breast cancer and high mortality rate of women who stricken by, appoint it among the most challenging subjects in the area of experiments. The two major types of breast cancer risks are objective and subjective factors. Objective breast cancer risk is defined as an estimated chance for bearing breast cancer based on scientifically established risk factors for the disease and is predictive of resultant health outcomes. Subjective breast cancer risk is identified as an individual's realization of her chance for getting breast cancer based on her own cognitive appraisal and is affected by depressive conditions. Objective BC risk had a limited but significant relationship with immune response and natural killer cell activity (NKCA), whereas Subjective risk was highly associated with psychological distress but was not associated with NKCA also the results are still controversial (4).

Many factors including prenatal conditions, diet, physical activity, estrogen exposure, body mass index, depression and quality of life have been mentioned as breast cancer risk factors. A positive family history is the main risk factor. Diet with high amounts of alcohol, fat, caffeine and red meat is a positive risk factor for bearing breast cancer, whereas phytoestrogens and high amounts of calcium/vitamin D can be effective to reduce it (5,6).

Hormonal conditions stand among the most important factors. Prolonged exposure to and higher concentrations of endogenous estrogen; which is controlled and modulated by menarche, pregnancy, and menopause; increase the risk of breast cancer. Testosterone level has also showed some parallelism with higher rate of breast cancer in some studies, although not in all of them. Younger age of menarche and older age of first full-term pregnancy are associated with a higher risk of breast cancer. The data about the effects of oral contraceptives on breast cancer risk are controversial. Some studies show an increased risk of breast cancer in oral contraceptive users, whereas in some other researches, no significant difference was seen. The two newer researches didn't give any data which show that oral contraceptives cause any increase in breast cancer risk. Long term use of post-menopausal hormone therapy is associated with higher risk of breast cancer. In contrast, short-term HT appears not to increase the risk significantly, although it may make mammographic detection more difficult. Environmental toxic agents such as Organochlorines include polychlorinated biphenyls (PCB's), dioxins, and organochlorine pesticides such as DDT are weak estrogens with high lipophilic properties and as a result, can store in adipose tissues. Some studies suggest that exposure to these chemicals will increase the risk of bearing breast cancer, however the data are controversial and more researches should be done.

Age and gender are among the strongest risk factors for breast cancer. Breast cancer occurs 100 times more frequently in women than in men. Incidence rates increase with age until about the age of 45 to 50.

Ethnic difference is another factor affecting breast cancer prevalence. For example, in United States, breast cancer is more common among whites. Much of these differences arise from lifestyle factors and social conditions. Furthermore, there are marked variations in breast cancer incidence and mortality among countries Women with higher educational, occupational and economic level are at greater risk because of their reproductive pattern including age of parity and age of first birth. Ethnic differences in estrogen and progesterone receptor subtypes have been also determined as important factors that affect the probability of breast cancer (7). In a Multiethnic Cohort Study, various status of estrogen receptor (ER)/progesterone receptor (PR) including ER-/PR-, ER+/PR+, ER-/PR+ and ER+/PR- have been reported and ER/PR status varied significantly across racial/ethnic groups even within the same tumor stage. Compared to whites, the high prevalence of hormone receptor-negative tumors in African-American women may contribute to their high breast cancer mortality (8).

2. Breast cancer classification

Nowadays, beside conventional use of grade, histology, and immunohistochemical analysis, changes in gene expression during bearing tumors are used as an instrument to classify breast cancer. Molecular profiling make us capable for better understanding of breast cancer, more precision in determining subtypes and better prediction of clinical outcome and response to therapy. New instruments like microarray kits provide the possibility for simultaneous studying of the expression of thousands of genes in a breast cancer cells and finding out the Gene expression profile. Future applications will take the same approach to proteins (proteomics), genome-wide germline variability (single nucleotide polymorphisms), or cellular metabolism (metabolomics). Based on these methods, several distinct breast cancer subtypes have been identified including two main subtypes of estrogen receptor (ER)-negative tumors and basal-like and human epidermal growth factor receptor-2 (HER2)-enriched, and two subtypes of ER-positive tumors including luminal A and luminal B. These subtypes differ markedly in prognosis and in the therapeutic targets they express.

The luminal cancers, luminal A and luminal B, so called because they are characterized by expression of genes also expressed by normal breast luminal epithelial cells, have overlap with ER-positive breast cancers. There are also several subtypes characterized by low expression of hormone receptor-related genes (ER-negative), one of which is called the "HER2-enriched" subtype (previously called HER2+/ER-) and another called the "basal-like" subtype. The basal-like subtype is named because it expresses many genes characteristic of normal breast basal epithelial cells.

3. Luminal subtypes

The name "luminal" derives from similarity in expression between these tumors and the luminal epithelium of the breast; they typically express luminal cytokeratins 8 and 18. These are the most common subtypes, make up the majority of ER-positive breast cancer, and are characterized by expression of ER, PR, and other genes associated with ER activation.

3.1 Luminal A and luminal B traits
High expression of ER-related genes, low expression of the HER2 cluster of genes, and low expression of proliferation-related genes are the two main characters of Luminal A tumors. This kind has the best prognosis of all breast cancer subtypes. Whereas luminal B tumors have relatively lower (although still present) expression of ER-related genes, variable expression of the HER2 cluster, and higher expression of the proliferation cluster.
Luminal B tumors carry a worse prognosis than luminal A tumors. Unfortunately, this subtype has high probability of recurrence.

3.2 HER2-enriched subtype
The HER2-enriched subtype (previously the HER2+/ER- subtype) is characterized by high expression of the HER2 and proliferation gene clusters, and low expression of the luminal cluster. For this reason, these tumors are typically negative for ER and PR, and positive for HER2. It is important to note that this subtype comprises only about half of clinically HER2-positive breast cancer. The rest have high expression of both the HER2 and luminal gene clusters and fall in a luminal subtype. Promotion in HER2-directed therapy has improved the poor prognosis of this subtype.

3.3 Basal-like subtype
The name of "basal-like" subtype comes from the similarity in gene expression to that of the basal epithelial cells. This subtype shows lower expression of the luminal and HER2 gene clusters. Therefore, these tumors are typically ER-, PR-, and HER2-negative on clinical assays. Because of this reason, the name "triple negative" is also used to describe them. However, while most triple negative tumors are basal-like, and most basal-like tumors are triple negative, there is significant inconsistency (up to 30 percent) between these two classifications. Although any subtype can be triple negative on clinical assays, an interesting subtype found in non-basal triple negative breast cancers is the more newly described claudin-low subtype, which is uncommon but interesting because of its expression of epithelial-mesenchymal transition genes and characteristics reminiscent of stem cells (9).
Recently, many studies have focused on finding molecular pathways that play some roles in breast cancer pathogenesis. Mutation in oncogenes, pro-oncogenes and tumor suppressor genes has been remarked as potential elements in breast cancer. DNA amplification (mostly in proto -oncogenes, growth factors and their receptors) and DNA deletion (in tumor-suppressor genes) are repeatedly observed in breast tumors. Berouk him et al. found 76 amplifications and 82 deletions in 243 breast tumors, in regions containing new possible sensitive genes, such as MCL1 and BCL2L1 (apoptosis), Interleukin-1 receptor-associated

kinase1 (IRAK1), TNF receptor associated factor (TRAF) 6, IKBKG which codes NF-kappa-B essential modulator (NEMO) protein and IKBKB which codes inhibitor of nuclear factor kappa-B kinase subunit beta (IKK-β) protein in NK- kB signaling pathway. PIK 3CA, the gene encoding the catalytic subunit of phosphatidylinositol 3-kinase (PI3K), is mutated in about 20 – 30% of breast tumors. TP53 mutations are found in about 30 – 35% of cases (10).

Two newly identified genes, BRCA1 (Breast Cancer gene A1) and BRCA 2 (Breast Cancer gene A2), have been identified and categorized as human tumor suppressor genes. Mutations in these two genes have been found in the majority of hereditary breast cancer cases. Until the age of 70 women with mutated BRCA1 or BRCA2 genes faces to 45-85% increase in the risk of developing breast cancer. Several studies have demonstrated that patients with mutation in BRCA1 usually bear triple-negative kind breast tumors. In contrast, pathologic characteristics of BRCA2-mutant cases did not seem to be very different with non-carriers. Both these two genes play important roles in DNA repair in a common pathway. BRCA 1 is necessary for mammary stem cell differentiation, a function that could explain its tissue-specificity.

Mutations usually result in dysregulation of signal transduction pathways. Increased expression of specific receptor tyrosine kinases (RTKs) has been implicated in the genesis of a significant proportion of sporadic human breast cancers. Increased activity of some of tyrosine kinases can result in aberrant cell proliferation. This phenomenon may result in cell transformation. For example, amplification and overexpression of neu/erbB2 proto-oncogene is observed in 20–30% human breast cancer, and is inversely correlated with the survival of the patient.

The epidermal growth factor receptor (EGFR) family is a member of growth factor receptors which consists of four members: EGFR, ErbB2/Neu, ErbB 3, and ErbB 4. Increase ErbB2 expression, has been further associated with poor clinical outcome, is observed in 20 – 30% of sporadic breast tumors. The main reason is ErbB2 gene amplification (11). Increased level of tyrosine phosphorylated ErbB3 has been also reported. The important point is that ErbB3 is a bridge which links the phosphatidyl inositol-3 kinase (PI-3K) signaling molecule to Neu which has attracted much attention because of its potent transforming properties. This oncogene activates a number of common signaling pathways by providing specific binding sites for a variety of signaling molecules that include either Src Homology 2 (SH2) or phosphotyrosine binding/interacting domains. Co-expression of ErbB2 and ErbB3 RTKs is usually observed in common tumor progression (11,12).

 Mammary epithelial expression of Polyoma virus middle T (PyV mT) antigen, another tyrosine kinase involved in murine mammary tumorigenesis and metastasis, results in the rapid induction of multifocal metastatic mammary tumors. Since these tumors occur during early steps of mammary gland development and involve whole of the gland, expression of PyV mT will result in transformation of the primary mammary epithelium. This molecule is also associated with many signaling pathways via Src Homology 2 (SH2) or phosphotyrosine binding/interacting domains (13).

It has been shown that Activated growth factor receptors can interact with integrin receptors and control their biological function in cancerous cells. An example is the stimulation of a6ß1 integrin through association with activated members of the EGFR family which conversely results in activation of EGFR family phosphorylation. Induction of tumor by the PyV M T oncogene is also dependent on the presence of functional ß1-integrin. Lack of functional ß1-integrin makes tumor cells unable to enter the cell cycle. Although, these tumor cells are unable to proliferate, There are still viable and bears pathological tumor dormancy. Interesting point is that inhibition of integrin-mediated FAK signaling will also shows the similar pathological features. ß4integrin, other member of integrin family, has shown a clear role cell proliferation and invasion through association with Erb B2. Not all integrins, however, have a role in bearing cancer. Deficiency in ß3 or/an d ß 5 integrins did not produce much difference in tumor growth, tumor numbers or lung metastasis in the PyV MT mouse model , only a little increase in tumor onset was observed. Taken together, these observations give promising data for targeting integrin receptors and their associated signaling pathways as a new treatment of breast cancer (11).

Activation of the phosphatidyl inositol-3 kinase is also important in mammary tumor progression. Association of PI-3K links to PyV mT through its binding to phosphotyrosine residues (Tyr 315/322) within the PyV mT coding sequences. Association with Neu happens through recruitment to ErbB3 (ErbB, is derived from the name of a viral oncogene to which these receptors are homologous: Erythroblastic Leukemia Viral Oncogene). Activation of PI-3K and resultant production of phosphoinotide-3 lipids stimulates several members of serine kinase family. The final of these cascades will be the stimulation a number of antiapoptotic signaling molecules such as nuclear factor-kB (NF- κB) (14,15)

4. Role of NF- κB

Because of the wide range of activities of transcription factor NF- κB in apoptosis and cell survival and cell proliferation pathways as well as cell adhesion and angiogenesis it plays a remarkable role in tumorigeneses.

Regulatory influence of NF- κ B on the expression of various tumor-promoting molecules such as MMP, cycloxygenase 2, inducible nitric oxide synthase, chemokines, and inflammatory cytokines explain its significant effect on bearing cancer. NF- κB increased the expression of these molecules, all of which enhance tumoral cell invasion and angiogenesis. Other aspect of the role of NF- κB in tumorigeneses includes increasing expression of proto-oncogenes such as c- myc and cyclin D1 which directly stimulate proliferation. (14)

4.1 Adapter proteins

Adapter proteins do not exert any kinase activity, but they regulate protein – protein interaction and help the formation of protein complex which participate in signal transduction pathways. GRB2-associated-binding protein 2 (Gab2) is one of the adapter proteins which is overexpressed in breast cancer. It promotes signaling pathways by recruiting SH2 containing proteins such as PI3K, Shc, and Shp2 downstream of tyrosine kinase receptors. Although elevated expression of Gab2 in the mammary epithelium is unable to induce tumor development, it has been shown that tumor onset time will decrease in presence of Gab2 (16,17)

4.2 Activation of the Ras signaling pathway

Activation of the Ras signaling pathway is commonly observed in mammary tumor progression. Adapter proteins such as Shc and Grb2 create some specific complexes with activated forms of Neu and PyV mT. The co-operation of Grb2 and Shc with these activated oncoproteins will result in stimulation of Ras signaling. In contrast to PyV mT, which signals to Ras only through its association with Shc, Neu can activate Ras through Grb2, Shc and several other unidentified adapter proteins. Resultant phenomenon of Ras activation will be the recruiting of a number of downstream effector molecules including PI-3K, Raf serine kinase, GRB associated-binding protein (GAP) and Ras-related protein (Ral) (16). Figure 1 presents an overview of Ras/MAPKs signaling pathway.

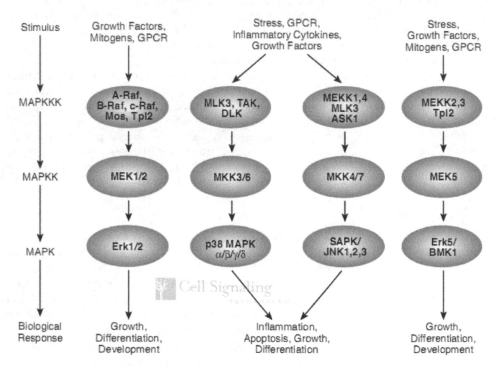

Fig. 1. MAPKs cascades Mitogen-activated protein kinases (MAPK) are a family of Ser/Thr protein kinases widely conserved among eukaryotes and are involved in many cellular programs such as cell proliferation, cell differentiation, cell movement, and cell death. MAPK signaling cascades are organized hierarchically into three-tiered modules. MAPKs are phosphorylated and activated by MAPK-kinases (MAPKKs), which in turn are phosphorylated and activated by MAPKK-kinases (MAPKKKs). The MAPKKKs are in turn activated by interaction with the family of small GTPases and/or other protein kinases, connecting the MAPK module to cell surface receptors or external stimuli. [Source: Pathway diagram reproduced courtesy of Cell Signaling Technology, Inc. (www.cellsignal.com).]

5. Dysregulation of cell cycle

Dysregulation of cell cycle can also results in malignant cell proliferation and Tumorigenesis. Cyclin D1, for example, has been reported to be overexpressed in human breast cancer (18). Observation has been confirmed in MMTV-Ras and MMTV-Neu mice deficit in Cyclin D1. Tumor development completely stops in these animals which show the critical role of Cyclin D1 in Ras-Neu transformation pathway..Although overexpression of

Cdc25b make mammary glands hyperplasic and more sensitive to carcinogenic chemicals, it does not directly induce tumorigeneses. Recently, inhibitor of nuclear factor kappa-B kinase (IKK a, a responsible kinase for activation of NF-k B, was identified as a necessary factor for Cyclin D1-associated epithelial proliferation in MMTV-Neu (but not in MMTV- Ra s) mice (11).

5.1 The role of extracellular matrix (ECM) enzymes
In addition to integrin family, which has discussed above, the role of other extracellular matrix (ECM) enzymes such as cathepsins and plasmin in tumorigensis and metastasis has attracted much attention (19,20)

Matrix metalloproteinases (MMP) are a family of matrix degrading enzymes associated with tumor progression, metastasis, and poor prognosis. A tumor cell must degrade the surrounding stroma to reach blood vessels. That's why it is thought that these degrading enzymes control the primary step in invasion and metastasis. The roles ofMMP2, MMP3,MMP7 and MMP9 have been established (21,22).

urokinase-type plasminogen activator (uPa) is another extracellular degrading enzyme which cleaves plasminogen into plasmin. The latter can degrade ECM directly or indirectly via activating MMPs. PyV MT -associated lung metastasis shows remarkable decrease was in plasminogen-deficient mice as well as in uPa-deficient mice (11,23).

5.2 Mutations in tumor suppressor genes
Transforming growth factor-ß (TGF- ß) is a secreted cytokine which induces s growth arrest in normal epithelium. It interacts with the TGF- ß type II receptor (T ß RII) which followed by recruitment and phosphorylation of TGF- ß type I receptor (Tß RI) and activation of downstream signaling cascade. The cytostatic effect of TGF- ß is also seen on early tumor progression and is mediated through the regulation of both apoptosis and cell proliferation. However, TGF-ß signaling increases lung metastasis in some transgenic mouse models. Breast carcinomas are well known for overexpressed TG F- ß. Induct ion of TGF- ß 1 after tumor initiation do not exert much effect on proliferation of tumor, but remarkably increase the lung metastasis. These data support the hypothesis that that TGF -ß 1 may no longer perform an inhibitory role in established tumors (24).

Another important tumor suppressor associated with mammary tumor development is p53. p53 is well-known for its involvement in a variety of cancer types. P53 gene is one of the most altered tumor suppressor genes in human breast cancer, such that around 50% of all breast cancers include mutated form of p53 gene (25).

It has been reported that Insulin-like Growth Factor (IGF) may have effect in breast cancer progression. It has been showed that Retinoic Acid (RA) mediate their inhibitory effects on cell growth of cancerous human breast cancer cells "MCF7" via selective reduction of Insulin Receptor Subtype-1 (IRS-1) and its activity which results in the selective down-regulation of IP3-kinase/ AKT. High levels of Irs-1 in human breast tumors correlate with elevated incidence of disease recurrence. Although the insulin receptor substrates (IRS) were primarily identified, as the name implied, as a substrate for the insulin receptor (IR), Nowadays it has been known that these adapter proteins, are involved in activation of downstream pathways of several growth factor receptors such as insulin-like growth factor-1 receptor (IGF-1R), vascular endothelial growth factor receptor (VEGF-R), cytokine

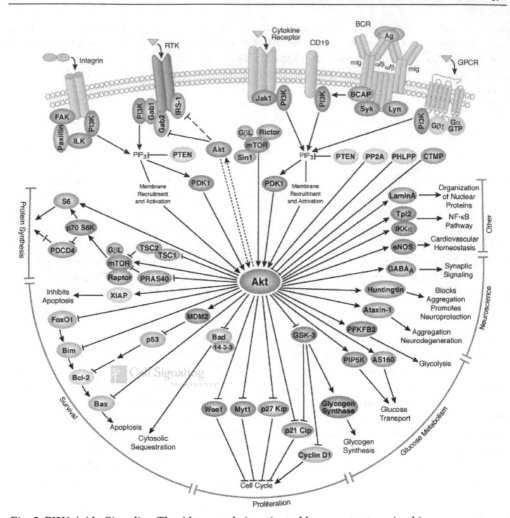

Fig. 2. PI3K / Akt Signaling. The Akt cascade is activated by receptor tyrosine kinases, integrins, B and T cell receptors, cytokine receptors, G protein coupled receptors and other stimuli that induce the production of phosphatidylinositol 3,4,5 triphosphates (PtdIns(3,4,5)P3) by phosphoinositide 3-kinase (PI3K). These lipids serve as plasma membrane docking sites for proteins that harbor pleckstrin-homology (PH) domains, including Akt and its upstream activator PDK1. There are three highly related isoforms of Akt (Akt1, Akt2, and Akt3) and these represent the major signaling arm of PI3K. For example, Akt is important for insulin signaling and glucose metabolism, with genetic studies in mice revealing a central role for Akt2 in these processes. Akt regulates cell growth through its effects on the mTOR and p70 S6 kinase pathways, as well as cell cycle and cell proliferation through its direct action on the CDK inhibitors p21 and p27, and its indirect effect on the levels of cyclin D1 and p53. Akt is a major mediator of cell survival through direct inhibition of pro-apoptotic signals such as Bad and the Forkhead family of transcription factors. T lymphocyte trafficking to lymphoid tissues is controlled by the expression of adhesion factors downstream of Akt. Figure 2 presents a

general map from the role of AKT and the signaling crosstalk which discussed above. In addition, Akt has been shown to regulate proteins involved in neuronal function including GABA receptor, ataxin-1, and huntingtin proteins. Akt has been demonstrated to interact with Smad molecules to regulate TGFβ signaling. Finally, lamin A phosphorylation by Akt could play a role in the structural organization of nuclear proteins. These findings make Akt/PKB an important therapeutic target for the treatment of cancer, diabetes, laminopathies, stroke and neurodegenerative disease. [Source: Pathway diagram reproduced courtesy of Cell Signaling Technology, Inc. (www.cellsignal.com).]

receptors, and some members of the integrin family. Interestingly, loss of either IRS -1 or IRS -2 did not show similar consequence on developing lung metastasis. Metastasis will increase in IRS -1-deficient tumors, IRS-2-deficient tumors shows decreased lung metastasis. It is thought that a compensatory mechanism which upregulate IRS-2 expression is involved in the increased metastasis seen in IRS-1-deficient tumors. These results are very similar to the ones seen with Akt1 and Akt2, where Akt1 was shown to inhibit invasion and metastasis while Akt2 perform in an opposite way. RA influence occurs at post-translational level by increase in ubiquitination and serine phosphorylation of IRS-1. The latter is protein-kinase C (PKC)-dependent, since PKC inhibitors block the process. Activation of PKC-δ by RA has also been reported. Activation of PI3K/PDK/Akt cascade also decreases sensitivity of MCF7 cells to anticancer drugs. Induction of Bcl-2 may contribute to this resistance (26,27). Figure 2 offers a comprehensive diagram which shows the role of PI3/Akt cascade in cellular functions. As it is seen, this pathway plays a vital role in cell proliferation and cell survival. Therefore, logically it is predictable that any signal disregulation in this cascade will be a risk factor for uncontrolled cell proliferation and malignancy.

In one of the recently-performed experiments, the increasing influence of estradiol (E2) on expression level of iNOS in breast cancer cell line T47D were identified as a result for resistance to tamoxifen. In these cells, administration of oligomycin-2 deoxy glucose (2DG) enhanced tamoxifen antiproliferative effects, which may be due to exacerbated ATP depletion following tamoxifen and oligomycin-2DG co-administration. Oligomycin-2DG neither changed iNOS expression nor affected its attenuated expression due to tamoxifen exposure, suggesting that ATP depletion-mediated sensitivity to tamoxifen is apart from iNOS (28).

6. Breast cancer stem cells

Recently, cancer stem cells (CSCs) have attracted a lot of attentions and some roles have been determined for estrogen and progesterone by affecting these cells. It has become clear that the normal and malignant breast contains stem cells (SCs) that play an essential role in the normal development o f the breast and are likely to play a significant role in the genesis and growth of human breast cancer. The CSC hypothesis introduced tissue-specific Stem Cells (SCs) and/or their early progenitors as the main causes of the malignant behavior of cancer. These cells are undifferentiated and, as a result, have the ability to divide into two daughter cells. But, division is asymmetrical and will cause an identical clone of the mother cell and another cell which can divide and fully differentiate into new cell line. This latter daughter cell is named a Progenitor. Physiological functions of breast SCs include producing the early milk ducts and the surrounding stroma at puberty and repair of damaged tissue and renovation the lost ductal and stromal cells during adult life.

In contrast to their progenitor and differentiated offspring, breast SCs are very long life and thus influences of the effect of chemicals and radiation. Since breast CSCs escape from the control of surrounding microenvironment, they are able to bear malignant progenitor offspring. The result will be the production of malignant daughter cells that create the bulk of the tumor.

As a rare phenomenon, some of breast CSCs are quiescent and, as it is expected, will be spared by current cancer therapies whose targets are rapidly divided cells (29-32)

6.1 Role of estrogens and progestins

It has been suggested that hormone therapy or oral contraception may increase the risk of breast tumor development because of proliferation of existing quiescent tumor cells. The estrogen receptor-alpha (ERa) has an important role in normal breast cell development. Genetic alterations in the ER a gene locus might therefore have important effects in breast carcinogenesis. Polymorphisms can also cause even more increase in estrogen-associated breast cancer risk. At least three polymorphisms, i.e. the G478T, A908G, and C975C have been put in this category (33).

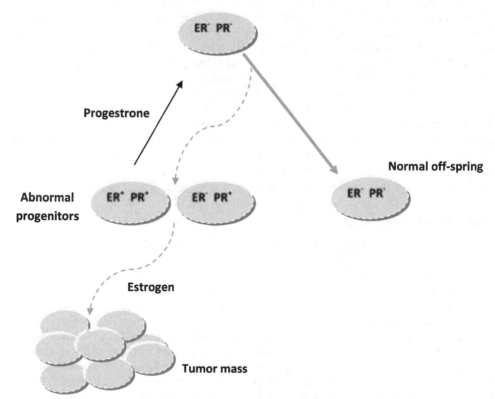

Fig. 3. Effect of Estrogens and progestines on breast CSCs. CSCs divide into abnormal off-spring which can differentiate to all types of breast tumoral cells

Progestins, on the other way, are able to upregulate growth factor and cytokine receptors at the cell surface. They are also involved in regulation of several intracellular effectors including Stat 5, and by potentiating mitogen-activated protein kinase (MAPK) and Janus kinase activities by increasing the levels and altering the subcellular compartmentalization of them at cytoplasmic level. Furthermore, growth factor-regulated nuclear transcription factors may have synergistic effect with PRs' agonists to regulate the function of key genes which are involved in breast cancer. (34)

Recently, the influence of estrogen, progesterone, and progestins on breast CSCs and their progeny has been found out. As it has been demonstrated in figure 3, although most of breast CSCs are estrogen receptor negative and progesterone receptor negative, some intermediate progenitor forms own hormone receptors, especially progesterone receptor. Progesterone and progestin specially work on these breast cancer stem intermediate forms, inducing them to return back to a more primitive breast CSC forms, thus increasing the pool of malignant SCs (29). These cells escape the microenvironment control. Estrogens, on the other hand, induce the proliferation of these abnormal progenitors, resulting in breast tumor. Figure 3 summarize this hypothesis.

7. P-glycoproteins and breast cancer resistance protein (Bcrp)

P-glycoproteins and breast cancer resistance protein (Bcrp) also play important roles in resistance and therapeutic outcome of breast cancer therapy and mutations in MDR genes (which codes p-glycoproteines) and influence the risk and resistance to treatment. Many drugs are substrates for this transporters and the reduction in their access to tissues can result in increase in metastasis and drug resistance. From glycoprotein family, glycoprotein non-metastatic B (GPNMB, also named as Osteoactivin) enhances breast cancer metastasis in an *in vivo* mouse model. It also has been studied as a prognostic indicator of recurrence. The data suggested this glycoprotein as a novel therapeutic target in breast cancer. GPNMB usually express in basal/triple-negative subtype of breast cancer and is associated with poor outcome (35).

Fetuin-A is another glycoprotein which its role in mammary tumorigenesis has been studied. It is a serum component protein which forms approximately 45% of non-collagenous glycoproteins which is synthesized by the liver and excreted into plasma. It is a conserved member of the cysteine protease inhibitors which contains the TGF-β receptor II homology 1 domain (TRH1). As a result, it is able to compete with epithelial cells for TGF- β. The possible sequestration of TGF β by fetuin-A could affect TGF β signaling in breast epithelial cells as previously reported for intestinal epithelial cells. Fetuin-A shows reduced incidence of mammary tumors for breast cancer by more than 60% and increases tumor onset. Another tumor-enhancer property of fetuin-A is its stabilizer effect matrix metalloproteinases in the extracellular matrix.

Consequently, they can drive the "tumor islands" to invade the stroma metastasize to other organs. Stronger TGF-ß signaling in the absence of fetuin-A exert suppressor effect on cell proliferation through increase in is ARF-p53 expression, whereas the sequestration of TGF-ß by fetuin-A, results in reduction of its signaling in epithelial cells and inactivation of ARF-p53 which is parallel with shortening the latency of mammary tumorigenesis and implications of breast cancer development (36).

7.1 Astrocyte Elevated Gene-1

Some newly reported show that elevation in expression level of astrocyte elevated gene-1(AEG-1, also known as Metadherin and lyric) in human breast cancer dramatically enhanced cell proliferation and their ability of anchorage-independent growth of breast cancer cells. These proliferative effects were significantly related to attenuation of two key cell-cycle inhibitors, p27Kip1 and p21Cip1, via Akt/ FOXO1 signaling pathway. FOXO1 is a transcription factor belonging to the Forkhead box-containing class O (FOXO) subfamily. Many biological functions have been shown to be related with FOXO1 including cell-cycle control, differentiation, stress response and apoptosis (37). FOXO proteins could act as tumor suppressors through induction of CDK inhibitors, including p21 Cip1, p27Kip1and p57 (38). Overexpression of AEG-1 increases migration and invasion of human glioma cells because of the presence of a lung-homing domain which facilitates breast tumor metastasis to lungs. Recent observations indicate that AEG-1 play this role by activating NF-κB pathway. Our recent observations indicate that, AEG-1 facilitates IκBa degradation, resulting in an increase in NF- κB DNA binding activity and NF- κB promoter activity in reporter assays These valuable findings are strengthen the idea which recommend AEG-1 as a crucial regulator of tumor progression and metastasis (39).

Another considerable role attributed to AEG-1 is mediating a broad-spectrum chemoresistance. In vitro and in vivo studies showed that knocking down AEG-1 makes several different breast cancer cell lines more sensetive to paclitaxel, doxorubicin, cisplatin, 4-hydroxy cylco phosphamide, hydrogen peroxide, and UV radiation mediated by the pro-survival pathways such as PI3K and NFκ B, or through other downstream genes of MTDH/AEG-1 that directly regulate chemoresistance. AEG-1 has also resulted in chemoresistance neuroblastoma and prostate cancer. In fact, MTDH/ AEG-1does not affect the uptake or retention of chemotherapy a. Instead,

it enhances chemoresistance by increasing cell survival after chemotherapy. Data gathered from Microarray analysis of breast cancer cells showed reduction of expression of chemoresistance genes ALDH3A1, MET, HSP90, and HMOX1, and increased expression of pro-apoptotic genes BNIP3 and TRAIL after MTDH/AEG-1knocking down. Among these genes, ALDH3A1 and MET were established to partially be associated with the chemoresistance role of MTDH/AEG-1 in MDA-MB-231 breast cancer cells. Some other genes also contribute to chemoresistance including drug-metabolizing enzymes for different chemotherapeutic agents, such as dihydropyrimidine dehydrogenase (DPYD), cytochrome P4502B6 (CYP2B6), dihydrodiol dehydrogenase (AKR1C2), and the ATP-binding cassette transporter ABCC11 for drug efflux (40). Roles of MTDH/AEG-1 have been simplified in figure 4.

There are some studies which suggest that Activated protein C (APC), an anticoagulant serine protease, is related to cell survival, cell migration, angiogenesis and breast cancer invasion. APC recruits EPCR, PAR-1, and EGFR in extracellular matrix in order to increase the invasive properties of MDA-MB-231 cells. Other mechanisms include activation of matrix metalloprotease (MMP) -2 and/or -9 and activation of ERK, Akt, and NF-κB (but not the JNK) pathways. APC does not employ the endogenous plasminogen activation system to increase invasion (41).

7.2 Role of STAT family

The Stat (Stands for signal transducer and activator of transcription) family of proteins are latent cytoplasmic transcription factors which are involved in cytokines signaling pathways. They are necessary for normal cell growth, survival, differentiation, and motility. STAT proteins need activation through tyrosine phosphorylation, which leads to dimerization via conserved structural features phosphotyrosine-SH2 (Src homology domain 2) of two Stat molecules. Fallowing activatin, Stats transport to the nucleus, where they bind to the

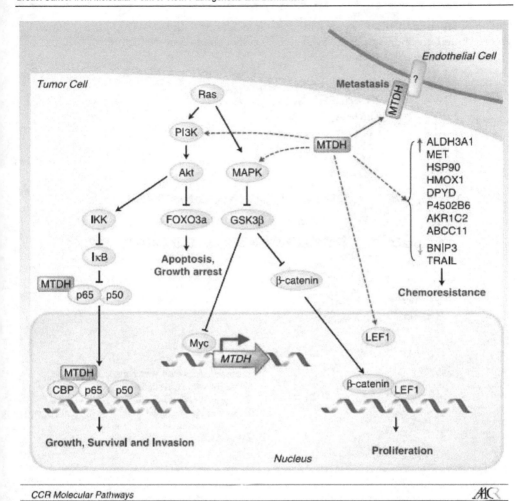

Fig. 4. MTDH/AEG-1 promotes tumor progression through the integration of multiple signaling pathways. Oncogenic Ha-Ras increases *MTDH/AEG-1* expression through the activation of the PI3K/Akt pathway, which phosphorylates and inactivates GSK3β, and subsequently enhances the stabilization and binding of c-Myc to the *MTDH/AEG-1* promoter. MTDH/AEG-1 can activate AKT, NFκB, and Wnt/β-catenin pathways to promote proliferation, survival, and invasion. Activation of NFκB signaling is in part mediated by the direct interaction of MTDH/AEG-1 with p65 and CBP, a general transcriptional co-activator. MTDH/AEG-1 activates the Wnt/β-catenin pathway through increasing the activity of MAPK kinases ERK and p38, which phosphorylates GSK3β and stabilized β-catenin. Furthermore, MTDH/AEG-1 increases the expression of LEF-1, a transcriptional cofactor for β-catenin. The prometastasis function of MTDH/AEG-1 is mediated by the interaction of the LHD of MTDH/AEG-1 with an unknown receptor in endothelial cells. The broad spectrum chemoresistance function of MTDH/AEG-1 is mediated by a number of downstream genes that promote the resistance to multiple

chemotherapeutic agents. Proteins with direct interactions with MTDH/AEG1 are shown in green. Dotted line indicates pathways yet to be fully validated or characterized. [Source: Figure 1 from Ref. 40] With permission

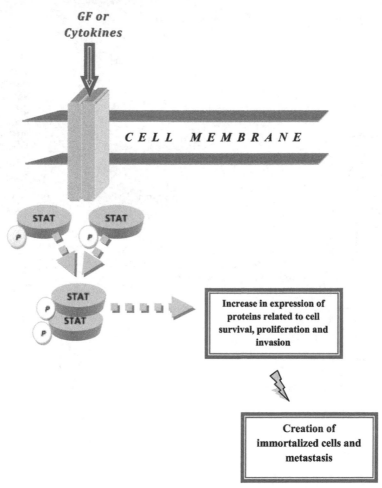

Fig. 5. Role of Stat3 signaling pathway to cancer metastasis. Activatin of STAT3 happens by recruitment to phosphotyrosine motifs within complexes of growth factor receptors (e.g., epidermal growth factor receptor), cytokine receptors (e.g., IL-6 receptor), or non-receptor tyrosine kinases (e.g., Src and BCR-ABL) through their SH2 domain. Stat3 is then phosphorylated on a tyrosine residue by activated tyrosine kinases in receptor complexes. Phosphorylated Stat3 forms homodimers and heterodimers and translocates to the nucleus. In the nucleus, Stat3 dimers bind to specific promoter elements of target genes and regulate gene expression. The Stat3 signaling pathway regulates cancer metastasis by regulating the expression of genes that are critical to cell survival, cell proliferation, invasion, angiogenesis, and tumor immune evasion.

promoter of target genes and activate their transcription. Dimerized status of STATs is transient in normal non-transformed cells. But in transformed cancerous cells, Stat proteins in particular, Stat3 are found in a permanent active dimerized manner. Activated form of STAT3 has been found in more than 50% of primary breast tumors and tumor-derived cell lines. It has been reported that expression of a constitutively active form of Stat3 (Stat3C) is sufficient for promoting cellular transformation and bearing an immortalized breast cell line. Since the IL-6/gp130/Jak signaling pathway has a crucial role in Stat3 activation in human breast cancer, blockade of this pathway may be an important therapeutic plan in breast cancer therapy (42). Role of STAT3 has been shown in figure 5

As it is mentioned above, dysregulation protein expression can result in increased metastatic properties of breast cancer. As a fact, reduction in cell adhesion and increased cell motility is necessary for tumor metastasis. Therefore, cell adhesion molecules have roles in promoting and inhibiting metastasis. Specific families of adhesion molecules including selectins, integrins, lectins, and cadherins have been established to be associated with metastasis (43-47). The cells have to pass the basement membrane to reach the surrounding vessels and spread to other sites. This process involves proteolysis and motility and need proteolytic enzymes to work. Three major categories of proteolytic enzymes including the matrix metalloproteinases (48), serine proteinases, and cathepsins (discussed above) are implicated in metastasis. Cell motility is another factor which cells need to be able to metastasize to other tissues. Several factors are necessary for cellular motility, including the autocrine motility factor, autotaxin, and hepatocyte growth factor (HGF). HGF will result in developing more as well as larger axillary lymph node metastases (24).

Chemoattractants and their corresponding receptors are the other factors affecting metastasis rocess. Osteonectin (a glycoprotein secreted by osteoblasts in bone, initiating mineralization and promoting mineral crystal formation) engages breast and prostate cancer cells to bone. Recently presented data indicate that chemokine receptors CXCR4 and CCR7 express in breast carcinoma cells predisposed for metastasis to lymph nodes and bone (24).

Metastasis-associated protein 1 (MTA1) mRNA expression is parallel to metastatic potential. Function of the MTA1 gene product in tumor progression and metastasis is still unknown, although it is thought that MTA1 is found in the chromatin remodeling histone deacetylase complex (24).

Osteopontin was identified as a metastasis associated gene. Osteopontin appears to be useful for prognosis in that elevated plasma levels and immunohistochemical staining of tumor cells are found in metastatic breast cancer patients. It is important, however, to note that not all studies show correlations. For example, immunohistochemical staining showed no correlation with lymph node involvement or histological grade (24).

8. Metastasis suppressor genes

8.1 E-cadherin

E-cadherin (a member of the cadherin superfamily of Ca^{2+}-dependent adhesion cell surface molecules, expressed predominantly in epithelial tissues) has been demonstrated to correlates negatively with the potential of tumor invasion. Reduction and/or loss of E-cadherin expression in carcinomas will result in increased tumor metastasis because of the reduction in tumor cell adhesiveness and increased cell motility (49)

Tissue Inhibitors of Metalloproteinases

The role of metalloproteinases (TIMPs) is inhibiting the activity of matrix proteinases (MMPs). As a result, they suppress tumor metastasis. An interesting paradox is that increased TIMPs are associated with progression to metastatic disease in some studies. One proposed explanation is that the balance between MMPs and TIMPs is important than the expression of each protein (50).

8.2 Maspin
Maspin (belonging to the serpin family of serine protease inhibitors) is a tumor suppressor gene which has been established to be involved at least in breast and prostate cancer. Loss of maspin expression has been established during immunohistochemical studies (51).

8.3 Kai1
Kangai 1 (from Chinese kang ai meaning anticancer) or Kai1 is a member of the Transmembrane-4 superfamily of adhesion molecules and is involved in lymphocyte differentiation and function. It was originally described as a metastasis suppressor in prostate cancer but its role has been established as a general suppressor of the metastatic phenotype in many cancer types including breast cancer, although KAI1 does not affect primary tumor growth (52).

8.4 BRMS1
Breast cancer metastasis-suppressor 1 (BRMS1) decreases metastatic potential of tumor cells, although tumorigenicity do not affected. The mechanism underlying BRMS1 tumor suppression is not yet known, but some data suggest that this role may be mediated by enhanced immune recognition, altered transport, and/or secretion of metastasis-associated proteins (53).

8.5 MKK4
This gene encodes a dual specificity protein kinase that belongs to the Ser/Thr protein kinase family. This kinase is a direct activator of MAP kinases in response to various environmental stresses or mitogenic stimuli. It has been shown to activate MAPK8/JNK1, MAPK9/JNK2, and MAPK14/p38, but not MAPK1/ERK2 or MAPK3/ERK3. This kinase is phosphorylated, and thus activated by MAP3K1/MEKK (54).

8.6 Role of micro-RNAs
A newly opened window in cancer studies is the discovery of microRNAs (mi RNAs). It has been noticed that alteration of non-coding genes, including miRNAs is related to cancer pathogenesis. Mi RNAs modulate the expression of many genes through cleaving mRNA molecules or inhibiting their translation. As a result, they are involved in a variety of physiological and pathological processes, including development, differentiation, cellular proliferation, programmed cell death, cancer initiation and metastasis. It is important to note that a single miRNA can influence the expression of hundreds of proteins. Early studies showed that compared to normal breast human tissues, miRNAs are extensively deregulated in breast tumors. MiRNAs exert their influences at several steps of tumor development and metastasis. Cancer cell adherence, migration, invasion, motility, and angiogenesis are all affected by these modulators. "Metastamir" is the name which has been applied for the class of miRNAs which are involved in metastasis associated processes.

Profiling of metastamirs in human breast cancer has been resulted in to find the new molecular mechanisms in metastatic process. Significant increase in expression of some of miRNAs has been identified in breast tumors and some others have shown some correlation with biopathological features such as Her2, ER and PR status, tumor stage, and response to treatments. The most important miRNAs involved in different steps of developing breast tumor are miR-335, miR-17/20, and miR-146 (involved inmicroenvironment modification), let-7, miR-200 and miR-30 (BCSC phenotype formation); miR-21,miR- 12 6, miR-373, and miR-520 (local invasion), miR-7, miR-661 and miR-17/20 (survival in vasculature) and miR-200 and let-7 (proliferation at distant sites).

Chemoresistance is also affected by miRNAs. Some miRNAs which play some roles in this step are miR-125b, miR-21, and miR -128. The mechanisms underlying miRNAs dysregulation in breast cancer development, whether dysregulated miRNA is a cause or consequence of pathological and many other questions remain to be explored (55). Some of the most important miRNAs have been mentioned in table 1.

miRNA involved	Protein inhibited	Function influenced
miR-7	EGFR	Anoikis resistance
miR-30	Ubc 9	Anoikis resistance
miR-520	CD 44	Local invasion
miR-373	CD 44	Local invasion
miR-21	Bcl-2	Colonization
miR-145	IRS-1	Colonization
miR-17/20	Cyclin D1	Colonization
MiR-205	VEGF	Angiogenesis
MiR-9	E-cadherin	Angiogenesis

Table 1. miRNAs and their function in cancer

9. Biomarkers

Identifying biomarkers in early stages of breast cancer as helpful instruments for increasing breast cancer survival has opened an important window in researches. Immunohistochemical testing of tumor samples for estrogen receptor(ER), progesterone receptor (PR) and human epidermal growth factor receptor 2 (HER 2) is a common method which is widely used (56,57). Biomarkers in biological fluids are more useful because they don't need biopsy and invasive methods. Four metabolic biomarkers including Homovanillate, 4-hydroxyphenylacetate, 5-hydroxyindoleacetate and urea have been shown to be different in urine samples of cancer subjects, compared to control group (58). The intraductal sampling including samples of nipple aspiration, ductal lavage, and duct endoscopy, is newly used for direct access to the microenvironment surrounding the breast cells that are undergoing malignant transformation (59).

Serum antigens and autoantibody profiling is another approach for early detection and diagnosis of breast cancer. Elevation in level of two antigens, CA 15-3 and CA 27.29, has been reported. Another way is detection of serum autoantibodies against tumor suppressor genes. Studying the changes appeared in level of several autoantibodies instead of only one antibody appears preferable to achieve more accuracy.

BRCA1/2 mutation or functional losses are the other markers will likely serve as a useful predictive biomarker for diagnosis as well as of response to treatment with PARP inhibitors. REGγ (also known as PA28γ, PSME3 or Ki antigen) is a member of the REG or 11S family of proteasome activators which bind to 20S proteasome and facilitate the related degradation of its intracellular protein substrates. REGγ is one of the potential markers in breast cancer whose expression is associated with breast cancer development and the presence of ER, CerBb-2 and lymph node metastasis. It has been reported that REGγ could facilitate the growth of breast cancer cells. Abnormal high expression of REGγ has been observed in breast cancer and its metastatic lymph nodes (60).

BCL2 has been introduced as an independent biomarker for prognosis of all types of early-stage breast cancers. Immunohistochemical studies have been introduced BCL2 expression as a new diagnostic instrument in breast cancer studies although further work should be done to ascertain the exact way to apply BCL2 testing for risk estimation and to find a standard protocol for BCL2 immunohistochemistry (61).

Ki-67, MI, PCNA, and LI have been reported as markers for poor prognosis, although the most important one has not been established yet (62). Serum associated tumor markers have been newly introduced for breast cancer diagnosis. Carbohydrate antigen (CA) 15-3 and carcinoembryonic antigen (CEA) are the most well-known markers. The noticeable point is that the elevation of CA 15-3 between 4 and 6 weeks after initiation of a new therapy, i.e. spurious early rise (surge), indicates poor prognosis. However, American Society of Clinical Oncology (ASCO) guidelines don't recommend CA 15-3 alone as a marker for either diagnosis or detection of early recurrence of breast cancer. CEA expression level has been not also confirmed as a marker for diagnosis or routine surveillance after primary therapy. The ASCO recommend CEA level measurement as supplementary information (63).

Overexpression of cathepsin B (CTSB) - which is involved in proteolytic pathways that lead to the degradation of ECM proteins - and caveolin-1 (cav-1) - which is correlated with increased expression of RhoC and resultant increase in cell motility and invasion - have been established in Inflammatory breast cancer (IBC) compared to non-IBC tissues. Furthermore, CTSB expression level has shown a significant positive correlation with the number of positive metastatic lymph nodes in IBC (and not in non-IBC patients). IBC is the most invasive and fatal form of primary breast cancer, the 3-year survival rate for this kind of breast cancer is 40% which compared to 85% for non- IBC, is very poor. Distinct clinical features of this form include a rapid onset, erythema, edema of the breast and a "peaud' orange" appearance of the skin. High metastatic behavior, rapid invasion into blood and lymphatic vessels and formation of tumor emboli within these vessels are also major characteristics of IBC which make this form the most dangerous kind of breast cancer (64).

MTDH/AEG-1overexpression or genomic amplification can also be used as biomarker to identify subgroups of patients with requirement for more aggressive treatment, although more studies should be done (40).

PKC (a family of serine/threonine kinases involved in several cellular signaling pathways including proliferation, differentiation, apoptosis, and migration) is a marker associated with poor prognosis of breast cancer. Although most breast cancers are PKCa -negative, the small PKCa-positive ratio shows more aggressiveness (65).

S100A4 protein expression appears to be elevated in early and advanced stages of breast cancer compared to normal breast, although its role in different stages of breast cancer seems to be complex. Compared to early stage, S100A4 protein has been observed to down regulate in more advanced stages of breast cancer (66).

Aldehyde dehydrogenase 1 (ALDH1) tumor cell expression is an independent predictor of BRCA1 mutation status. Since BRCA1 related breast cancers consist of increased cancer stem cell components, these hereditary tumors shows significantly elevated expression of ALDH1. ALDH1 positive population of breast cancer cells show high tumorigenic capacity through serial passages *in vitro*, compared with A LDH1 negative population. ALDH1 tumor cell expression has been introduced as an independent predictor of BRCA1 mutation status. Furthermore, ALDH1 might be useful as a BRCA1 biomarker and therapeutic target (67). High saturated to monounsaturated fatty acid ratio measured in blood is another indicator associated with breast cancer risk. Low activity or reduced expression of stearoyl-CoA desaturase-1 will result in a decreased breast cancer risk. The suppression of stearoylCoA desaturase expression leads to reduction of cell proliferation and invasion in vitro, and impairs tumor formation and growth which could not be overcome by use of exogenous monounsaturated fatty acids. Since high saturated to monounsaturated fatty acid ratiois related to the activity of this enzyme, it can be used as a new marker to assume breast cancer risk, although more studies should be done.

Since SCD-1 expression is regulated by dietary and lifestyle factors, new nutritional strategies for cancer prevention could be focused on SCD1 function (68).

Newly introduced Metastamirs assume to be useful biomarkers for prediction of progression and prognosis of breast cancer and in identification of the novel targets for therapeutic intervention in future breast cancer diagnosis and treatment (55).

Taken together, our knowledge about molecular pathways involved in breast cancer and prognostic and diagnostic markers are much more than before, although many works remain to be done.

10. References

[1] Uptodate.
        http://www.uptodate.com/contents/an-overview-of-breast-
        cancer?source=search_result&selectedTitle=1~150
[2] Rodriguez A.O., Chew H., Cress R., Xing G., McElvy S., Danielsen B., et. Al. Evidence of
        poorer survival in pregnancy associated breast cancer. Obstetrics and Gynecology
        2008;112(1):71-8
[3] Uptodate.
        http://www.uptodate.com/contents/epidemiology-and-risk-factors-for-breast-
        cancer?source=see_link
[4] Park N.J., Kang D.H., Weaver N.T. Objective and Subjective Breast Cancer Risk. Cancer
        Nursing 2010; 33(6):411-20

[5] Press D.J., Pharoah P. Risk Factors for Breast Cancer; A Reanalysis of Two Case-control Studies From 1926 and 1931. Epidemiology 2010;21:566-572

[6] Ruder E.H., Dorgan J.F., Kranz S., Kris-Etherton P.M., Hartman T.J. Examining Breast Cancer Growth and Lifestyle Risk Factors: Early Life, Childhood, and Adolescence. Clinical Breast Cancer 2008;8(4):334-342.

[7] Uptodate.
http://www.uptodate.com/contents/meningioma-epidemiology-risk-factors-and-pathology?source=search_result&selectedTitle=32~150

[8] Setiawan V.W., Monroe K.R., Wilkens L.R., Kolonel L.N., Malcolm C.P., Henderson B.E. Breast Cancer Risk Factors Defined by Estrogen and Progesterone Receptor Status, the Multiethnic Cohort Study. American Journal of Epidemiology 2009;169(10):1251-1259

[9] Uptodate.http://www.uptodate.com/contents/molecular-intrinsic-subtypes-of-breast-cancer?source=search_result&selectedTitle=18~150

[10] Bie`che I., Rosette L. Genome-based and transcriptome-based molecular classification of breast cancer. Current Opinion in Oncology 2011;23:93-99

[11] Marcotte R., Muller W.J. Signal Transduction in Transgenic Mouse Models of Human Breast Cancer-Implications for Human Breast Cancer. Journal of Mammary Gland Biology and Neoplasia 2008;13:323-335

[12] D'Alessio A., De Luca A., Maiello M.R., Lamura L., Rachiglio A.M., et. al. Effects of the combined blockade of EGFR and ErbB-2 on signal transduction and regulation of cell cycle regulatory proteins in breast cancer cells. Breast Cancer Research and Treatment 2010;123:387–396

[13] Reese D.M., Slamon D.J. HER-2/neu Signal Transduction in Human Breast and Ovarian Cancer. Stem Cells 1997;15:1-8

[14] Shen Q., Brown P.H. Novel Agents for the Prevention of Breast Cancer:Targeting Transcription Factors and Signal Transduction Pathways. Journal of Mammary Gland Biology and Neoplasia 2003;8(1):45-73

[15] Bhat-Na kshatri P., Sweeney C.J., Nakshatri H. Identification of signal transduction pathways involved in constitutive NF-kB activation in breast cancer cells. Oncogene 2002;21:2066-2078

[16] Andrechek E.R., Muller W.J. Tyrosine kinase signalling in breast cancer. Tyrosine kinase-mediated signal transduction in transgenic mouse models of human breast cancer. Breast Cancer Research 2000;2:211–216

[17] Rauh M.J., Blackmore V., Andrechek E.R., Tortorice C.G., Daly R., Lai V.K., et al. Accelerated mammary tumor development in mutant polyoma virus middle T transgenic mice expressing elevated levels of either the Shc or Grb2 adapter protein. Molecular Cell Biology 1999;19(12):8169-79

[18] Arnold A., Papanikolaou A. Cyclin D1 in Breast Cancer Pathogenesis. Journal of Clinical Oncology 2005;23(18):4215-4224

[19] Chappuis P.O., Dieterich B., Sciretta V., Lohse C., Bonnefoi H., Remadi S., et al. Functional evaluation of Plasmin formation in primary breast cancer. Journal of Clinical Oncology 2001;19(10):2731-8

[20] Nomura T., Katunuma N. Involvement of cathepsins in the invasion, metastasis and proliferation of cancer cells. The Journal of Medical Investigation 2005;52:1-9

[21] Mendes O., Kim H.T., Stoica G. Expression of MMP2, MMP9 and MMP3 in breast cancer brain metastasis in a rat model. Clinical and Experimental Metastasis 2005;22(3):237-46

[22] Voorzanger-Rousselot N., Juillet F., Mareau E., Zimmermann J., Kalebic T., Garnero P. Association of 12 serum biochemical markers of angiogenesis, tumor invasion and bone turnover with bone metastases from breast cancer: a cross-sectional and longitudinal evaluation. British Journal of Cancer. 2006;95(4):506–514

[23] Han B., Nakamura M., Mori I., Nakamura Y., Kakudo K. Urokinase-type plasminogen activator system and breast cancer (Review). Oncology Reports 2005;14(1):105-12.

[24] Debies M.T., Welch D.R. Genetic Basis of Human Breast Cancer Metastasis. Journal of Mammary Gland Biology and Neoplasia 2001;6(4): 441-51

[25] Lacroix M., Toillon R.A., Leclercq G. P53 and breast cancer, an update. Endocrine-Related Cancer 2006;13:293-325

[26] Del Rincón, S.V. Molecular interactions between insulin-like growth factor signal transduction and retinoids in breast cancer cells. Partial fulfillment of the requirements of the degree of Doctor of Philosophy. Department of medicine, Division of experimental medicine, McGill University, Canada. http://digitool.Library.McGill.CA:80/R/-?func=dbin-jump-full&object_id=85148&current_base=GEN01

[27] Navolanic P.M. Sensitivity of MCF-7 breast cancer cells to anticancer drugs is decreased by activation of PI3K/PDK/AKT signal transduction pathway. Partial fulfillment of the requirements of the degree of Doctor of Philosophy. Faculty of Interdisciplinary program in Biological Sciences. East California University, 2004

[28] Ostad S.N., Maneshi A., Sharifzadeh M., Azizi E. Effect of 17-ß Estradiol on the Expression of Inducible Nitric oxide Synthase in Parent and Tamoxifen Resistant T47D Breast Cancer Cells. Iranian Journal of Pharmaceutical Research 2009; 8(2):125-133

[29] Eden J.A. Human breast cancer stem cells and sex hormones a narrative review. Menopause 2010;17(4):801-810

[30] Luo J., Yin X., Ma M., Lu J. Stem Cells in Normal Mammary Gland and Breast Cancer. The American Journal of the Medical Sciences 2010;339(4):366-370

[31] Lawson J.C., Blatch G.L., Edkins A.L. Cancer stem cells in breast cancer and metastasis. Breast Cancer Research and Treatment. 2009; 118:241-254

[32] Molyneux G., Regan J., Smalley M.J. Mammary stem cells and breast cancer. Cellular and Molecular Life Sciences. 2007;64:3248 – 3260

[33] Kang H.J., Kim S.W., Kim H.J., Ahn S.J., Bae J.Y., et. al. Polymorphisms in the estrogen receptor-alpha gene and breast cancer risk. Cancer Letters 2002; 178:175–180

[34] Lanari C., Molinolo A.A. Progesterone receptors – animal models and cell signalling in breast cancer. Diverse activation pathways for the progesterone receptor: possible implications for breast biology and cancer. Breast Cancer Research 2002;4(6):240-243

[35] Salphati L., Lee L.B., Pang J., Plise E.G., Zhang X. Role of P-glycoprotein and breast cancer resistance protein-1 in the brain penetration and brain pharmacodynamic activity of the novel phosphatidylinositol 3-kinase inhibitor GDC-0941. Drug Metabolism and Disposition 2010;38(9):1422-6

[36] Guillory B, Sakwe AM, Saria M, Thompson P, Adhiambo C, Koumangoye R, et. Al. Lack of fetuin-A (alpha2-HS-glycoprotein) reduces mammary tumor incidence and prolongs tumor latency via the transforming growth factor-beta signaling pathway in a mouse model of breast cancer. The American Journal of Pathology, Vol. 177, No. 5, November 2010: 2635-44

[37] Frescas D., Pagano M. Deregulated proteolysis by the F-box proteins SKP2 and beta-TrCP: tipping the scales of cancer. Nature Reviews Cancer 2008;8(6):438-49

[38] Li J, Yang L., Song L., Xiong H., Wang L., et. al. Astrocyte elevated gene-1 is a proliferation promoter in breast cancer via suppressing transcriptional factor FOXO1. Oncoge ne 2009;28:3188–3196

[39] Emdad L., Sarkar D., Su Z., Lee S.G., Kang D.C., et.al. Astrocyte elevated gene-1: Recent insights into a novel gene involved in tumor progression, metastasis and neurodegeneration. Pharmacology & Therapeutics2007;114:155-170

[40] Hu G., Wei Y., Kang Y. The Multifaceted Role of MTDH/AEG-1 in Cancer Progression. Clinical Cancer Research 2009;15(18):5615-20

[41] Mark W. Gramling M.W, Beaulieu L.M., Church F.C. Activated protein C enhances cell motility of endothelial cells and MDA-MB-231 breast cancer cells by intracellular signal transduction. Experimental Cell Research 2010;316(3):314-328

[42] Berishaj M., Gao S.P., Ahmed S., Leslie K., Al-Ahmadie H. Stat3 is tyrosine-phosphorylated through the interleukin-6/glycoprotein 130/Janus kinase pathway in breast cancer. Breast Cancer Research 2007; 9(3): R32.

[43] Krause T., Turner G.A. Are selectins involved in metastasis? Clinical & Experimental Metastasis 1999;17:183-192.

[44] Kumar C.C. Signaling by integrin receptors. Oncogene 1998;17:1365-1373.

[45] A. Raz A., Lotan R. Endogenous galactoside-binding lectins: A new class of functional tumor cell surface molecules related to metastasis. Cancer Metastasis Review 1987 6:433-452.

[46] Perl A.K., Wilgenbus P., Dahl U., HSemb H., Christofori G. A causal role for E-cadherin in the transition from adenoma to carcinoma. Nature 1998;392:190-193

[47] Akimoto T., Kawabe S., Grothey A., Milas L. Low E-cadherin and beta-catenin expression correlates with increased spontaneous and artificial lung metastases of murine carcinomas. Clinical and Experimental Metastasis 1999;17:171-176.

[48] Konjevic G., Stankovic S. Matrix metalloproteinases in the process of invasion and metastasis of breast cancer. Archive of Oncology 2006;14(3-4):136-40.

[49] Kowalski P.J., Rubin M.A., Kleer C.G. E-cadherin expression in primary carcinomas of the breast and its distant metastases. Breast Cancer Research 2003; 5(6): R217–R222.

[50] Ree A.H., Florenes V.A., Berg J.P., Maelandsmo G.M., Nesland G.M., Fodstad O. High levels of messenger RNAs for tissue inhibitors of metalloproteinases (TIMP-1 and TIMP-2) in primary breast carcinomas are associated with development of distant metastases. Clinical Cancer Research. 1997;3(9):1623-8.

[51] Maass N., Hojo T., Rösel F., Ikeda T., Jonat W., Nagasaki K. Down regulation of the tumor suppressor gene maspin in breast carcinoma is associated with a higher risk of distant metastasis. Clinical Biochemistry 2001;34(4):303-7.

[52] Malik F.A., Sanders A.J., Kayani M.A., Jiang W.G. Effect of expressional alteration of KAI1 on breast cancer cell growth, adhesion, migration and invasion. Cancer Genomics and Proteomics. 2009;6(4):205-13.

[53] Seraj M.J., Samant R.S., Verderame M.F., et. al. Functional Evidence for a Novel Human Breast Carcinoma Metastasis Suppressor BRMS1, Encoded at Chromosome 11q13. Cancer Research 2000; 60:2764-69

[54] Kim H. L., Van der Griend D. J., Yang X., Benson D. A., Dubauskas Z., Yoshida B. A., Met. al. Mitogen-activated protein kinase kinase 4 metastasis suppressor gene expression is inversely related to histological pattern in advancing human prostatic cancers. Cancer Research 2001;61:2833-2837.

[55] Shi M., Liu D., Duan H., Shen B., Guo N. Metastasis-related miRNAs, active players in breast cancer invasion , and metastasis. Cancer Metastasis Review 2010;29:785-799

[56] Sparano J.A., Fazzari M., Kenny P.A. Clinical Application of Gene Expression Profiling in B reast Cancer. Surgical Oncology Clinics of North America 2010,19:581-606

[57] Hung T, Wolber R, Garratt J, Kalloger S, Gilks CB. Improved breast cancer biomarker detection through a simple, high frequency, low cost external proficiency testing program. Pathology 2010;42(7):637-42.

[58] Nam H., Chung B.C., Kim Y., Lee K., Lee D. Combining tissue transcriptomics and urine metabolomics for breast cancer biomarker identification. Bioinformatics 2011;25:3151-57

[59] Dua RS, Isacke CM, Gui GP. The Intraductal Approach to Breast Cancer Biomarker. Journal of Clinical Oncology. 2006;24(7):1209-16.

[60] Wang X., Tu S., Tan J., Tian T., et. al. REG gamma: a potential marker in breast cancer and effect on cell cycle and proliferation of breast cancer cell. Medical Oncology. Middlesex: 2011; 28(1) pg. 31

[61] Dawson S.J., Markets N., Blows F.M., Driver K.E., et al. BCL2 in breast cancer: a favourable prognostic marker across molecular subtypes and independent of adjuvant therapy received. The British Journal of Cancer. London: 2010;103(5)pg. 668-74

[62] Stuart-Harris R., Caldas C., Pinder S.E., Pharoah P. Proliferation markers and survival in early breast cancer: A systematic review and meta-analysis of 85 studies in 32,825 patients. The Breast 2008;17:323-334

[63] Hashimoto K., Yonemori K., Katsumata N., et. al. Prediction of progressive disease using tumor markers in metastatic breast cancer patients without target lesions in first-line chemotherapy. Annals of Oncology 2010;2:2195–2200

[64] Mohamed A Nouh M.A., Mohamed M.M., Mohamed El-Shinawi, Shaalan M.A., Cavallo-Medved D. Khaled H.M., Bonnie F Sloane. Cathepsin B: a potential prognostic marker for inflammatory breast cancer. Journal of Translational Medicine 2011;9:1

[65] Lønne G.K., Cornmark L., Zahirovic I.O., Landberg G., Jirström K., Larsson C. PKC a expression is a marker for breast cancer aggressiveness. Molecular Cancer 2010, 9:76

[66] Ismail N., Kaur G., Hashim H., Hassan M.S. S100A4 overexpression proves to be independent marker for breast cancer progression. Cancer Cell International 2008, 8:12

[67] Marise R., Voss H.V., Groep P.V., Bart J., Wall E.V., Diest P.J. Expression of the stem cell marker ALDH1 in BRCA1 related breast cancer. Cellular Oncology 2011;34:3-10

[68] Chaje`s V., Joulin V., Clavel-Chapelon F. The fatty acid desaturation index of blood lipids, as a biomarker of hepatic stearoyl-CoA desaturase expression, is a predictive factor of breast cancer risk. Current Opinion in Lipidology 2011; 22(1):6-10

6

Remarks in Successful Cellular Investigations for Fighting Breast Cancer Using Novel Synthetic Compounds

Farshad H. Shirazi[1,2] et al.[*]
*1Department of Pharmaco-Toxicology, SBMU Pharmacy School, Tehran,
2SBMU Pharmaceutical Research Center, Tehran,
Iran*

1. Introduction

Breast cancer is one of the most life threatening risks in women's life. In spite of considerable progress in its understanding and challenges, treatment is not yet the correct word to apply on this disease and losing life is the most foreseeing adventure in many patients. Although new gene therapy based approaches are looking for the cure of breast malignant cells, but using cytotoxic agents is currently the main chemotherapy approach to fight this problem. Effective chemotherapy treatment of breast cancer requires targeting the pathways that support the cell growth and proliferation. A good *in vitro* investigational model is essential to understand the process of carcinogenesis, risk and hazard mechanism of carcinogens, protection from carcinogens, mode of action and efficacy of novel and even in practice chemotherapeutic agents. The main part for any of these laboratory models is suitable cell lines to properly address the problem and goal of investigation.

Estrogen Receptor (ER) is considered to cause different growth responses in ER-positive, normal, preneoplastic and neoplastic cells (DuMond et al., 2001; Roy & Cai, 2002; Welshons et al., 2003). One of the most significant researches in cancer treatment has been based on designing and studying the ER-antagonism effects of molecules on cells. This is important to select suitable cell lines for *in vitro* drug discoveries studies. Table 1 shows a list of epithelial breast cell lines with different expression in estrogen receptor.

Intracellular enzymes responsible for the different consequences of receptors stimulations and signaling cascades are also under big considerations in fighting breast cancer cells. Dihydrofolate reductase (DHFR; tetrahydrofolate dehydrogenase; 5,6,7,8-tetrahydrofolate-NADP+ oxidoreductase) is an example of pivotal importance in biochemistry and medicinal chemistry. DHFR catalyzes the reduction of folate or 7,8-dihydrofolate to tetrahydrofolate and intimately couples with thymidylate synthase (TS). Reduced folates are carriers of one-

[*] Afshin Zarghi[3], Farzad Kobarfard[3], Rezvan Zendehdel[1], Maryam Nakhjavani[1], Sara Arfaiee[3], Tannaz Zebardast[3], Shohreh Mohebi[3], Nassim Anjidani[1], Azadeh Ashtarinezhad[1] and Shahram Shoeibi[4]
1Department of Pharmaco-Toxicology, SBMU Pharmacy School, Tehran, Iran
3Department of Medicinal Chemistry, SBMU Pharmacy School, Tehran, Iran
4Food and Drug Organization, Ministry of Health Treatment and Medical Education, Tehran, Iran

Cell line	Suitable growth media	Kinds of receptor	Oncogene considerations
ZR-75-1	RPMI-1640 & 10% FBS	Estrogen receptor	
MCF-7	DMEM:F12 & 10% FBS	-Estrogen receptor	
UACC-3199	Leibovitz's L-15 & 10% FBS	-Epidermal growth factor receptor expressed -Estrogen receptor negative, -Progesterone receptor negative	
HCC1954	RPMI-1640 & 10% FBS	-Estrogen receptor -Progesterone receptor	her2/neu + (over expressed)
HCC1500	RPMI-1640 & 10% FBS	-Estrogen receptor -Progesterone receptor	Negative for expression of Her2-neu, positive for expression of p53
HCC70	RPMI-1640 & 10% FBS	-Progesterone receptor negative	Negative for expression of Her2/neu, positive for expression of p53
HCC1008	DMEM:F12 & 10% FBS	-Estrogen receptor negative, -Progesterone receptor negative	Positive for expression of Her2-neu, positive for expression of p53
HCC1143	RPMI-1640 & 10% FBS	-Estrogen receptor negative, -Progesterone receptor negative	Negative for expression of Her2/neu, positive for expression of p53
HCC38	RPMI-1640 & 10% FBS	-Estrogen receptor negative, -Progesterone receptor negative	Negative for expression of Her2/neu, positive for expression of p53
UACC-893	Leibovitz's L-15 & 10% FBS	-Estrogen receptor negative -Progesterone receptor negative -P glycoprotein negative	The cells exhibit a 20 fold amplification of the HER-2/neu oncogene sequence
HCC1395	RPMI-1640 & 10% FBS	-Estrogen receptor negative, -Progesterone receptor negative	Negative for expression of Her2/neu, Positive for expression of p53
HCC1419 & HCC202	RPMI-1640 & 10% FBS	-Estrogen receptor negative, -Progesterone receptor negative	Positive for expression of Her2/neu, Negative for expression of p53
HCC1806 & HCC1599	RPMI-1640 & 10% FBS	-Progesterone receptor negative, -Estrogen receptor negative	Negative for expression of Her2-neu, Negative for expression of p53
HCC1937	RPMI-1640 & 10% FBS	-Estrogen receptor negative -Progesterone receptor negative	BRCA1 (mutated, insertion C at nucleotide 5382), Negative for expression of Her2-neu, Negative for expression of p53

Cell line	Suitable growth media	Kinds of receptor	Oncogene considerations
HCC2157	ACL-4 medium & 10% FBS	-Estrogen receptor negative, -Progesterone receptor negative	Positive for expression of Her2-neu , Positive for expression of p53

Table 1. List of breast cell lines with different expression in estrogen receptor.

carbon fragments; hence they are important cofactors in the biosynthesis of nucleic acids and amino acids. The inhibition of DHFR or TS activity in the absence of salvage leads to 'thymineless' death.

There are some other enzymes which came into special consideration in cancer development, particularly in the breast cancer. Cyclooxygenase-2 is an example that over expresses in several epithelial tumors including breast cancer. Preclinical evidence favors an anti tumor role for COX inhibitors in breast cancer because there is a clear relationship between tissue prostaglandin levels in human breast tumors and the development of metastasis and patient survival (Arun & Goss, 2004). Selective COX-2 inhibitors can prevent mammary tumors from developing cancer in experimental animals. Celecoxib (a COX-2 inhibitor) has proven to minimize the progression of carcinogen-induced mammary tumors (Arun et al., 2001). A good cell line to clearly address alterations in above mentioned systems is also critical for challenging breast cancer cells *in vitro*.

A trustable measurement approach to detect results of the application of under-investigation agents on cells is very much important. Different methods have been applied to investigate cell alterations and ultimately cell death resulted from cancer chemotherapy and cytotoxic agents. Each of them has advantages and disadvantages in different situations and for different purposes. Misuse of any of these methods for the detection of the cytotoxicity of different agents on different cell lines is one of the main problems of many publications for years. These techniques usually look at the viability, morphology and/or biochemical function of various cellular functions. Table 2 lists some of the most popular methods used to measure the cytotoxicity of agents in cellular experiments.

A precise and accurate investigation is one that selects the best possible measurement method on the best possible cell line in the most optimal situation for the best possible conclusion. Cellular investigations to look for new anti-breast cancer agents rely on these bases. MCF-7 proves to be a suitable model cell line for breast cancer investigations worldwide. This is a well known breast cancer cell line derived from a 69 years old Caucasian female. MCF-7 cell line presents most of characteristics of differentiated mammary epithelium tissues including those of expressing estradiol and estrogenic receptors features (Brandes & Hermonat, 1983). Here, we are summarizing some of our results using this cell line to search for novel anti-breast cancer agents, with emphasis and conclusive remarks on the good laboratory practice.

2. Targeting estrogen receptors

Estrogens are known to play an important role in the regulation of the development and maintenance of the female reproductive system, in particular of the uterus, ovaries and breast. Moreover, estrogens are involved in the growth and/or function of several other tissues such as bone, liver, brain, and the cardiovascular system (Ciocca & Roig, 1995).

Method	Measurement criteria	Sample methodology references
Vital dyes (Methylene blue, Trypan blue, Phenol red, ...)	Cell membrane integrity	(Shirazi et al., 2005; Shokrzadeh et al., 2006)
Clonogenic assay, cell numbers	Cellular proliferation	(Shirazi & Eftekhari, 2004; Shirazi et al., 1996)
MTT and XTT	Function of mitochondrial enzymes	(Shirazi et al., 2004; Tamaddon et al., 2007)
Thymidine assay, Bromodeoxyuridine	Cellular DNA synthesis	(Hammers et al., 2002; Maghni et al., 1999; Raaphorst et al., 1998; Yokochi & Gilbert, 2007)
Blotting techniques	DNA, RNA and Protein synthesis machinery	(Ko et al., 1993; Singh et al., 2008; Skliris et al., 2002)
Flowcytometry	Population based cell cycle analysis, Individual cell content and biophysical status	(Lukyanova et al., 2009; Niknafs & Shirazi, 2002; Skliris et al., 2002;)
Light and electron microscopes	Cellular morphology and structural features	(Lukyanova et al., 2009; Russo et al., 1977; Vic et al., 1982)

Table 2. Different popular methods to measure cellular alterations after exposure to cytotoxic agents.

Figure 1 represents the general effects of estradiol (as a proliferative estrogen receptor stimulant agent) and tamoxifen (as an estrogen receptor blocking agent) on the growth curve of MCF-7 cell line. To obtain this, 50,000 cells were seeded in four series of cell culture petri dishes and incubated in phenol red-free RPMI media supplemented with 10% fetal bovine serum for 7 days. From the beginning, three different series of petri dishes were selected for the experiments; estradiol was added into the media of one series, tamoxifen was added to the media of the second series and a mix of these two agents was added to the third series of petri dishes. Cells in each perti dish were counted for seven consecutive days as the presentation of cell proliferation in control, estradiol exposed, tamoxifen exposed, and affected by both of estradiol and tamoxifen agents. As is seen in figure 1, estradiol has a significant effect to promote the growth of MCF-7 breast cancer cells compared to the control cells. MCF-7 cells, however, are arrested for at least five days before being able to start a significant proliferation after the exposure to the estrogen-blocking agent of tamoxifen. This block is effective enough to prevent the stimulating effect of estradiol when cells are exposed to both agents simultaneously. This experiment would further emphasize on the stimulating effect of estrogen receptors in breast cancer progression.

Several studies have established that estrogens are predominantly involved in the initiation and proliferation of breast cancer. Lots of efforts are now being devoted to block estrogen formation and action as an anticancer strategy (Clemons & Goss, 2001; Jensen et al., 2001; Nelson et al., 2009). This has led to the development of compounds termed Selective

Estrogen Receptor Modulators (SERMs), which function as estrogen agonists in some tissues (bone, brain and the cardiovascular system) but as antagonists in others (uterus and breast). Estrogen action is mediated through two Estrogen Receptor (ER) subtypes, ERα and ERβ, which have distinct target tissue distributions and functional activities (Gustafsson et al., 2003; Matthews & Gustafsson, 2003; Välimaa et al., 2004). ERα is predominantly found in the uterus, bone, cardiovascular tissue, and liver and is the predominant ER expressed in breast cancer. ERβ is expressed in many tissues including prostate, breast, vascular endothelium, and ovary. The precise function of ERβ and its role in breast is not clear (Fox et al., 2008; Novelli et al., 2008). Recent studies indicate that ERβ expression may have a potential protective effect on normal cells against ERα induced hyperproliferation (Bardin et al., 2004).

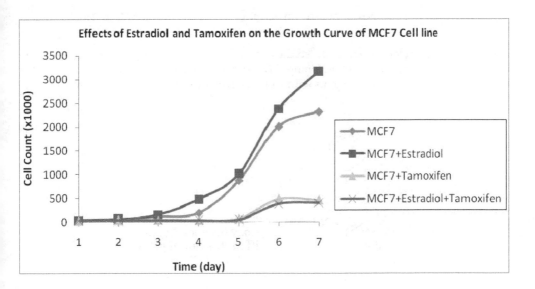

Fig. 1. Stimulation and inhibition of MCF-7 breast cancer cell line exposed to estradiol, tamoxifen and mix of these two agents for 7 days in phenol red-free RPMI media incubated in 37°C and 5% CO_2 humified incubator.

Estrogen receptors can bind a variety of steroidal and non-steroidal ligands. Tamoxifen was the first SERM approved for the treatment of breast cancer (Jordan, 1988). The search for better SERMs has driven efforts to increase the chemical diversity of these compounds, especially the non-steroidal ones (Meegan & Lloyd, 2003). Figure 2 shows the structures of tamoxifen and other known SERMs such as ralolxifen and rasofoxifen.

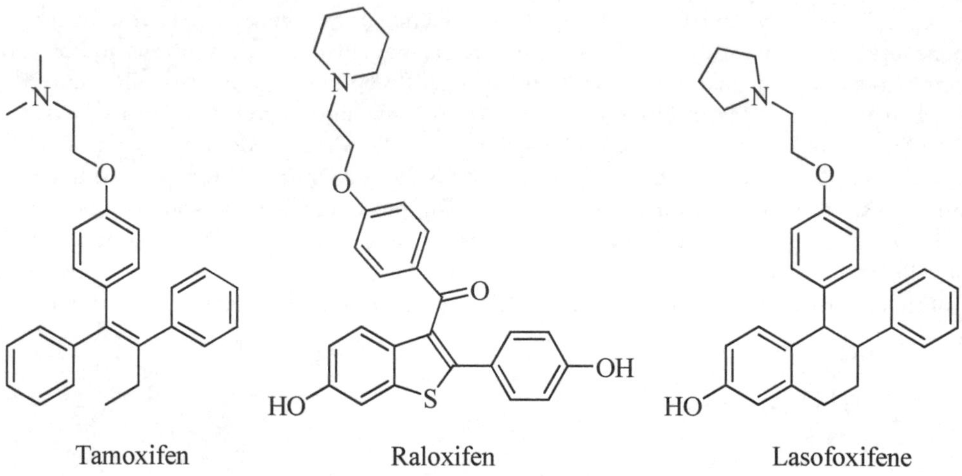

Tamoxifen   Raloxifen   Lasofoxifene

Fig. 2. Chemical structures of some known Selective Estrogen Receptor Modulators (SERMs).

Structure-activity relationship (SAR) studies and molecular modeling studies center lead to the design of novel structures containing 1,2,3-triarylpropenone scaffold to act as potential SERMs and anti breast cancer agents with a unique structure as is shown in Figure 3.

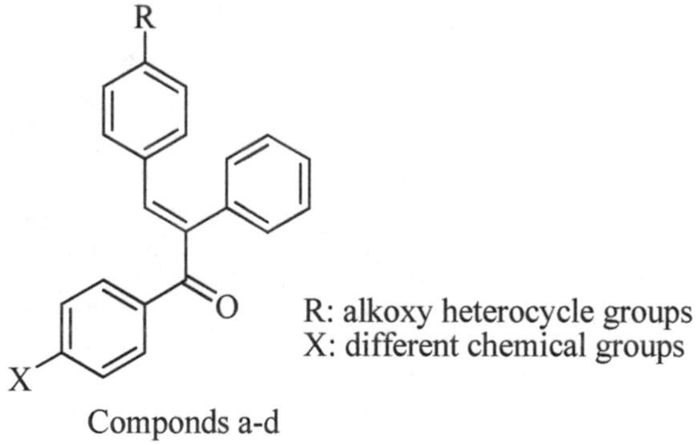

R: alkoxy heterocycle groups
X: different chemical groups

Componds a-d

Fig. 3. The general model of 1,2,3-triarylpropenone scaffold as a novel potential SERMs and anti breast cancer agents.

The compounds a to d have been synthesized and undergone biological evaluations in an *in vitro* cellular system using MCF-7 breast cancer cell line as the model. The anti-proliferative activities of these compounds were determined using MTT assay. To do so, a ten thousands cells were seeded in phenol red-free RPMI-1640 medium supplemented with 10% FBS in each well of 96-well micro culture plates and incubated for 24 hours at 37 °C in a 5% CO_2 incubator. Different concentrations of each compound were added to the wells with respective vehicle control for 72 hours. Media were then removed and MTT (3-(4,5-dimethylthiazol-2-yl)-2,5-diphenyl tetrazolium bromide) was added to each well. Formazon crystals were dissolved in 200 μL of DMSO after 4.5 hours incubation and the dye absorbance for each well was measured at 540 nm. A comparison of absorbance in each well containing different concentrations of each compound to the control wells could easily represent the number of live cells in that well as a result of the cell mitochondrial function (Zhu et al., 2006).

The results of anti-proliferative MTT assays of compounds a to d on MCF-7 breast cancer cells are shown in the graphs below (Figure 4). Start point (time 0) is shifted in each set of figures for a better clarification of the shape and trends of graphs in case of compounds a, b and d. These graphs show the comparative cytotoxic and antiproliferative effects of all of these compounds on MCF-7 cell line.

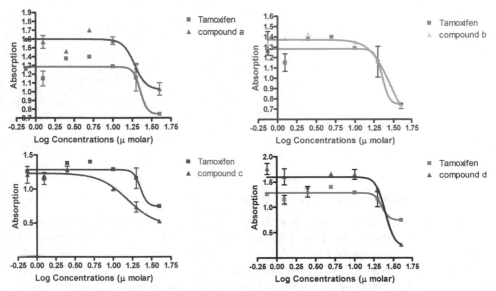

Fig. 4. Cytotoxic effects of tamoxifen and compounds a to d on MCF-7 cell line presents a comparable antiproliferative effects on cancer cells.

Estrogen receptor binding studies were carried out for the compounds with ERα and ERβ using a fluorescence polarization procedure to prove the stimulatory and inhibitory mechanism being through the estrogenic receptors (data not shown). The compounds were active on ERα at nanomolar concentrations and on ERβ at micromolar concentrations. Therefore compounds a to d selectively bind to ERα.

Interestingly, clonogenic assays on MCF-7 cell line after exposure to these compounds fail to present solid and reliable growth inhibitory effects. Figure 5 shows some graphs resulted from the same exposure strategy of above-mentioned compounds on MCF-7, but using the clonogenic methodology to compare the results. A clear weakness is evident in these graphs preventing from any conclusive interpretation of results. We will further discuss this finding at the end of this chapter.

3. Targeting COX-2 enzyme

There is considerable evidence to suggest that prostaglandins play an important role in the development and growth of cancer. The enzyme cyclooxygenase (COX) catalyses the conversion of arachidonic acid to prostaglandins (Abou-Issa et al., 2001). There has been a considerable amount of interest in recent years to take advantage of COX inhibitors specifically COX-2 inhibitors in prevention and treatment of malignancies (Talley et al., 2000; Zarghi et al., 2006). Majority of COX-2 inhibitors belong to a class of diaryl heterocycles that possess vicinal diaryl substitution attached to mono, bicyclic or tricyclic central rings (Penning et al., 1997; Prasit et al., 1999; Riendeau et al., 2001).

As a part of ongoing program to design new types of selective COX-2 inhibitors, our center has synthesized novel COX-2 inhibitor derivatives having a new tricyclic central ring scaffold and different substituents at the N-3 as is shown in figure 5.

R1=SO2Me
R2=H,F,Cl
X=N,NH

Fig. 5. Central structure of novel COX-2 inhibitors.

The nature and size of substituent attached to N-3 influenced both selectivity and potency for COX-2 inhibitory activity. Two different compounds of C1 and C2 with different N-3 substituent have been applied to MCF-7 cell line for the evaluation of anticancer effects, using clonogenic assay. MCF-7 cells were seeded for the clonogenic assay in 12-well plates at 150 cells per well for 24 hours. These cells were then exposed to C1 and C2 derivatives for 24 hours. Media was then changed to fresh media without these compounds and plates remained in incubator for couple of days until most of colonies in the control wells contained more than 50 cells. Media was then excluded and cells were fixed with 96% ethanol and stained using trypan blue. Plates were washed and percentages of colonies in different wells were compared to controls (Shirazi et al., 2005).

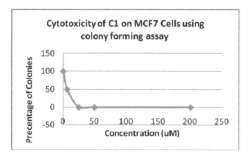
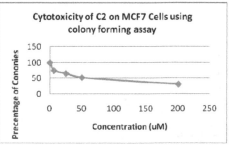

Fig. 6. Cytotoxicity of two novel COX-2 inhibitors of C1 and C2 on MCF-7 cell line using clonogenic assay.

As is shown in figure 6, both compounds have acceptable cytotoxicity effects with C1 being stronger. However, the same experiment has been conducted using the same cell line and the same concentrations of C1 and C2 compounds but using MTT assay. MTT failed to present any cytotoxicity for these compounds on MCF-7 cell line as is shown in figure 7.

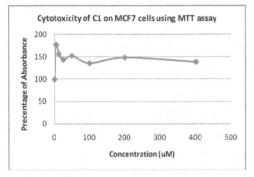
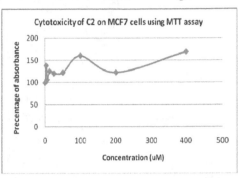

Fig. 7. MTT based cytotoxicity measurement of two novel COX-2 inhibitors of C1 and C2 on MCF-7 cell line.

Failure of one experiment using a technique in spite of success for the other technique in acquiring result is a considerable phenomena in cellular investigation on cytotoxic agents and will be discussed later on in this chapter.

4. Targeting dihydrofolate reductase (DHFR) enzyme

Inhibitors of DHFR are classified as either 'classical' or 'non-classical' antifolates. The 'classical' antifolates are characterized by a p-aminobenzoylglutamic acid side-chain in the molecule and thus closely resemble folic acid itself. Methotraxate (MTX) is the most well known drug among the 'classical' antifolates. Compounds classified as 'non-classical' inhibitors of DHFR do not possess the p-aminobenzoylglutamic acid side-chain but rather have a lipophilic side-chain. MTX serves as an antimetabolite, which means that it has a similar structure to that of a cell metabolite, resulting in a compound with a biological activity that is antagonistic to that of the metabolite, which in this case is folic acid (Barnhart et al., 2001; Takemura et al., 1997).

New, more lipophilic antifolates have been developed in an attempt to circumvent the mechanisms of resistance, such as decreased active transport, decreased polyglutamation, DHFR mutations and so on (Assaraf, 2007; Gangjee et al., 2006; Takemura et al., 1997). In a series of synthesized compounds for this purpose in our center the pyrimidine ring remained (figure 8) and the side-chain attachment at the position 2 was replaced with different substituent.

Fig. 8. The central structure of novel DHFR inhibitors.

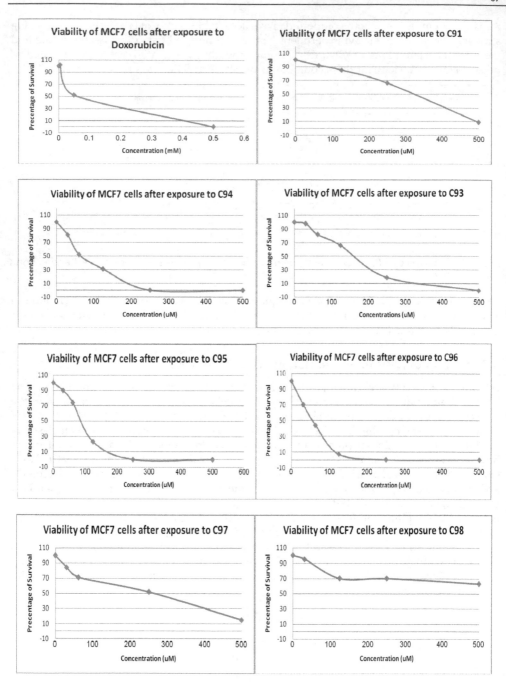

Fig. 9. Cytotoxicity measurement of seven selected DHFR inhibitors on MCF-7 cell line resulted from clonogenic assay.

These modified antifolates differ from the traditional 'classical' analogues by increased potency, greater lipid solubility, or improved cellular uptake. Although being very effective as inhibitors, problems still remain with respect to the issue of toxicity due to the lack of selectivity (Cody et al., 2003; Graffner-Nordberg et al., 2004; McGuire, 2003). To evaluate the cytotoxic potency of these compounds, we have used the clonogenic assay. MCF-7 cells were plated in 6-well plates (200 cells/well) for 24 hours before treatment with the test compounds to allow the attachment of cells to the wells surface. Seven different concentrations of each compound, doxorubicin (as reference), and 0.5% DMSO (applied solvent to dissolve the compound) were added to the monolayer cells in triplicates. The plates were then incubated for 10 days at 37 °C in atmosphere of 5% CO_2. The media were removed after 10 days and the colonies were stained with a solution of 0.5% crystal violet in ethanol for 10 minutes and the number of colonies containing more than 50 cells was counted under microscope. The relation between the number of the colonies (as a percentage to the control containing 0.5% DMSO) and the concentrations of each compound were plotted to get survival curve of the tumor cell line and IC_{50} values were calculated. Cellular viability test results for some examples of this series of novel DHFR inhibitors are presented in figure 9.

5. Discussion

Human mammary gland adenocarcinoma MCF-7 cell line (ATCC HTB-22™) is proven to be a good breast tissue model for anticancer drugs investigations in our experiments. However, selection of a suitable cell line is only a part of a successful and meaningful in vitro cellular examination of potential anticancer agents. Many different factors might very much influence the final outcome of the evaluation of a medication in a cellular experiment, among them are the cell culture media and its components during the time of drug exposure and afterward, exposure time, drug solvent, volume of drug solution to be added to the cell culture media, the proper use of agonists and antagonists for the purpose of elaborations on the results and making a meaningful conclusion, methodology of cellular viability assessment, and the most important factor; the personnel who run the experiment. We are not going to extensively discuss all of these parameters and their specific influences on the final result and conclusion, but the limited examples presented in this chapter may be sufficient to raise awareness for a good cellular practice.

The importance of a suitable protocol for the measurement of survival percentage (live versus death) of cells is underestimated in many of experiments. Selection of the method in many instances is easily a matter of facility, budget and distributing companies' advertisements in the region. However, one should notice that for many known and unknown reasons, various methods of MTT, XTT, SRB, fluorescence dye staining and so on might work or not for different experiments. The main reason might well be the cellular measurement criteria for any of these methods. One should keep in mind that although mitochondria is the heart of cellular energy system, but MTT and XTT experiments would only measure the functionality of a mitochondrial enzyme (Cody et al., 2003; Marshall et al., 1995; Scudiero et al., 1988) and would not necessarily reflect the cell viability. The same is very much true for many of staining methods e.g Annexin V which is an indication of cell membrane flip-flop that would most properly occur during the process of apoptosis (Kolodgie et al., 2003; Van Heerde et al., 2000). Both of these methods are extensively used for the measurement of the cytotoxicity of many different agents. The chemical structure of under investigation compound, its solvent, its cellular site of action, the exposure time, the lag time from the beginning of exposure to the start of measurement, and even the selection of cell line might dramatically alter the final survival curve. Methotrexate is a good example of MTT limitation in cytotoxicity measurement (Haber et al., 1993) and colleagues have shown that MTT protocol is not able to assess the cytotoxicity of this anticancer agent on various cells including MCF-7. Our experiments on other novel DHFR inhibitors have also proven the same conclusion when MTT results were not conclusive while the clonogenic g assay could easily provide a meaningful dose-response result. Figure 10 shows a comparison of MTT versus clonogenic assay for the measurement of methotrexate as well as some other novel DHFR inhibitors. As is shown in this figure, clonogenic assay was more successful in determining the LD_{50} of these compounds in MCF-7 cell line, but not the MTT protocol. Alteration of the exposure time and lag time between the addition of drugs and start of MTT assay, media components and calculation method were not helpful to provide a conclusive survival curve using this method (Data are not shown).

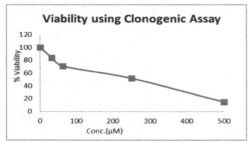 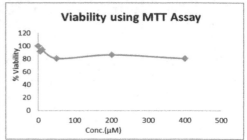

Fig. 10. Comparison of clonogenic versus MTT assays for the measurement of methotrexate and some other novel DHFR inhibitors.

Clonogenic assay is usually considered as a final answer for drugs cytotoxicity because of its long waiting time to acquire result. A minimum of five to six cellular doubling times to look at results in clonogenic assay might well overcome all cellular adventures of arrest, repair, detoxification and exertion pumps influences on drug cellular mortality which might affect the result of cross sectional measurement methods like MTT and Annexin V. Figure 7 is another example of the limitation of these type of experiments in some instances in comparison with the clonogenic assay. Clonogenic assay, however, would surprisingly fail to present a meaningful graph of cytotoxicity after exposure to some compounds.

There are many different mechanisms which might cause these differences in the result of the viability measurement using different methodologies. Cellular target of the test compound and the cellular repair system are two of the most possible explanation. Rosenberg confusion about the effects of electric field on the cells resulted in cisplatin identification and later use as a very important and most used anticancer drug in many different kinds of malignancies including the breast cancer (Rosenberg et al., 1969). Cells in Rosenberg set up did not die, rather changed shape and remained alive for a long time (Rosenberg, 1985, 1977). Cisplatin, like many other anti-mitotic agents, does not kill cells right after exposure. Its principle mechanism of action is on the DNA and thus while stopping DNA synthesis and cell proliferation, won't affect the mitochondrial action and cell membrane integrity. That is why, while the thymidine assay and cell cycle progression based techniques like the flowcytometery, as well as proliferation based measurements like the clonogenic assay present good results, cell membrane integrity and mitochondrial enzyme function based assays have a significant lag time before the presenting of measurable alterations. A successful cellular repair event during this lag time may change the final conclusion dramatically. One needs to be aware of these possibilities in interpretation of cytotoxicity test results. Figure 11 represents the measurement of cisplatin cytotoxicity effect on MDCK cell line using MTT assay. As is shown in this figure, a 48 hours exposure time difference is needed to acquire a reasonable survival curve using this method.

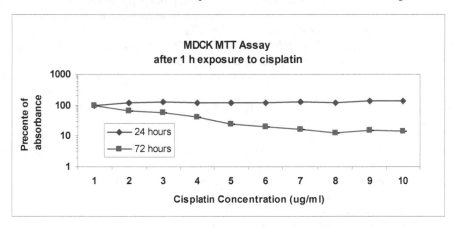

Fig. 11. The lag time required to get a good MTT result on the cytotoxicity of cisplatin on MDCK cell.

A discrepancy analysis to measure the cytotoxicity of many of novel anticancer drugs developed in our center under the same condition on the same cell line using two different methods of clonogenic assay and the neutral red assay, did not show agreement with a clear horizontal line and 95% confidence interval of about 1. It would further prove the importance of the selection and application of a suitable survival measurement system in the analysis of various anticancer candidates.

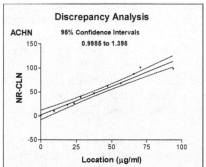
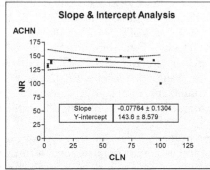

Fig. 12. A comparison of clonogenic versus neutral red assay for the measurement of cell survival after exposure to various novel anticancer drugs, using a discrepancy analysis method.

A good cellular practice on anticancer drugs requires the best selections of cell line and model system, the best matched measurement methodology, and the most optimized lag time to look at the result for acquiring the most precise and accurate conclusion.

6. References

Abou-Issa, HM.; Alshafie, GA.; Seibert, K.; Koki, AT.; Masferrer, JL. & Harris, RE. (2001). Dose-response effects of the COX-2 inhibitor, celecoxib, on the chemoprevention of mammary carcinogenesis. *Anticancer Res.* Vol.21, No.5, pp. 3425-3432

Arun, B.; Zhang, H, & Mirza, NQ. (2001). Growth inhibition of breast cancer cells by celecoxib. *Breast cancer Res treat.* Vol.69, p. 234

Arun, B. & Goss, P. (2004). The role of COX-2 inhibition in breast cancer treatment and prevention. *Semin Oncol.* Vol.31, Suppl. 7, pp. 22-29

Assaraf, YG. (2007). Molecular basis of antifolate resistance. *Cancer Metastasis Rev.* Vol.26, No.1, pp. 153-181.

Bardin, A.; Boulle, N.; Lazennec, G.; Vignon, F. & Pujol, P. (2004). Loss of ERbeta expression as a common step in estrogen-dependent tumor progression. *Endocr Relat Cancer,* Vol.11, No.3, pp. 537-551

Barnhart, K.; Coutifaris, C. & Esposito, M. (2001). The pharmacology of methotrexate. *Expert Opin Pharmacother.* Vol.2, No.3, pp. 409-417

Brandes, LJ. & Hermonat, MW. (1983). Receptor status and subsequent sensitivity of subclones of MCF-7 human breast cancer cells surviving exposure to diethylstilbestrol. *Cancer Res.* Vol.43, No.6, pp. 2831-2835

Ciocca, DR. & Roig, LM. (1995). Estrogen receptors in human nontarget tissues: biological and clinical implications. *Endocr Rev.* Vol.16, No.1, pp. 35-62

Clemons, M. & Goss, P. (2001). Estrogen and the risk of breast cancer. *N Engl J Med. Vol.*344, No.4, pp. 276-285

Cody, V.; Luft, JR.; Pangborn. W. & Gangjee, A. (2003). Analysis of three crystal structure determinations of a 5-methyl-6-N-methylanilino pyridopyrimidine antifolate complex with human dihydrofolate reductase. *Acta Crystallogr D Biol Crystallogr.* Vol.59, No.9, pp. 1603-1609

DuMond, JWJ.; Singh, KP. & Roy, D. (2001). Regulation of the growth of mouse Leydig cells by the inactive stereoisomer, 17alphaestradiol: Lack of correlation between the elevated expression of ERalpha and difference in sensitivity to estradiol isomers. *Oncol Rep,* Vol.8, No.4, pp. 899-902

Fox, EM.; Davis, RJ. & Shupnik, MA. (2008). ERbeta in breast cancer--onlooker, passive player, or active protector? Steroids. Vol.73, No.11, pp. 1039-1051

Gangjee, A.; Yang J. & Queener SF. (2006). Novel non-classical C9-methyl-5-substituted-2,4-diaminopyrrolo[2,3-d]pyrimidines as potential inhibitors of dihydrofolate reductase and as anti-opportunistic agents. *Bioorg Med Chem.* Vol.14, No.24, pp. 8341-8351

Graffner-Nordberg, M.; Kolmodin, K.; Aqvist, J.; Queener, SF. & Hallberg, A. (2004). Design, synthesis, and computational affinity prediction of ester soft drugs as inhibitors of dihydrofolate reductase from Pneumocystis carinii. *Eur J Pharm Sci.* Vol.22, No.1, pp. 43-54

Gustafsson, JA. (2003). What pharmacologists can learn from recent advances in estrogen signalling. *Trends Pharmacol Sci.* Vol.24, No.9, pp. 479-485

Haber, M.; Madafiglio, J. & Norris, MD. (1993). Methotrexate cytotoxicity determination using the MTT assay following enzymatic depletion of thymidine and hypoxanthine . *J Cancer Res Clin Oncol*. Vol.119, No.6, pp. 315-317

Hammers, HJ.; Saballus, M.; Sheikzadeh, S. & Schlenke, P. (2002). Introduction of a novel proliferation assay for pharmacological studies allowing the combination of BrdU detection and phenotyping. *J Immunol Methods*. Vol.264, No.1-2, pp. 89-93

Jensen, EV.; Cheng, G.; Palmieri, C.; Saji, S.; Mäkelä, S.; Van Noorden, S.; Wahlström, T.; Warner, M.; Coombes, RC. & Gustafsson, JA. (2001). Estrogen receptors and proliferation markers in primary and recurrent breast cancer. *Proc Natl Acad Sci USA*. Vol.98, No.26, pp. 15197–15202

Jordan, VC. (1988). The development of tamoxifen for breast cancer therapy: a tribute to the late Arthur L. Walpole. *Breast Cancer Res Treat*. Vol.11, No.3, pp. 197–209

Ko, Y.; Totzke, G.; Graack, GH.; Heidgen, FJ.; Meyer zu Brickwedde, MK.; Düsing, R.; Vetter, H. & Sachinidis A. (1993). Action of dihydropyridine calcium antagonists on early growth response gene expression and cell growth in vascular smooth muscle cells. *J Hypertens*. Vol.11, No.11, pp. 1171-1178

Kolodgie, FD.; Petrov, A.; Virmani, R.; Narula, N.; Verjans, JW.; Weber, DK.; Hartung, D.; Steinmetz, N.; Vanderheyden, JL.; Vannan, MA.; Gold, HK.; Reutelingsperger, CP.; Hofstra, L. & Narula, J. (2003). Targeting of apoptotic macrophages and experimental atheroma with radiolabeled annexin V: a technique with potential for noninvasive imaging of vulnerable plaque. *Circulation*. Vol.108, No.25, pp. 3134-3139.

Lukyanova, NY.; Rusetskya NV.; Tregubova, NA. & Chekhun, VF. (2009). Molecular profile and cell cycle in MCF-7 cells resistant to cisplatin and doxorubicin. *Exp Oncol*. Vol.31, No.2, pp.87-91

Maghni, K.; Nicolescu, OM. & Martin, JG. (1999). Suitability of cell metabolic colorimetric assays for assessment of CD4+ T cell proliferation: comparison to 5-bromo-2-deoxyuridine (BrdU) ELISA. *J Immunol Methods*. Vol.223, No.2, pp. 185-194

Marshall, NJ.; Goodwin, CJ. & Holt, SJ. (1995). A critical assessment of the use of microculture tetrazolium assays to measure cell growth and function. *Growth Regul*. Vol.5, No.2, pp. 69–84

Matthews, J. & Gustafsson, JA. (2003). Estrogen signaling: a subtle balance between ER α and ER β. *Mol Interv*.Vol.3, No.5, pp. 281–292

McGuire, JJ. (2003). Anticancer antifolates: current status and future directions. *Curr Pharm Des*. Vol.9, No.31, pp. 2593-2613

Meegan, MJ. & Lloyd, DG. (2003). Advances in the science of estrogen receptor modulation. *Curr Med Chem*. Vol.10, No.3, pp. 181-210

Nelson, HD.; Fu, R.; Griffin, JC.; Nygren, P.; Smith, ME. & Humphrey, L. (2009). Systematic review: comparative effectiveness of medications to reduce risk for primary breast cancer. *Ann Intern Med*.Vol.151, No.10, pp. 703–715

Niknafs, B. & Shirazi, F.H. (2002). Human Ovarian Carcinoma OV2008 Cell Cycle Analysis After Exposure to Cisplatin. *J. Gilan Medical University*, Vol.42, pp. 7-13.

Novelli, F.; Milella, M.; Melucci, E.; Di Benedetto, A.; Sperduti, I.; Perrone-Donnorso, R.; Perracchio, L.; Venturo, I.; Nisticò, C.; Fabi, A.; Buglioni, S.; Natali. PG. & Mottolese, M. (2008). A divergent role for estrogen receptor-beta in node-positive and node-negative breast cancer classified according to molecular subtypes: an observational prospective study. *Breast Cancer Res* Vol.10, No.5, R74

Penning, TD.; Talley, JJ.; Bertenshaw, SR.; Carter, JS.; Collins, PW.; Docter, S.; Graneto, MJ.; Lee, LF.; Malecha, JW.; Miyashiro, JM.; Rogers, RS.; Rogier, DJ.; Yu, SS.; Anderson, GD.; Burton, EG.; Cogburn, JN.; Gregory, SA.; Koboldt, CM.; Perkins, WE.; Seibert, K.; Veenhuizen, AW.; Zhang, YY. & Isakson, PC. (1997). Synthesis and biological evaluation of the 1,5-diarylpyrazole class of cyclooxygenase-2 inhibitors: identification of 4-[5-(4-methylphenyl)-3-(trifluoromethyl)-1H-pyrazol-1-yl]benze nesulfonamide (SC-58635, celecoxib). *J Med Chem.* Vol.40, No.9, pp. 1347-1365

Prasit, P.; Wang, Z.; Brideau, C.; Chan, CC.; Charleson, S.; Cromlish, W.; Ethier, D.; Evans, JF.; Ford-Hutchinson, AW.; Gauthier, JY.; Gordon, R.; Guay, J.; Gresser, M.; Kargman, S.; Kennedy, B.; Leblanc, Y.; Léger, S.; Mancini. J.; O'Neill, GP.; Ouellet, M.; Percival, MD.; Perrier, H.; Riendeau, D.; Rodger, I. & Zamboni, R. (1999). The discovery of rofecoxib, [MK 966, Vioxx, 4-(4'-methylsulfonylphenyl)-3-phenyl-2(5H)-furanone], an orally active cyclooxygenase-2-inhibitor. Bioorg Med Chem Lett. Vol.9, No,13, pp. 1773-1778.

Raaphorst, G.P.; Mao, J.; Yang, H.; Goel, R.; Niknafs, B.; Shirazi, F.H.; Yazdi, M.H. & Ng, C.E. (1998). Evaluation of apoptosis in four human tumour cell lines with differing sensitivities to cisplatin. *AntiCancer Research.* Vol.18, No.4C, pp. 2945-2951.

Riendeau, D.; Percival, MD.; Brideau, C.; Charleson, S.; Dubé, D.; Ethier, D.; Falgueyret, JP.; Friesen, RW.; Gordon, R.; Greig, G.; Guay, J.; Mancini, J.; Ouellet, M.; Wong, E.; Xu, L.; Boyce, S.; Visco, D.; Girard, Y.; Prasit, P.; Zamboni, R.; Rodger, IW.; Gresser, M.; Ford-Hutchinson, AW.; Young, RN.; Chan, CC. (2001). Etoricoxib (MK-0663): preclinical profile and comparison with other agents that selectively inhibit cyclooxygenase-2. . *J Pharmacol Exp Ther.* Vol.296, No.2, pp. 558-566

Rosenberg, B. (1977). Noble metal complexes in cancer chemotherapy. *Adv Exp Med Biol.* Vol.91, pp. 129-150

Rosenberg, B. (1985). Fundamental studies with cisplatin. *Cancer,* Vol.55, No.10, pp. 2303-2316

Rosenberg, B.; VanCamp, L.; Trosko, JE.; & Mansour, VH. (1969). Platinum compounds: a new class of potent antitumour agents. *Nature,* Vol.222, No.5191, pp. 385-386

Roy, D. & Cai, Q. (2002). Estrogen, immunoactivation, gene damage, and development of breast, endometrial, ovarian, prostate, and testicular cancers. *Recent Res Devel Steroid Biochem Mol Biol.* Vol.3, pp. 1-32

Russo, J.; Bradley, R.H.; McGrath, C. & Russo, I.H. (1977). Scanning and transmission electron microscopy study of a human breast carcinoma cell line (MCF-7) cultured in collagen-coated cellulose sponge. *Cancer Res.* Vol.37, pp. 2004-2014

Scudiero, DA.; Shoemaker, RH.; Paull, KD.; Monks, A.; Tierney, S.; Nofziger, TH.; Currens, MJ.; Seniff, D. & Boyd, MR. (1988). Evaluation of a soluble tetrazolium/formazan assay for cell growth and drug sensitivity in culture using human and other tumor cell lines. *Cancer Res.* Vol.48, No.17, pp. 4827–4833

Shirazi, F.H. & Eftekhari, M. (2004). Cellular toxicity of cisplatin in Chiness hamster ovarian (CHO) cell line. *Pajohandeh.* Vol.9, No.40, pp. 191-197

Shirazi, F.H.; Ahmadi, N. & Kamalinejad, M. (2004). Evaluation of northern Iran Mentha pulegium on cancer cells. *Journal of Daru,* Vol. 12, No. 3

Shirazi, F.H.; Molepo, M.; Stewart, D.J. & Goel, R. (1996). Cisplatin and its metabolites cytotoxicity, accumulation and efflux in human ovarian carcinoma cells. *Toxicology and Applied Pharmacology*. Vol.140, pp. 211-218

Shirazi, F.H.; Shokrzadeh, M. & Hossinzadeh, L. (2005) Cellular cytotoxicity of arsenic and its association with cellular glutathione. *Chemistry: An Indian Journal*, Vol.1, No.10, pp. 689-692.

Shirazi, F.H.; Shokrzadeh, M.; Abdollahi, M.; Rahimi, FB.; & Hossinzadeh, L. (2005). Relationship of cellular glutathione concentration with the cytotoxicity of acetaminophen in different cell lines. *Int. J. Biol. Biotech.*, Vol.2, No.2, pp. 397-402.

Shirazi, F.H.; Yazdanpanah, H.; Khoshjoo, F. & Hossinzadeh, L. (2006). Pistachio extracts effects on the aflatoxin B1 cytotoxicity in HepG2 cells. *Int. J. Pharmacology*, Vol.2, No.2, pp. 233-239.

Shokrzadeh, M.; Shirazi, F.H.; Abdollahi, M.; Abadi, A.G. & Asgarirad, H. (2006). Relationship of glutathione concentrations with cytotoxicity of cisplatin in different cell lines after confront vitamin C and E. *Pakistan Journal of Biological Sciences*, Vol.9, No.15, pp. 2734-2742

Singh, B.; Cook, KR.; Vincent, L.; Hall, CS.; Berry, JA.; Multani, AS. & Lucci, A. (2008). Cyclooxygenase-2 induces genomic instability, BCL2 expression, doxorubicin resistance, and altered cancer-initiating cell phenotype in MCF7 breast cancer cells. *J Surg Res*. Vol.147, No.2, pp. 240-246

Skliris, GP.; Parkes, AT.; Limer, JL.; Burdall, SE.; Carder, PJ. & Speirs, V. (2002). Evaluation of seven oestrogen receptor beta antibodies for immunohistochemistry, western blotting, and flow cytometry in human breast tissue. *J Pathol*. Vol.197, No.2, pp. 155–162.

Takemura, Y.; Kobayashi, H. & Miyachi, H. (1997). Cellular and molecular mechanisms of resistance to antifolate drugs: new analogues and approaches to overcome the resistance. *Int J Hematol*. Vol.66, No.4, pp. 459-477

Talley, JJ.; Brown, DL.; Carter, JS.; Graneto, MJ.; Koboldt, CM.; Masferrer, JL.; Perkins, WE.; Rogers, RS.; Shaffer, AF.; Zhang, YY.; Zweifel, BS. & Seibert, K. (2000). 4-[5-Methyl-3-phenylisoxazol-4-yl]- benzenesulfonamide, valdecoxib: a potent and selective inhibitor of COX-2. *J Med Chem*. Vol.43, No.5, pp. 775-777

Tamaddon, A.M.; Shirazi, F.H. & Moghimi, H.R. (2007). Preparation of oligodeoxynucleotide encapsulated cationic liposomes and release study with models of cellular membranes. *Journal of Daru*, Vol.15, No.2, pp. 61-69

Välimaa, H.; Savolainen, S.; Soukka, T.; Silvoniemi, P.; Mäkelä, S.; Kujari, H.; Gustafsson, JA. & Laine, M. (2004). Estrogen receptor-β is the predominant estrogen receptor subtype in human oral epithelium and salivary glands. *J Endocrinol*. Vol.180, No.1, pp. 55–62.

Van Heerde, WL.; Robert-Offerman, S.; Dumont, E.; Hofstra, L.; Doevendans, PA.; Smits, JF.; Daemen, MJ. & Reutelingsperger, CP. (2000). Markers of apoptosis in cardiovascular tissues: focus on Annexin V. *Cardiovasc Res*. Vol.45, No.3, pp. 549-559.

Vic, P.; Vignon, F.; Derocq, D. & Rochefort H. (1982). Effect of Estradiol on the Ultrastructure of the MCF7 Human Breast Cancer Cells in Culture. *Cancer Res*. Vol.42, No.2, pp. 667-673

Welshons, WV.; Thayer, KA.; Judy, BM.; Taylor, JA.; Curran, EM. & Vom Saal, FS. (2003). Large effects from small exposures. I. Mechanisms for endocrine-disrupting chemicals with estrogenic activity. *Environ Health Perspect.* Vol.111, No.8, pp. 994-1006.

Yokochi, T. & Gilbert. DM. (2007). Replication labeling with halogenated thymidine analogs. *Curr Protoc Cell Biol.*, Chapter.22, Unit.22.10

Zarghi, A.; Zebardast, T.; Hakimion, F.; Shirazi, F.H.; Rao, P.N. & Knaus, E.E. (2006). Synthesis and biological evaluation of 1,3-diphenylprop-2-en-1-ones possessing a methanesulfonamido or an azido pharmacophore as cyclooxygenase-1/-2 inhibitors. *Bioorg Med Chem.* Vol.14, No.20, pp. 7044-7050

Zhu, Y.; Sullivan, LL.; Nair, SS.; Williams, CC.; Pandey, A.; Marrero, L.; Vadlamudi, RK. & Jones, FE. (2006). Coregulation of estrogen receptor by estrogen-inducible ERBB4/HER4 establishes a growth promoting autocrine signal in breast cancer. *Cancer Res.* Vol.66, No.16, pp. 7991-7998

Part 2

Breast Cancer and Microenvironment

7

Novel Insights Into the Role of Inflammation in Promoting Breast Cancer Development

J. Valdivia-Silva[3,], J. Franco-Barraza[4],
E. Cukierman[4] and E.A. García-Zepeda[1,2]
[1]CBRL,
[2]Departamento de Inmunología, Instituto de Investigaciones Biomédicas, Universidad Nacional Autónoma de México,
[3]Life Science & Astrobiology Division, NASA Ames Research Center, Moffett Field, CA,
[4]Cancer Biology Program, Fox Chase Cancer Center, Philadelphia, PA,
[1,2]México
[3,4]USA

1. Introduction

In the past decades the major focus of cancer research has been the transformed tumor cells itself, while the role of cellular microenvironment in tumorigenesis has not been widely explored. Several studies have demonstrated the ability of stroma to regulate the growth and differentiation state of breast cancer cells, and the invasive behaviour, and polarity of normal mammary epithelial and breast carcinomas are influenced by tumor microenvironment, immune and stromal cells (Bissell, et al., 2002, Radisky & Radisky, 2007, Tlsty, 2001, Tlsty & Hein, 2001). In addition, genetic abnormalities, such as loss of heterozygosity, occur not only in cancer cells, but in stromal cells as well (Kurose, et al., 2002, Kurose, et al., 2001, Moinfar, et al., 2000).

It is believed that a better understanding of the tumor microenvironment could help render more accurate diagnostics or assist in predicting tumor aggressiveness (i.e., bad prognosis) thus facilitating the design of personalized treatments.

By the end of the nineteenth century, the English surgeon S. Paget suggested the idea that, in order for breast cancer to develop, a specific "seeding" process must occur and, for this primary onset to metastasize to a specific distant organ, particular stromal features would be required postulating his "seed and soil" hypothesis (Paget, 1889). His work greatly contributed to somewhat earlier observations by T. Langhans who first used the word stroma to describe the connective tissue, vessels and other components between tumors (Langhans, 1879) and to the theory postulated by R. Virchow suggesting a possible origin of cancer at sites of chronic inflammation (Balkwill& Mantovani, 2001). A century later, researchers such as B. Mintz and K. Illmensee in general, as well as M. Bisell, in breast cancer in particular, pointed to the tumor milieu as an essential component of neoplasias, not only for cancer evolution but also for cancer instigation (Mintz & Illmensee, 1975; Lochter & Bissell, 1995). Together these and additional findings had painted a broad picture of the complexity of tumor microenvironment, where diverse stromal cells interact with each other and with the cancer cells playing important roles in tumorigenesis (Soto & Sonnenschein, 2004; Egeblad et al., 2010).

It is clear now that metastatic tumors represent the greatest threat to cancer patient mortality. Indeed, when breast cancer is diagnosed early and metastases are not present, 5-year survival is >88%; however, if metastases are also present, long-term survival is significantly diminished (~10%) (Jemal, et al., 2011). Thereby, the major cause of mortality of breast cancer and different types of cancer is due to metastasis to distant organs, such as lung, bone, liver and brain (Lu & Kang, 2007). A notable feature of this process is the variation in metastatic organ tropism displayed by different types of cancer (Chambers, et al., 2002, Fidler, 2002). A classic view has proposed that purely mechanical factors regulate the fate of blood-borne metastasis tumor cells (MacDonald, et al., 2002); however, this does not fully explain the non-random distribution and distinct pattern of metastasis in each tumor type (Lu & Kang, 2007). However, tumor microenvironment has also shown an important role in the regulation of this process (Valdivia-Silva, et al., 2009). A number of different molecules present in the microenvironment have been associated to the metastasis of breast cancer, among them, chemokines, which have been associated with regulation of cell migration and invasion of tumor cells into specific organs (Muller, et al., 2001, Zlotnik, 2006). Chemokines are a superfamily of chemotactic cytokines characterized by their ability to induce directed migration of leukocytes, during haematopoiesis, lymphoid organ development, and in disease (Sallusto, et al., 2000); their expression may be inducible, primarily by pro-inflammatory cytokines such as TNF-a and IL-1-b (Ben-Baruch, 2003). Chemokine receptor expression in many cancer cells have shown to be a non-random process (Shields, et al., 2007, Zlotnik, 2006) and to have a role in organ-specific metastasis: for example, CXCR4 expression and metastasis to lung, bone and lymph nodes (Muller, et al., 2001), CCR7 to lymph nodes (Shields, et al., 2007), CX3CR1 to brain (Mourad, et al., 2005), CCR9 to liver and small bowel (Amersi, et al., 2008, Letsch, et al., 2004), and CCR5 and CXCR2 to lung, liver, vessel endothelial cells and bone (Gross & Meier, 2009, Keeley, et al., 2010, Miller, et al., 1998).

Here, we will discuss the ability of the chemokines to affect tumor cell–microenvironment interactions, increasing the invasive behaviour and metastasis, confirming the importance of the host inflammatory response that may differ between tumor types, disease stages, and/or many other host factors; and the role of stromal contribution of the inflammatory microenvironment to cancer progression and metastasis.

2. Inflammatory mediators as regulator of breast cancer development and metastasis

The link between inflammation and cancer has been observed over 150 years ago when Rudolf Virchow noted that cancers tend to occur at sites of chronic inflammation. Indeed, epidemiological studies indicate that inflammatory and infectious diseases are often associated with an increased risk of cancer (Coussens & Werb, 2002). The microenvironment of tumors mimics that of tissues during the height of an inflammatory response to injury (Joyce & Pollard, 2009). However, unlike the organized morphology of normal tissue, and the ultimate resolution of the inflammation that occurs during healing, tumors exist in a state of chronic inflammation characterized by the presence of cancer cells, immune cells, aberrant vascular cells, and the persistence of inflammatory mediators, such as cytokines and chemokines.

The presence and significance of leukocyte infiltrates in developing neoplasms is now undisputed (Allen, et al., 2007, Moser & Loetscher, 2001, Moser & Willimann, 2004). It has been demonstrated that leukocyte infiltration in developing tumors is one of the host's main immune mechanisms to eradicate malignant cells. However, while some leukocytes certainly have this potential, i.e., cytotoxic T lymphocytes (CTLs) and natural killer (NK) cells (Luster, 1998), other leukocyte cell types, most notably innate immune cells, i.e., mast cells (MCs), immature myeloid cells, granulocytes, and macrophages, instead potentiate tumor progression (Baggiolini, et al., 1997, Chen, et al., 2006, Joyce & Pollard, 2009), and enhance neoplastic cell survival. Upon entry into the neoplastic microenvironment, infiltrating leukocytes become alternatively activated and manifest a pro-tumor phenotype as defined by activation of cellular programs involved in immune tolerance and tissue remodelling (Mishra, et al., 2011, Strieter, et al., 2006). During premalignant progression, a consequence of alternative activation of leukocytes is promotion and elaboration of a microenvironment rich in extracellular matrix (ECM) remodelling proteases, and increased presence of pro-survival, pro-growth and pro-angiogenic factors that further enhance proliferative and invasive capacities of neoplastic cells (Li, et al., 2007, Orimo, et al., 2005). Such pro-tumor inflammatory microenvironments promote not only malignant conversion and development of solid tumors, but also dissemination of neoplastic cells into blood vasculature by driving invasive capacity of malignant cells, expansion of angiogenic vasculature, and neoplastic cell entry into blood vessels (and lymphatics) (Keeley, et al., 2010).

Breast carcinomas are highly infiltrated by different types of host leukocytes, including primarily T cells, and monocytes that differentiate into tumor-associated macrophages (TAM) at the tumor site (Ben-Baruch, 2003, Crowther, et al., 2001). The presence of the cellular infiltrate in breast tumors was initially regarded as evidence for the potential activity of immune mechanisms against the growing neoplasm. As explained above, several studies suggest that T-cell antitumor responses are impaired in advanced stages of breast carcinoma, and there is no definite conclusion regarding the efficacy of T-cell-dependent immune mechanisms, or regarding the correlation between the type of T-cell infiltration and tumor progression in most subtypes of breast carcinoma (Hsiao, et al., 2010). The only exception is the relatively infrequent type of medullary carcinoma, in which favourable prognosis was correlated with intensive lymphoid infiltration (Hadden, 1999). In contrast to T lymphocytes, large evidence suggests that high levels of TAM are correlated with poor prognosis in breast carcinoma. Many studies have shown a positive relationship between high levels of TAM and lymph node metastases, and suggested that the density of TAM is associated with clinical aggressiveness (Crowther, et al., 2001, O'Sullivan & Lewis, 1994). Again, the potential contribution of TAM to tumor elimination, in view of several potential antimalignant activities that may be exerted by these cells, such as antigen presentation, cytotoxicity, or/and phagocytosis, was contradictory with the promalignant activities of TAM in breast carcinoma. These promalignant activities of TAM are the result of their ability to express numerous tumor-promoting mediators, such as growth factors for breast tumor cells, angiogenic molecules, ECM degrading enzymes, inflammatory cytokines, and chemokines (Balkwill & Mantovani, 2001, Colotta, et al., 2009). In addition, TAM might contribute to tumor progression by the release of reactive oxygen intermediates, which may induce mutagenic changes that could result in increased DNA damage and generation of new subtypes of cancer cells within the tumor (Colotta, et al., 2009). A major TAM-derived inflammatory cytokine shown to be highly expressed in breast carcinomas is tumor necrosis factor alpha (TNF-a) (Leek, et al., 1998), which is a multifactorial cytokine. Tumor necrosis factor alpha was first isolated as an anti-cancer cytokines more than two decades ago (Aggarwal, 2003). However, these effects may depend on multiple factors, such as estrogen therapy and the expression of members of the epidermal growth factor receptor family. The fact that TNF-a activities vary under different physiological conditions and in a cell-type-dependent manner contributes to a sense of ambiguity regarding its antitumor effects (Kanoh, et al., 2001, Offersen, et al., 2002). A number of reports indicate that TNF-a induces cellular transformation, proliferation, and tumor promotion (Balkwill & Mantovani, 2001, Li, et al., 2007). A interesting study reported that human TNF-a is more effective than the chemical tumor promoters okadaic acid and 12-O-tetradecanoylphorbol-13-acetato in inducing cancer (Komori, et al., 1993).

The number of cells expressing TNF-a in inflammatory breast carcinoma has been correlated with increasing tumor grade and node involvement (Ben-Baruch, 2003, Leek, et al., 1998). Furthermore, patients with more progressed tumor phenotypes were shown to have significantly higher TNF-a and IL-2 serum concentration (Tesarová, et al., 2000). The tumor-promoting functions of TNF-a may be mediated by its ability to induce pro-angiogenic functions, to promote the expression of matrix metalloproteinases (MMP) and endothelial adhesion molecules, and to cause DNA damage via reactive oxygen, the overall effect of which is promotion of tumor-related processes (Garg & Aggarwal, 2002).

In addition, several inflammatory interleukins have been linked with carcinogenesis and tumor progression. Among these, IL-6 and IL-1 have been widely studied in breast carcinoma. In different types of cancer, IL-1 promotes growth and confers chemoresistance (Arlt, et al., 2002, Woodworth, et al., 1995). Furthermore, IL-1 secretion into the tumor milieu also induces several angiogenic factors from tumor and stromal cells that promotes tumor growth through hyperneovascularization (Zhou, et al., 2011). IL-6 may act as a paracrine growth factor for multiple myeloma, non-Hodgkin's lymphoma, bladder cancer, colorectal cancer, and renal carcinoma (Angelo, et al., 2002, Landi, et al., 2003, Okamoto, et al., 1995, Voorzanger, et al., 1996). However, contradictory studies suggested that elevated levels of IL-6 might contribute to breast cancer progression (Karczewska, et al., 2000, Kurebayashi, 2000). Initial analyses regarding IL-1b indicated that its levels were significantly higher in invasive carcinoma than in ductal carcinoma *in situ* or in benign lesions, implying that elevated levels of IL-1b are directly correlated with a more advanced disease (Jin, et al., 1997). Of interest is the fact that the two cytokines (IL-6 and IL-1b) and TNF-a are interrelated and may act in an additive manner, suggesting that these three cytokines form a network of related factors that may affect tumor cell progression in a cooperative manner.

Cyclooxygenase (COX)-2, an inducible enzyme with expression regulated by NF-kb, mediates tumorigenesis. COX-2, the inducible isoform of prostaglandin H synthase has been implicated in the growth and progression of a variety of human cancers, and its expression can be induced by various growth factors, cytokines, oncogenes, and other tumor factors. IL-1 has been reported to upregulate COX-2 expression in human colorectal cancer cells via multiple signalling pathways (Liu, et al., 2003). COX-2 is expressed at an intermediate or high level in epithelial cells of invasive breast cancers (Chang, et al., 2005, Half, et al., 2002). Expression of COX-2 in breast cancer correlates with poor prognosis, and COX-2 enzyme inhibitors reduce breast cancer incidence in humans. COX-2 overexpression has also been found in the mammary gland of transgenic mice induced mammary cancer (Kundu & Fulton, 2002).

Hypoxia is also an important cellular stressor that triggers a survival program by which cells attempt to adapt to the new environment. This primarily involves adaptation of metabolism and/or stimulation of oxygen delivery. These cell-rescuing mechanisms can be conducted rapidly by a transcription factor that reacts to hypoxic conditions, the hypoxia-inducible factor-1 (HIF-1a) (Semenza & Wang, 1992). HIF-1a stimulates processes such as angiogenesis, glycolysis, and erythropoiesis (Jiang, et al., 1996) by activating genes that are responsible for these processes. Cancer cells are able to survive and proliferate in extreme microenvironmental conditions and show changes in oncogenes and tumor suppressor genes. Hypoxia and HIF-1a have been implicated in carcinogenesis and in clinical behaviour of tumors. Upregulation of HIF-1a was noted during breast carcinogenesis (Bos, et al., 2001) especially in the poorly differentiated pathway. Hypoxia is related to poor response to therapy in various cancer types. In invasive breast cancer, high HIF-1a concentrations were associated with poor survival in lymph node-negative patients (Bos, et al., 2003). As prognosis in breast cancer is closely related to proliferation rate (van Diest & Baak, 1991) and poorly differentiated tumors usually exhibit high proliferation and HIF-1a overexpression, the prognostic value of HIF-1a might well be explained by a close association between HIF-1a and proliferation. Additionally, HIF-1a has shown to be a master regulator for surviving hypoxia interacting with cell cycle-related proteins. High concentrations of HIF-1a are associated with overexpression of p53 and markers of proliferation during the late SG2 phase of the cell cycle (Bos, et al., 2004).

3. Role of chemokines and their receptors in breast cancer progression and metastasis

While most evidence presented above suggests that proinflammatory cytokines and enzymes play an important role in mediating tumorigenesis, and tumor progression, the molecular mechanisms of metastasis and its relationship with the organotropism of cancer cell remain unclear. However, recent studies focused on the chemokines and their receptors, and the different interactions with inflammatory cytokines in the tumor microenvironment have provided additional information that might better explain the non-random patterns of organotropism during metastasis, including atypical metastasis to rare organs (Franco-Barraza, et al., 2010, Valdivia-Silva, et al., 2009).

Chemokine activities in different malignancy including breast cancer are mediated primarily by their ability to induce chemotaxis of leukocytes, endothelial cells, and/or the tumor cells. Chemokines induce migration of leukocyte subpopulations to tumor sites that may promote antitumor activities (such as Th1 cells or natural killer cells), while other chemokines are responsible for large quantities of deleterious tumor-associated macrophages (TAM) at tumor sites (Allavena, et al., 2008, Ben-Baruch, 2008, Soria & Ben-Baruch, 2008) as discussed above. Moreover, specific chemokines upregulate endothelial cell migration and proliferation, and promoting angiogenesis, whereas other chemokines have powerful angiostatic properties (Strieter, et al., 2006, Struyf, et al., 2011). Another very important activity of chemokines is induction of tumor cell invasion and migration, thereby playing key roles in dictating site-directed metastasis formation (Ben-Baruch, 2008, Zlotnik, 2006). Chemokines and their receptors can execute such multifaceted roles in malignancy because cells of the tumor microenvironment, and in many cases also by the tumor cells themselves express them. As such, they can affect through autocrine pathways the ability of the cancer cells to express tumor-promoting functions, and can also act in paracrine manners on host cells, thereby influencing their roles in malignancy.

Breast cancer metastasis is the result of several sequential steps and represents a highly organized, non-random and organ selective process dependent on intricate stroma-stroma interactions at the target organ (Ben-Baruch, 2006, Lu & Kang, 2007), causing high mortality by invasion of vital organs, such as bone, lung, brain and liver. Important evidence suggests that chemokines have an important role in regulating trafficking and metastasis (Bagley, et al., 2010). Indeed, breast cancer cells express chemokine receptors in a non-random manner, and these observations pointed to several chemokine/ receptor pairs that control cell–cell migration (Zlotnik, 2008). Association of chemokine receptors with various cancers including breast carcinoma has been widely documented (Ali & Lazennec, 2007, Karnoub & Weinberg, 2006, Koizumi, et al., 2007, Ruffini, et al., 2007). Accumulative evidence, in particular from clinical retrospective studies, presents a compelling picture indicating that the experimental evidence derived from *in vitro* experiments and animal models pointing to a pivotal role of chemokine receptors in cancer metastasis. CXCR4 and CCR7 are the most widely expressed in many different cancers, and the expression of CXCL12 and CCL21, their specific ligands, respectively, are highest in lung, liver bone marrow for the first one and lymph nodes for both (Nevo, et al., 2004, Schimanski, et al., 2008). Additionally, the expression of CCR7 in patients with several types of cancer has an excellent correlation with the ability of the tumor to spread to the lymph nodes (Takanami, 2003, Wang, et al., 2005). Other chemokine receptors may participate in the regulation of metastasis of specific cancers and in tumor progression. CX3CR1 is involved in homing metastasis to brain for glioblastoma and breast cancer (Andre, et al., 2010, Lavergne, et al., 2003) and to bone and bone marrow endothelial cell for prostate cancer (Shulby, et al., 2004). CCR9/CCL25 axis was found in melanoma (Letsch, et al., 2004), ovarian cancer (Johnson-Holiday, et al., 2007), prostate cancer (Singh, et al., 2004), nasopharyngeal carcinoma (Ou, et al., 2006), acute lymphoblastic leukaemia (Annels, et al., 2004) and probably breast cancer (Johnson-Holiday, et al., 2011); most of the cases are related to metastatic lesions in the gastrointestinal tract included the liver. Additionally, elevated expression levels of CXCR2 and CCR5 and their ligands, CXCL8 and CCL5, respectively, in breast carcinoma and other neoplasias were significant associated with increased malignancy, advance disease, early relapse and poor prognosis (Ben-Baruch, 2006, Yaal-Hahoshen, et al., 2006). Moreover, it has been demonstrated that tumor cells can generate autocrine gradients of ligands of chemokine receptors (i.e., CCR7) that guide their migration in direction of a physiological level of interstitial flow towards functional lymphatics, even if lymphatic endothelial cells are absent; although the effect is greatly amplified when both flow and cells are present (Shields, et al., 2007). This data suggests that the chemokine–chemokine receptor interaction is of particular importance in the metastatic destination of many cancers.

However, a couple of questions are very important to make in this point: Is the chemokine receptor expression in cancer cells constant? Or might the tumor microenvironment or inflammation regulate the chemokine receptor expression in cancer cells? Interestingly, these questions, which are product of logic thinking on the tumor microenvironment, were not made until recently by our group (Valdivia-Silva, et al., 2009). Indeed, the chemokine receptor expression has not been thoroughly studied under inflammatory conditions.

Although there are reports demonstrating that tumor and leukocytes increase expression of chemokines and cytokines during disease progression, it is not clear what are the chemokine receptors involved in regulation of metastasis. Most of the previously reported studies had focused in analysing chemokine receptors expressed in different neoplasias without evaluating their phenotypic changes and functionality during the progress of the disease (Ben-Baruch, 2008). However, it has not been clearly demonstrated any type of regulation of the microenvironment in these changes. Finally, the chemokine receptors expressed under non-stimulated conditions by cancer cells were considered biomarkers to specific homing to organs, but it does not explained atypical metastasis of cancer to rare organs (Charalabopoulos, et al., 2004, Johnson, 2010, Kilgore, et al., 2007, Saisho, et al., 2005).

Within the tumor microenvironment, chemokines and their receptors play different roles in modulating several functions as described above, and through these processes, help to define the progression of the cancer. Stromal, and immune cells, including leukocytes differentiating into tumor-associated macrophages (TAM) at the tumor site, express numerous promoting factors, such as growth factors, angiogenic mediators, extracellular matrix-degrading enzymes, inflammatory cytokines, and more chemokines (Polyak & Kalluri, 2010). Interestingly, pro-inflammatory cytokines like IL-1, IL-6, IFN-g and TNF-a, which are important modulators of chemokine receptors expression in different tissues, have demonstrated to regulate their expression in cancer cells in a non–random manner (Valdivia-Silva, et al., 2009). Similar to cytokines regulate for CXCR4 and CCR5 in astrocytes (Croitoru-Lamoury, et al., 2003), CXCR2 in human mesangial cells(Schwarz, et al., 2002), and CX3CR1 in smooth muscle cells (Chandrasekar, et al., 2003), synovium (Nanki, et al., 2002), and different epithelial cells (Fujimoto, et al., 2001, Matsumiya, et al., 2001); different doses and times of exposition allowed the expression of specific type of chemokine receptor in several breast cancer cell lines and the change of their phenotypes into more invasiveness ones (Franco-Barraza, et al., 2010).

We have analysed the human breast carcinoma MCF-7 cell line as a model of pre-invasive stage to demonstrate the regulation by an inflammatory microenvironment on chemokine receptor expression and functionality (Valdivia-Silva, et al., 2009). The comparison of the expression of CXCR4, CX3CR1, CXCR2, CCR9 and CCR5 at the transcriptional, protein, and functional levels under two different *in vitro* conditions (basal versus cytokine- stimulation) showed clearly the regulation of the specific cytokine over specific chemokine receptor, independently of the genetic background of MCF-7, which presents very low levels of these receptors under basal conditions. This was also observed in the highly metastatic MDA-MB-231, MDA-MB-361 and in the poorly metastatic T47D breast cancer cell lines; although the levels of expression observed after cytokine stimulation were different than those obtained in the MCF-7 cell line. A direct suggestion of these results, affirms that basal expression of a given chemokine receptor is not by itself a good marker of homing or aggressiveness and is subject to change by the microenvironment. Another important outcome in that work was the absence of correlation between the functionality of the receptor and their expression (gen or protein). For example, an increase in CXCR2 expression in MCF-7 cell line does not correlates with an increase in the migration index. In contrast, CX3CR, induced by TNF-a, had a small but significant increase at the protein level, which had an impact on their chemotactic activity. A considerable increase of chemokine receptors was found in non-migratory cancer cells indicating that that chemokine receptor expression does not necessarily result in migration response to a chemoattractant ligand. It also suggests that only a fraction of the cells have the potential to form metastases and capable to invade different organs. In fact, genetic analysis of the MDA-MB-231 breast cancer cell line subpopulations, obtained from *in vivo* experiments, identified a gene set whose expression pattern is associated to metastasis to bone but not adrenal medulla (Kirschmann, et al., 1999, Xu, et al., 2010). Interestingly this signature is retained through repeated passage of the metastatic cell population both in vitro and in vivo. Therefore, breast cancer cells with a defined tissue-specific metastatic ability pre-exist in the parental tumor cell population and may have a distinctive metastasis gene expression signature. Thus, these data suggested that inflammatory stimulation in the tumor microenvironment might affect cancer cells migration by different mechanisms. Importantly, not all cancer cell population, including cell lines, had the same behaviour under the same cytokine stimulation. Finally, other important finding in this study suggested that cancer cells require constant inflammatory stimuli by the microenvironment to trigger their invasive and metastatic activity, because of after a short time without stimuli (hours to days), the cells diminished their specific-stimuli chemokine receptor expression.

Altogether, these data allowed us to propose that exist sub-populations expressing different levels of chemokine receptor expression, which under a particular stimuli in the host microenvironment, change their expression levels and thus their aggressiveness. Then, atypical metastasis of breast cancer to others organs, which are relatively rare, could fall under this scheme. The biological inflammatory global response in the tumor microenvironment might be triggering the expression of different chemokine receptors and determining a new homing for these cancer cells. More broadly, these observations strongly support the overall model where chemokines determine the metastatic destinations of cancer cells (Fig 1.)

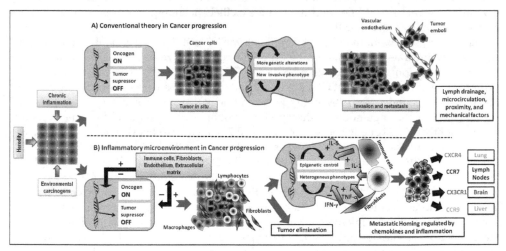

Fig. 1. Microenvironment and cancer progression.

Two theories have been proposed to explain this process, a conventional theory based on genetic alterations and a second view that involves participation of an inflammatory microenvironment. A) Initially, susceptible cells to different carcinogenic factors (e.g., genetic susceptibility obtained by inheritance) suffer specific DNA mutations that trigger tumorigenesis. The conventional theory is focused on the view that cancer progression is initially dependent on a sequence of genetic alterations and, finally, purely mechanical factors regulate the fate of blood-borne metastasis tumour cells (e.g. proximity, microcirculation, direction of lymph or circulation drainage, etc.). B) A second view, based on the participation of an inflammatory microenvironment, takes into account constant interactions between tumor cells and surrounding cells during the different stages of cancer development. Therefore, the final response is the result of positive and negative effects and not only dependent on internal genetic changes in cancer cells but on interactions and epigenetic control of multiple inflammatory into molecules released into the tumor microenvironment. Therefore, the final metastatic homing, which is mediated by expression of chemokines and chemokine receptors, will be dependent on the deregulation of the host immune response

4. Targeting chemokines for breast cancer metastasis

As a consequence of studies focusing almost exclusively on cancer cells, nearly all of the currently used cancer therapeutic agents target the cancer cells that, due to their inherent genomic instability, frequently acquire therapeutic resistance (Rajagopalan, et al., 2003). In part due to frequent therapeutic failures during the course of treatment of advanced stage tumors, increasing emphasis has been placed on targeting various stromal cells, particularly endothelial cells, via therapeutic interventions. Since these cells are thought to be normal and genetically stable, they are less likely to develop acquired resistance to cancer therapy. Thus, isolating, and characterizing each cell type (epithelial, myoephitelial, and various stromal cells) comprising non-malignant and cancerous breast tissue would not only help us to understand the role these cells play in breast tumorigenesis, but would likely give us new molecular targets for cancer intervention and treatment.

There is now an abundant literature documenting the associations of chemokine receptors with various types of cancer (Zlotnik, 2006) and their importance to mediate the establishment or development of metastatic foci. In fact, some anticancer drugs currently in use -like Herceptin- may involve the downregulation of chemokine receptors as part of their mechanism of action (Li, et al., 2004). This would provide the ultimate validation of the hypothesis, and would also point to future opportunities for therapeutic intervention as we discussed below. Current therapies such as surgery, radiotherapy and chemotherapy are primarily concerned with destruction of cancer. Targeting chemokines and chemokine receptors will allow limiting angiogenesis or metastasis and may enable such therapies to act as chemotherapeutic agents alone or in synergism with conventional agents. The up-regulation of certain chemokine molecules in tumor as compared with normal cells offers a potential avenue — where cancer cells and their metastases can be specifically targeted. This selective destruction of cells is also pre-requisite of non-toxic treatment regimens.

Manipulation of the tumor microenvironment by treatment with chemokines can be used to recruit either immature dendritic cells for the initiation of anti-tumor responses or effector cells for cytotoxic responses. Intratumoral delivery of CCL21 using pox virus vaccine into established tumors derived from murine colon cancer line, CT26 results in enhanced infiltration of CD4 T cells which correlated with inhibition of tumor growth (Flanagan, et al., 2004). Non-immunogenic murine breast carcinoma is rejected after transducing cells with CCL19. The rejection of tumor was mediated by activated NK and CD4+ cells (Braun, et al., 2000). Adenoviral delivery of the CCL16 is able to inhibit growth of mammary tumors and prevent metastatic growth (Okada, et al., 2004). Importantly, in treatment involving delivery of chemokines to the tumor environment, there is a major problem of heterogeneity of the tumor cells. Chemokines may have dual effects, can be beneficial to one patient might be harmful to another. However, this problem can be circumvented by chemokine typing every tumor prior to deciding on an appropriate therapy regime. They may be used as an adjunct to increase the efficacy of currently available therapies. Targeting specific chemokines can also modulate tumor infiltrating leukocytes or angiogenesis. High CXCL8 expression levels render tumor cells highly tumorigenic, angiogenic and invasive (Chavey, et al., 2007, Freund, et al., 2003, Freund, et al., 2004). In a murine model of breast cancer treatment with Met-CCL5, an antagonist of CCR1 and CCR5 led to a reduction in the total number of infiltrating inflammatory cells, in particular a decrease in macrophage infiltration and reduced growth of tumors (Liang, et al., 2004, Robinson, et al., 2003). The 7-transmembrane structure of chemokine receptors makes them attractive targets for small molecule inhibitors (Seaton, et al., 2009).

In summary, the exploration and manipulation of the chemokine network has just started and is likely to improve efficiency of current tumor therapies. However, since these chemotactic cytokines are also utilized in a plethora of normal interactions, caution is needed especially when extrapolating *in vitro* data into the clinical situation. Differences amongst tumor entities are obvious and the same chemokine/chemokine-receptor system seems to have divergent functions in different tumor entities. A more in-depth analysis of the real players in tumor immunosuppression, for example characterization of the subtypes of infiltrating immune cells and thorough analysis of the cytokine and chemokine milieu of primary tumors, will be necessary to pave the way for more efficient therapeutic interventions.

5. Tumor stroma: A permissive substrate for breast cancer development and progression

The stroma of carcinomas is an intricate ecosystem where heterogeneous cell populations coexist. This structural and functional connective tissue niche is inhabited by immune and inflammatory cells such as macrophages and monocytes, mesenchymal bone marrow-derived stem cells, endothelial and pericyte cells, lipocytes, additional smooth muscle cells and activated fibroblastic cells known as myofibroblasts, which are believed to be responsible for producing and maintaining the altered extracellular matrix (ECM) (Beacham & Cukierman, 2005; Li et al., 2007; Xouri & Christian, 2010). It is well accepted that the altered and excessive deposition of ECM, which is part of a process named desmoplasia, is directly associated with rapid progression and bad prognosis in carcinomas such as breast, pancreas, colon and prostate to name a few (Beacham & Cukierman, 2005; Arendt et al., 2010; Franco et al., 2010). In fact, we and others have suggested that stroma progression could be staged (analogously to classic tumor staging) into discrete stromagenic stages (Bissell et al., 2002; Mueller & Fusenig, 2002; Beacham & Cukierman, 2005; Quiros et al., 2008; Castello-Cros et al., 2009). Briefly, under normal (i.e., homeostatic) conditions, the breast stroma maintains the tissue architecture where a specialized ECM rich in collagen IV and laminin-1 known as basement membrane (BM) demarks a barrier between epithelium and the mesenchyme (Gudjonsson et al., 2002). A particular feature of the glandular epithelium in breast tissue is that both alveolar and ductal epithelial cells are not in direct contact with the BM. Instead, they are supported by a monolayer of myoepithelial cells that resides in between. Myoepithelial cells play an important role in supporting epithelial cell differentiation and controlling proliferation and cell polarity. These cells secrete the BM proteins and together with adjacent stromal fibroblasts maintain the integrity of this specialized gland (Gudjonsson et al., 2002; Polyak & Kalluri, 2010). Under physiological conditions, a normal stroma preserves and drives regular breast tissue morphogenesis (Kuperwasser et al., 2004) and, at the same time, suppresses the transformation of epithelial cells thus preventing the development of breast carcinoma *in situ* (CIS) and inhibiting progression towards invasive cancer (Hu et al., 2008). Although not much information is available to describe the mechanistic events responsible for normal stroma prevention of carcinoma progression, recent data suggests that the tumor microenvironment lacks the regulatory mechanisms that are necessary to maintain a normal epithelial phenotype (Postovit et al., 2008). As shown by interesting work conducted by Mintz and Illmensee in 1975 where they observed that a normal embryo microenvironment is repressive of teratoma tumorigenesis (Mintz & Illmensee, 1975), more recent work by Postovit *et al* looking at specific human embryonic stem cells-secreted factors also concluded that embryonic microenvironments can control and sustain a normal behaviour of invasive tumor cells (Postovit et al., 2008). In summary, one could state that the normal stroma is a natural barrier or a non-permissive environment for tumor progression.

In an effort to understand premature events that occur during stroma progression (i.e., stromagenesis (Cukierman, 2009)), researchers have used animal models where they have shown stromal cells alterations at early stages of tumorigenesis. For example, prostate smooth muscle cells, known to support homeostasis and epithelium differentiation and considered to be analogous to normal myoepithelial cells in breast, have been shown to undergo alterations during early tumorigenesis (Wong & Tam, 2002). Similar to myoepithelial cells, smooth muscle cells are also lost in advanced stages of tumor progression, but prior to this they lower the expression levels of differentiation markers such as myosin, desmin, and laminin (Wong & Tam, 2002). This fact strongly suggests the advent of a discrete intermediate state between normal and activated stroma. To this end, the up-regulated expression of proteins, such as fibroblast activation protein, has been suggested as potential markers of this intermediate or primed stromal stage (Mathew et al., 1995; Huber et al., 2003; Santos et al., 2009). Another such molecule is tenascin-C, an ECM protein expressed in breast cancer at early stages of the tumorigenesis, which has been shown to have a diagnostic value (Adams et al., 2002; Guttery et al., 2010).

Once the stroma becomes activated, many histological features are evident. This stage is commonly described by pathologists as desmoplasia and is characterized by increased interstitial ECM-deposition. The desmoplastic ECM is believed to be produced by a highly proliferating fibroblastic and alpha-smooth muscle actin (α-SMA) expressing myofibroblastic cell population. It is common in many cancers including breast, and it can constitute up to 50% of the tumor mass (Kunz-Schughart & Knuechel, 2002a, b; Desmouliere et al., 2004). The altered architecture of the desmoplastic stroma reaction is characterized by the over expression of ECM proteins such as collagen I and differential spliced fibronectin isoforms such as EDA and EDB (Matsumoto et al., 1999; Desmouliere et al., 2004). The desmoplastic ECM is highly organized in a parallel fiber pattern, which is clearly oriented *in vivo* perpendicular to the tumor border (Provenzano et al., 2006). In fact, this particular feature of the tumor associated-ECM (TA-ECM) has been suggested to facilitate migration of breast cancer cells *in vitro*, in a β1-integrin dependent manner (Castello-Cros et al., 2009). Moreover, there is evidence to suggest that TA-ECM can induce a phenotypic switch upon naïve fibroblasts thus inducing a myofibroblastic (or activated) conformation (Amatangelo et al., 2005). To this end, in a xenograft model of human breast cancer, it was shown that activated fibroblasts influence the local microenvironment to promote invasion (Orimo et al., 2005; Hu et al., 2008).

6. Tumor- or carcinoma-associated fibroblasts: A bad myofibroblastic influence

Fibroblasts are the main cellular component of the stroma and responsible for producing the mesenchymal (i.e., interstitial) ECM. These cells have been described as non-epithelial, non-inflammatory and non-vascular semi-differentiated connective tissue cells (Tarin & Croft, 1969). They are best known for their role in maintaining the tissue's integrity while they become quickly activated (e.g., myofibroblastic) and can modify the plasticity of the resident's tissue under conditions that alter the homeostatic equilibrium such as during wound healing, organogenesis, cancer and other pathological and inflammatory conditions (Kalluri & Zeisberg, 2006) . In fact, fibroblasts are known as tissue remodelers capable of renovating ECMs while, at the same time, facilitating access to ECM stored growth factors, such as transforming growth factor-beta (TGF-b), through a tightly regulated release and activation of matrix digestive enzymes such as matrix metalloproteinases (MMPs) (Jodele et al., 2006).

The fibroblastic cell population, known as carcinoma-associated fibroblasts (CAFs) or tumor-associated fibroblasts (Barsky et al., 1984), presents a myofibroblastic phenotype that is very similar to the one observed in activated fibroblasts during wound healing (Barsky et al., 1984). CAFs are the main stromal cell component of solid epithelial carcinomas (Shao et al., 2000). In addition to a characteristic, high proliferation rate and increased ECM deposition, the development of contractile cell features affects the physico-chemical characteristics of TA-ECM (Tomasek et al., 2002; Butcher et al., 2009; Cukierman & Bassi, 2010). Interestingly, CAFs are capable of establishing interactions with inflammatory, endothelial, and tumor cells by means of cytokines/chemokines secretions such as interleukin (IL)-1β, IL-6, CXCL-8, stromal derived factor-1 (SDF-1), also known as CXCL-12, and the monocyte chemotactic protein (MCPs/CCLs) among others (Silzle et al., 2004; Mishra et al., 2011). In an effort to find a discrete set of CAF specific markers, proteins such as γ- and α-SMA (Brouty-Boye et al., 1991; Kunz-Schughart & Knuechel, 2002b; Desmouliere et al., 2004; Xouri & Christian, 2010) specific isoforms of the actin binding protein palladin, (Ronty et al., 2006; Goicoechea et al., 2010; Gupta et al., 2011) as well as the intermediate filament proteins vimentin and desmin (Schmid et al., 1982) have been suggested. Furthermore, the specific breast cancer microenvironmental niche has been shown to contain increased levels of expression of ECM stabilizing (e.g., cross-linking) enzymes such as prolyl-4 hydroxylase (Orimo et al., 2005) and lysyl oxidase (Chang et al., 2005; Levental et al., 2009; Barry-Hamilton et al., 2010). Additional proteins have been shown to be specifically overexpressed at the tumor-associated stroma such as fibroblast activation protein (LeBeau et al., 2009; Lee, 2011), endosialin (Becker et al., 2008; Christian et al., 2008) S100A4 (Ambartsumian et al., 1996; Ryan et al., 2003; Katoh et al., 2010), and a plethora of MMPs, among others (Rasanen & Vaheri, 2010). In fact, some of these have already been proposed to serve as stromal monitoring or prognostic markers (Erkan et al., 2008; Gupta et al., 2011).

Nevertheless, this hardly consistent signature of myofibroblastic markers strongly suggests that the tumor stroma is a heterogeneous milieu (Sugimoto et al., 2006). The variety of myofibroblastic phenotypes is also suggestive of the eliciting of different roles played by these cell populations at the tumor stroma. Interestingly, this heterogeneity could have been originated (i.e., differentiated) by the multiple cell lineages known to produce myofibroblastic CAFs. These are: local fibroblasts (Kalluri & Zeisberg, 2006), bone marrow recruited mesenchymal cells (Ishii et al., 2003; Goldstein et al., 2010), as well as endothelial and tumor (i.e., epithelial) cells (Petersen et al., 2003; Kalluri & Zeisberg, 2006; Zeisberg et al., 2007), among others. In all these cases, TGF-β has been closely associated with tumor-induced myofibroblastic activation or differentiation (Zeisberg et al., 2007; Hinz, 2010; Taylor et al., 2010). The myofibroblastic differentiation is a complex and not yet fully understood process that is believed to play a central role during breast tumorigenesis (Cukierman, 2004; McAllister & Weinberg, 2010). Even though a plethora of molecules has been implicated in regulating fibroblastic activation, the specific desmoplastic response in breast cancer is believed to be driven by four main groups of inducers; i) growth factors, ii) TA-ECM, iii) acute inflammation and iv) microenvironmental stress denoted by nutrient and oxygen depravation as well as low pH.

i.   Specific growth factor presence at the tumor microenvironment may constitute the most studied aspect believed to trigger a myofibroblastic switch of the otherwise quiescent homeostatic fibroblasts. Determined mainly *in vitro* by an increment in proliferation rate, induction of α-SMA expression, and an up-regulation of ECM components, the growth factors most commonly implicated in this process are TGF-α, TGF-β, insulin-like growth factors I and II (TGF-I and TGF-II), the platelet-derived growth factor (PDGF), and the basic fibroblast growth factor (bFGF) (Beacham & Cukierman, 2005; Kalluri & Zeisberg, 2006; Rasanen & Vaheri, 2010; Xouri & Christian, 2010). Although many questions remain regarding specific triggers for breast cancer desmoplasia, work from Walker and Dearing implicated TGF-β_1, TGF-β_2 and TGF-β receptor as vital contributors of breast tumorigenesis associated with a stromal increment of fibronectin and tenascin in the tumor stroma (Walker & Dearing, 1992; Walker et al., 1994). Moreover, TGF-β known to induce myofibroblastic differentiation and to increase collagen I deposition during the wound healing process (Desmouliere et al., 2005), has also been implicated as a main factor in inducing breast cancer associated bone marrow-derived myofibroblasts differentiation (Goldstein et al., 2010). Similarly, PDGF has been shown to increase the breast myofibroblastic population by 30% while greatly increasing the amount of interstitial collagen I *in vivo* (Shao et al., 2000). In the context of epithelial to mesenchymal transition (EMT)-derived myofibroblasts, hepatocyte growth factor (HGF) and epidermal growth factor (EGF), in addition to the above-mentioned PDGF and TGF-β, have also been implicated (Mimeault & Batra, 2007; Kalluri & Weinberg, 2009).

ii. Breast TA-ECMs' features are known to become altered in both their molecular composition (Chen, S.T. et al., 2008; Levental et al., 2009; Ronnov-Jessen & Bissell, 2009) and their architectural characteristics (Provenzano et al., 2006). Together these two altered features can modulate tumorigenic behaviours of cancer cells and promote or delay the evolution of carcinomas in a permissive or restrictive manner (Ronnov-Jessen & Bissell, 2009; Cukierman & Bassi, 2010). In addition, it has been suggested that the physico-chemical characteristics of the ECM also affect the behaviour of mesenchymal cells (Discher et al., 2005). Fibroblasts are influenced by stromal stiffness, which exerts mechanical forces that modulate their cell behaviour. Thus, it has been demonstrated that as the substrate stiffness increases, fibroblastic cells change exhibiting three discrete phenotypic switch stages: normal or naive fibroblasts, intermediate or proto-myofibroblastic and activated myofibroblastic (Hinz, 2010). The phenotype transition induced by the increased tension in the substratum is also accompanied by the maturation or elongation of focal adhesions, together with cytoskeletal changes known to build-up contractile stress fibers (Hinz, 2010). Interestingly, studies of normal breast revealed a relatively limp tissue composition (0.15 kPa, expressed in E values of a Young modulus) compared to the stiffer and highly desmoplastic ~4 kPa tissue that has been affected by breast cancer (Butcher et al., 2009). The altered (i.e., myofibroblastic) phenotype of fibroblasts is linked to the stiffer ECM during tumor progression as these cells are responsible for the production of the TA-ECM (Cukierman & Bassi, 2010). Indeed increments of mammographic density, suggesting excessive collagen deposition, have been associated with higher risk in breast cancer (Boyd et al., 1998). Moreover, increases in cross-linked collagen due to over expression of LOX together with patterned linearization of the TA-ECM and specific ECM receptor, integrin, clustering and enhanced phosphoinositide 3-kinase (PI3K) activity, have all been correlated with breast cancer progression (Levental et al., 2009). Additionally, it has been shown that the interstitial ECM can function as a reservoir for diffusible molecules, such as the above-mentioned TGF-β which is secreted by both stromal and tumor cells in its inactivated form (Wipff & Hinz, 2008), but can be both activated and released due to the intrinsic myofibroblastic forces that increase the tension of TA-ECM's fibrils (Wipff et al., 2007; Tenney & Discher, 2009).

iii. Recently, an inflammatory microenvironment has been suggested as the seventh hallmark of cancer (Colotta et al., 2009). This cancer hallmark is also believed to play an important role in desmoplasia as a fibroblast phenotypic-switch activator. To this end, it has been demonstrated that stromal inflammatory responses that result from wounding can trigger tumorigenesis (Arwert et al., 2010). The importance of an inflammatory component has also been suggested for the breast cancer stroma (Hu & Polyak, 2008), and its repercussion in inducing or promoting cancer aggressiveness and metastasis has been highlighted in numerous occasions (Pantschenko et al., 2003; Elaraj et al., 2006; Valdivia-Silva et al., 2009; Franco-Barraza et al., 2010; Goldberg & Schwertfeger, 2010). However, our current knowledge regarding fibroblastic responses to inflammatory cytokines in breast cancer remains relatively modest. Work conducted at the Polyak laboratory suggested that cytokines could participate in triggering a fibroblast phenotypic switch at the breast cancer microenvironment (Hu et al., 2009). This work and the work of others has opened up the possibility of targeting inflammatory cytokines for the treatment of neoplasias as in the case of COX-2 and arachidonic acid inhibitors (Chen, X. et al., 2006; Hu et al., 2009). In fact, in the kidney, it has been shown that collagen I regulates COX-2 expression in a pro-proliferative type of response (Alique et al., 2011). Interestingly, CAFs are known to promote inflammation in an NFκ-b dependent manner, suggesting a vicious cycle between inflammation and stromal activation during tumorigenesis (Erez et al., 2010). Moreover, it has been shown that CAFs effectively suppress anti-tumor inflammation while, at the same time, maintaining acute inflammatory (pro-tumor) conditions (Kraman et al., 2010).

As established before, the cytokine/growth factor TGF-β imparts a pleiotropic and decisive role in the promotion of the desmoplastic tumor microenvironment thus supporting tumor progression (Yang et al., 2010). In addition, this same factor plays an additional important stromal role in inducing the expression of NADPH oxidase family protein, Nox4 (Bondi et al., 2010). Nox4 is a potent regulator of reactive oxygen species (ROS) (Barnes & Gorin, 2011) and has been shown to induce the accumulation of ROS in damaged tissues while transactivation of fibroblasts into myofibroblasts (Cucoranu et al., 2005; Rocic & Lucchesi, 2005). In breast cancer, the oxidative stress present at the tumor stroma is also considered to be an inductor for myofibroblastic differentiation, as recently shown in a JunD deficient mouse model, where the absence of this transcription factor allowed the accumulation of Ras-mediated production of ROS with the subsequent conversion of fibroblasts into myofibroblasts and shortening of the tumor free survival rate (Toullec et al., 2010).

iv. It is well known that as tumors progress increased regions of nutrient deprivation, low pH and low oxygen tension (hypoxia) are evident. Under these hypoxic stress conditions, breast cancer tissues are known to up-regulate the expression of hypoxia-inducible family (HIF) genes such as HIF-1α (Chen, C.L. et al., 2010). HIF proteins are known to participate in many cellular events such as angiogenesis, through the induction of vascular endothelium growth factor (VEGF), angiopoietin-2, PDFG and FGF (Allen & Louise Jones, 2011) which in turn can also activate stromal myofibroblastic differentiation in breast cancers (Shao et al., 2000). Finally, other molecules known to be induced by HIF-1α in carcinomas (and other fibrotic conditions) are the above mentioned ECM-cross-linkers (i.e., LOX) which have been associated with aggressive breast tumorigenesis (Chang et al., 2005; Levental et al., 2009; Barry-Hamilton et al., 2010).

7. Fibroblasts as moderators of signals at the tumor microenvironment

At the tumor microenvironment, intercellular communications resemble a social network emitting signals (either static or diffusible molecules) that in turn are collected, processed and emitted to additional cells. Using this analogy, it seems that CAFs play a decisive role during cancer progression acting as microenvironment signals moderators that sense extracellular signals and, after intracellular processing, emit new ones that in turn modulate both stromal and neoplastic neighbouring cells' behaviours (Bhowmick et al., 2004). In fact during cancer progression, CAFs constitute a very important source of the exogenous stimulants such as the above-mentioned TGF-β (Kalluri & Zeisberg, 2006). To this end, using an elegant humanized stromal reconstruction model of human breast cancer in mouse, Kuperwasser et al demonstrated that CAFs facilitate tumor development in a fibroblastic TGF-β- and HGF-dependent manner (Kuperwasser et al., 2004). Additionally, recent findings have demonstrated that epigenetic changes induced by mesenchymal cells on breast cancer cells that are regulated by the TGF-β/TGF-βR/Smad2 signalling axis provoke the silencing of critical epithelial genes resulting in the pro-tumorigenic EMT process (Papageorgis et al., 2010). To this end, in support of the above proposed vicious cycle effect, it is interesting to note that following quiescent fibroblasts transdifferentiation into CAFs, these cells support an invasive phenotype of mammary carcinomas where they secrete inflammatory cytokines (Powell et al., 1999; Buckley et al., 2001; Silzle et al., 2004) thus activating NF-κb and promoting EMT as well as promoting aggressiveness of breast cancer cells (Sullivan et al., 2009; Wu et al., 2009). An ever more complicated interplay between CAFs, cytokines and neoplastic cells has recently been proposed in breast cancers where, due to the presence of an altered TA-ECM, an integrin-dependent activation of Src family kinases results in the increase of NF-κB activity which blocks the production of certain microRNAs such as Let-7. Under these conditions, IL-6 production is promoted resulting in the increased secretion of this pro-tumorigenic cytokine, which in turn induces or promotes a positive feedback in tumor cells (Iliopoulos et al., 2009). Moreover, activated myofibroblastic and cancer cells are known to remodel the stromal ECM by means of increased secretion of MMPs and urokinase-type plasminogen activator (uPA). These enzymes cleave the ECM molecules to release fragments that contain chemotactic properties called matrikines that activate leukocytes to also release inflammatory cytokines (Maquart et al., 2004; Silzle et al., 2004). For example, a special feature of MMP-2, -3 and -9 is that these proteases can increase the availability of IL-1b at the tumor microenvironment by cleavage of the pIL-1b (immature IL-1b) (Schonbeck et al., 1998). Also, analyses of co-cultures containing both breast cancer cells and CAFs have shown increases in stromal MMP-2 and MMP-9 expression (Singer et al., 2002). These observations concur with observations stemming from an immunohistochemical study where tissue arrays of breast cancer patients showed that intratumor stromal fibroblasts express MMP-2, -7, and -14, while fibroblast at the invasive front highly express MMP-9. What is more, this specific profile of stromal MMPs staining was found to be a predictor of future distant metastases occurrences (Del Casar et al., 2009). Another uncovered effect of released MMPs into the tumor stroma is the capacity of these molecules to promote a permissive environment that supports epithelial tumorigenic progression including the promotion of genomic alterations (Radisky, E.S. & Radisky, 2007). In the mammary glands of transgenic mice, the overexpression of MMP-3 has been shown to be sufficient to stimulate myofibroblastic presence, increased fibrosis, epithelial hyperplasia, and development of mammary carcinoma (Thomasset et al., 1998). What is more, mammary epithelial cells exposed to stromal MMP-3 showed activation of a genotoxic metabolic pathway, where the over expression of the spliced variant Rac1b produced DNA-damaging superoxide radicals and induced EMT (Radisky, D.C. et al., 2005). Interestingly, the epithelial genomic alterations induced by stromal MMPs *in vitro,* suggest a possible mechanism to understand the presence of areas with genomic imbalance patterns detected in histologically normal tissues adjacent to the tumor stroma (Ellsworth et al., 2004; Holliday et al., 2009).

8. Targeting fibroblasts as an anti-cancer therapy

Various aspects of the tumor microenvironment have been explored as putative therapeutic targets in the fight against cancer (Andre et al., 2010; Cukierman & Khan, 2010; Allen & Louise Jones, 2011). Since a desmoplastic reaction is an ECM component-rich substratum and some of the TA-ECM components are believed to be specific for discrete types of carcinomas, they constitute a promising basis for therapeutics (i.e., inhibitory functional antibodies). For example, in glioblastoma patients an iodine-131 radiolabeled anti-tenascin-C monoclonal antibody has produced encouraging results in phase II trials (Reardon et al., 2006). Similarly, the development of radioactive or bioactive molecules coupled to antibodies against TA-ECM specific EDB, the L-19 antibody, showed encouraging results when tested in various carcinomas (Kaspar et al., 2006). The TA-ECM has been considered as both a target as well as a means to attract anti-tumoral drugs. For example, as albumin binds efficiently to the TA-ECM protein osteonectin (also known as SPARC), known to be upregulated in a plethora of cancer stromas and often associated with bad prognosis (Tai &

Tang, 2008), paclitaxel delivered through nanoparticles conjugated to albumin (nab-paclitaxel) are being tested (Vishnu & Roy, 2010; Robert et al., 2011; Volk et al., 2011). Moreover inhibition of the serine protease activity of the CAF specific fibroblast activation protein has been suggested as a therapeutic target in a plethora of cancers including breast (Mersmann et al., 2001). In fact, antibodies against fibroblast activation protein induced a marked decrease in desmoplastic collagen I expression resulting in an increased (up to 70%) increment in chemotherapeutic drugs uptake (Loeffler et al., 2006). Therefore, it is not surprising that fibroblast activation protein has been suggested as a tumor targeting molecule for the delivery of peptide protoxins (amongst others) thus diminishing non-tumoral side effect toxicities (LeBeau et al., 2009).

Pro-inflammatory molecules have also been used as effective targets. For example TNF-α antagonists have been shown to have good results preventing disease acceleration in a considerable number of breast cancer patients (Madhusudan et al., 2004; Brown et al., 2008). The SDF-1α/CXCR4 chemokine axis has been proposed as a general target for anticancer strategies (Guleng et al., 2005), and recently a compound derived from marine organisms that blocks CXCR4 has been shown effective as well (He et al., 2008). Antibodies blocking the TGF-β signalling pathway have been developed and showed promising synergistic effects when added to known chemotherapeutics and, thus, have been regarded as anti angiogenesis-depending tumor stromal agents in breast cancer (Takahashi et al., 2001). Finally, it was recently shown that eliminating pro-tumorigenic macrophages in pancreas causes desmoplastic shrinkage and subsequent tumor stalling (Beatty et al., 2011). We believe that these types of treatments, together with similar novel ones, could provide increased hope in the common fight against breast cancers.

9. Acknowledgment

A DGAPA Grant IN214611-2 from Universidad Nacional Autonoma de Mexico to EGZ and CA113451 from NIH/NCI to EC and JFB supported this work.

10. References

Adams, M.;Jones, J.L.;Walker, R.A.;Pringle, J.H. & Bell, S.C. (2002). Changes in tenascin-C isoform expression in invasive and preinvasive breast disease. Cancer research, Vol.62, No.11, pp. 3289-3297, ISSN 0008-5472

Ali, S. & Lazennec, G. (2007). Chemokines: novel targets for breast cancer metastasis. Cancer metastasis reviews, Vol. 26, No. pp. 401-420,

Alique, M.;Calleros, L.;Luengo, A.;Griera, M.;Iniguez, M.A.;Punzon, C.;Fresno, M.;Rodriguez-Puyol, M. & Rodriguez-Puyol, D. (2011). Changes in extracellular matrix composition regulate cyclooxygenase-2 expression in human mesangial cells. Am J Physiol Cell Physiol, Vol.300, No.4, pp. C907-918, ISSN 1522-1563

Allavena, P.; Sica, A.; Solinas, G.; Porta, C. & Mantovani, A. (2008). The inflammatory micro-environment in tumor progression: The role of tumor-associated macrophages. Critical reviews in oncology/hematology, Vol. 66, No. 1, pp. 1-9, 1040-8428

Allen, M. & Louise Jones, J. (2011). Jekyll and Hyde: the role of the microenvironment on the progression of cancer. The Journal of pathology, Vol.223, No.2, pp. 162-176, ISSN 1096-9896

Allen, S.J.; Crown, S.E. & Handel, T.M. (2007). Chemokine: receptor structure, interactions, and antagonism. Annual review of immunology, Vol. 25, No. pp. 787-820,

Amatangelo, M.D.;Bassi, D.E.;Klein-Szanto, A.J. & Cukierman, E. (2005). Stroma-derived three-dimensional matrices are necessary and sufficient to promote desmoplastic differentiation of normal fibroblasts. The American journal of pathology, Vol.167, No.2, pp. 475-488, ISSN 0002-9440

Ambartsumian, N.S.;Grigorian, M.S.;Larsen, I.F.;Karlstrom, O.;Sidenius, N.;Rygaard, J.;Georgiev, G. & Lukanidin, E. (1996). Metastasis of mammary carcinomas in GRS/A hybrid mice transgenic for the mts1 gene. Oncogene, Vol.13, No.8, pp. 1621-1630, ISSN 0950-9232

Amersi, F.F.; Terando, A.M.; Goto, Y.; Scolyer, R.A.; Thompson, J.F.; Tran, A.N.; Faries, M.B.; Morton, D.L. & Hoon, D.S.B. (2008). Activation of CCR9/CCL25 in Cutaneous Melanoma Mediates Preferential Metastasis to the Small Intestine. Clinical cancer research, Vol. 14, No. 3, pp. 638-645, ISSN 1557-3265

Andre, F.; Berrada, N. & Desmedt, C. (2010). Implication of tumor microenvironment in the resistance to chemotherapy in breast cancer patients. Curr Opin Oncol, Vol. 22, No. 6, pp. 547-551, 1531-703X (Electronic)

Angelo, L.S.; Talpaz, M. & Kurzrock, R. (2002). Autocrine Interleukin-6 Production in Renal Cell Carcinoma. Cancer research, Vol. 62, No. 3, pp. 932-940,

Annels, N.E.; Williemze, A.J.; van der Velden, V.H.; Faaij, C.M.; E. van Wering, E.; Sie-Go, D.M.; R.M. Egeler, R.M.; van Tol, M.J. & Revesz, T. (2004). Possible link between unique chemokine and homing receptor expression at diagnosis and relapse location in a patient with childhood T-ALL. Blood, Vol. 103, No. pp. 2806-2808,

Arendt, L.M.;Rudnick, J.A.;Keller, P.J. & Kuperwasser, C. (2010). Stroma in breast development and disease. Seminars in cell & developmental biology, Vol.21, No.1, pp. 11-18, ISSN 1096-3634

Arlt, A.; Vorndamm, J.; Mfi?erkfi›ster, S.; Yu, H.; Schmidt, W.E.; Ffi›lsch, U.R. & Schfi?fer, H. (2002). Autocrine Production of Interleukin 1â? Confers Constitutive Nuclear Factor â¨B Activity and Chemoresistance in Pancreatic Carcinoma Cell Lines. Cancer research, Vol. 62, No. 3, pp. 910-916,

Arwert, E.N.;Lal, R.;Quist, S.;Rosewell, I.;van Rooijen, N. & Watt, F.M. (2010). Tumor formation initiated by nondividing epidermal cells via an inflammatory infiltrate. Proceedings of the National Academy of Sciences of the United States of America, Vol.107, No.46, pp. 19903-19908, ISSN 1091-6490

Baggiolini, M.; Dewald, B. & Moser, B. (1997). Human chemokines: an update. Annual review of immunology, Vol. 15, No. pp. 675-705,

Bagley, R.G.; Nannuru, K.C.; Singh, S. & Singh, R.K. (2010). Chemokines and Metastasis. In: Chemokines and MetastasisBook. pp. 601-631. Springer New York, 978-1-4419-6615-5

Balkwill, F. & Mantovani, A. (2001). Inflammation and cancer: back to Virchow? Lancet, Vol. 357, No. 9255, pp. 539-545, ISSN 0140-6736

Barnes, J.L. & Gorin, Y. (2011). Myofibroblast differentiation during fibrosis: role of NAD(P)H oxidases. Kidney international, ISSN 1523-1755

Barry-Hamilton, V.;Spangler, R.;Marshall, D.;McCauley, S.;Rodriguez, H.M.;Oyasu, M.;Mikels, A.;Vaysberg, M.;Ghermazien, H.;Wai, C.;Garcia, C.A.;Velayo, A.C.;Jorgensen, B.;Biermann, D.;Tsai, D.;Green, J.;Zaffryar-Eilot, S.;Holzer, A.;Ogg, S.;Thai, D.;Neufeld, G.;Van Vlasselaer, P. & Smith, V. (2010). Allosteric inhibition of lysyl oxidase-like-2 impedes the development of a pathologic microenvironment. Nature medicine, Vol.16, No.9, pp. 1009-1017, ISSN 1546-170X

Barsky, S.H.;Green, W.R.;Grotendorst, G.R. & Liotta, L.A. (1984). Desmoplastic breast carcinoma as a source of human myofibroblasts. The American journal of pathology, Vol.115, No.3, pp. 329-333, ISSN 0002-9440

Beacham, D.A. & Cukierman, E. (2005). Stromagenesis: the changing face of fibroblastic microenvironments during tumor progression. Seminars in cancer biology, Vol.15, No.5, pp. 329-341, ISSN 1044-579X

Beatty, G.L.;Chiorean, E.G.;Fishman, M.P.;Saboury, B.;Teitelbaum, U.R.;Sun, W.;Huhn, R.D.;Song, W.;Li, D.;Sharp, L.L.;Torigian, D.A.;O'Dwyer, P.J. & Vonderheide, R.H. (2011). CD40 agonists alter tumor stroma and show efficacy against pancreatic carcinoma in mice and humans. Science, Vol.331, No.6024, pp. 1612-1616, ISSN 1095-9203

Becker, R.;Lenter, M.C.;Vollkommer, T.;Boos, A.M.;Pfaff, D.;Augustin, H.G. & Christian, S. (2008). Tumor stroma marker endosialin (Tem1) is a binding partner of metastasis-related protein Mac-2 BP/90K. FASEB J, Vol.22, No.8, pp. 3059-3067, ISSN 1530-6860

Ben-Baruch, A. (2003). Host microenvironment in breast cancer development: inflammatory cells, cytokines and chemokines in breast cancer progression: reciprocal tumor-microenvironment interactions. Breast cancer research., Vol. 5, No. pp. 31-36,

Ben-Baruch, A. (2006). Inflammation-associated immune suppression in cancer: The roles played by cytokines, chemokines and additional mediators. Seminars in cancer biology, Vol. 16, No. 1, pp. 38-52, 1044-579X

Ben-Baruch, A. (2008). Organ selectivity in metastasis: regulation by chemokines and their receptors. Clinical and experimental metastasis, Vol. 25, No. 4, pp. 345-356,

Bhowmick, N.A.;Neilson, E.G. & Moses, H.L. (2004). Stromal fibroblasts in cancer initiation and progression. Nature, Vol.432, No.7015, pp. 332-337, ISSN 1476-4687

Bissell, M.J.;Radisky, D.C.;Rizki, A.;Weaver, V.M. & Petersen, O.W. (2002). The organizing principle: microenvironmental influences in the normal and malignant breast. Differentiation, Vol.70, No.9-10, pp. 537-546

Bondi, C.D.;Manickam, N.;Lee, D.Y.;Block, K.;Gorin, Y.;Abboud, H.E. & Barnes, J.L. (2010). NAD(P)H oxidase mediates TGF-beta1-induced activation of kidney myofibroblasts. Journal of the American Society of Nephrology : JASN, Vol.21, No.1, pp. 93-102, ISSN 1533-3450

Bos, R.; van der Groep, P.; Greijer, A.E.; Shvarts, A.; Meijer, S.; Pinedo, H.M.; Semenza, G.L.; van Diest, P.J. & van der Wall, E. (2003). Levels of hypoxia-inducible factor-1? independently predict prognosis in patients with lymph node negative breast carcinoma. Cancer, Vol. 97, No. 6, pp. 1573-1581, 1097-0142

Bos, R.; van Diest, P.; van der Groep, P.; Shvarts, A.; Greijer, A. & van der Wall, E. (2004). Expression of hypoxia-inducible factor-1alpha and cell cycle proteins in invasive breast cancer are estrogen receptor related. Breast Cancer Res, Vol. 6, No. 4, pp. R450 - R459, ISSN 1465-5411

Bos, R.; Zhong, H.; Hanrahan, C.F.; Mommers, E.C.; Semenza, G.L.; Pinedo, H.M.; Abeloff, M.D.; Simons, J.W.; van Diest, P.J. & van der Wall, E. (2001). Levels of hypoxia-inducible factor-1? during breast carcinogenesis. Journal of the national cancer institute, Vol. 93, No. pp. 309-314,

Boyd, N.F.;Lockwood, G.A.;Martin, L.J.;Knight, J.A.;Byng, J.W.;Yaffe, M.J. & Tritchler, D.L. (1998). Mammographic densities and breast cancer risk. Breast disease, Vol.10, No.3-4, pp. 113-126, ISSN 0888-6008

Braun, S.E.; Chen, K.; Foster, R.G.; Kim, C.H.; Hromas, R.; Kaplan, M.H.; Broxmeyer, H.E. & Cornetta, K. (2000). The CC Chemokine CKfiî-11/MIP-3fiî/ELC/Exodus 3 Mediates Tumor Rejection of Murine Breast Cancer Cells Through NK Cells. The Journal of Immunology, Vol. 164, No. 8, pp. 4025-4031,

Brouty-Boye, D.;Raux, H.;Azzarone, B.;Tamboise, A.;Tamboise, E.;Beranger, S.;Magnien, V.;Pihan, I.;Zardi, L. & Israel, L. (1991). Fetal myofibroblast-like cells isolated from post-radiation fibrosis in human breast cancer. Int J Cancer, Vol.47, No.5, pp. 697-702, ISSN 0020-7136

Brown, E.R.;Charles, K.A.;Hoare, S.A.;Rye, R.L.;Jodrell, D.I.;Aird, R.E.;Vora, R.;Prabhakar, U.;Nakada, M.;Corringham, R.E.;DeWitte, M.;Sturgeon, C.;Propper, D.;Balkwill, F.R. & Smyth, J.F. (2008). A clinical study assessing the tolerability and biological effects of infliximab, a TNF-alpha inhibitor, in patients with advanced cancer. Annals of oncology : official journal of the European Society for Medical Oncology / ESMO, Vol.19, No.7, pp. 1340-1346, ISSN 1569-8041

Buckley, C.D.;Pilling, D.;Lord, J.M.;Akbar, A.N.;Scheel-Toellner, D. & Salmon, M. (2001). Fibroblasts regulate the switch from acute resolving to chronic persistent inflammation. Trends in immunology, Vol.22, No.4, pp. 199-204, ISSN 1471-4906

Butcher, D.T.;Alliston, T. & Weaver, V.M. (2009). A tense situation: forcing tumor progression. Nature reviews. Cancer, Vol.9, No.2, pp. 108-122, ISSN 1474-1768

Castello-Cros, R.;Khan, D.R.;Simons, J.;Valianou, M. & Cukierman, E. (2009). Staged stromal extracellular 3D matrices differentially regulate breast cancer cell responses through PI3K and beta1-integrins. BMC Cancer, Vol.9, pp. 94, ISSN 1471-2407

Chambers, A.F.; Groom, A.C. & MacDonald, I.C. (2002). Dissemination and growth of cancer cells in metastatic sites. Nature review in cancer, Vol. 2, No. 8, pp. 563-572, ISSN 1474-175X

Chandrasekar, B.; Mummidi, S.; Perla, R.P.; Bysani, S.; Dulin, N.O.; Liu, F. & Melby, P.C. (2003). Fractalkine (CX3CL1) stimulated by nuclear factor kappaB (NF-kappaB)-dependent inflammatory signals induces aortic smooth muscle cell proliferation through an autocrine pathway. The biochemical journal, Vol. 373, No. 2, pp. 547-558,

Chang, H.Y.;Nuyten, D.S.;Sneddon, J.B.;Hastie, T.;Tibshirani, R.;Sorlie, T.;Dai, H.;He, Y.D.;van't Veer, L.J.;Bartelink, H.;van de Rijn, M.;Brown, P.O. & van de Vijver, M.J. (2005). Robustness, scalability, and integration of a wound-response gene expression signature in predicting breast cancer survival. Proceedings of the

National Academy of Sciences of the United States of America, Vol.102, No.10, pp. 3738-3743, ISSN 0027-8424

Chang, S.-H.; Ai, Y.; Breyer, R.M.; Lane, T.F. & Hla, T. (2005). The Prostaglandin E2 Receptor EP2 Is Required for Cyclooxygenase 2_Í„Mediated Mammary Hyperplasia. Cancer research, Vol. 65, No. 11, pp. 4496-4499,

Charalabopoulos, K.; Dalavaga, Y.; Stefanou, D.; Charalabopoulos, A.; Bablekos, G. & Constantopoulos, S. (2004). Direct endobronchial metastasis is a rare metastatic pattern in breast cancer. International Journal of Clinical Practice, Vol. 58, No. 6, pp. 641-644, ISSN 1742-1241

Chavey, C.; Bibeau, F.; Gourgou-Bourgade, S.; Burlinchon, S.; Boissiere, F.; Laune, D.; Roques, S. & Lazennec, G. (2007). Oestrogen receptor negative breast cancers exhibit high cytokine content. Breast Cancer Research, Vol. 9, No. 1, pp. R15, 1465-5411

Chen, C.L.;Chu, J.S.;Su, W.C.;Huang, S.C. & Lee, W.Y. (2010). Hypoxia and metabolic phenotypes during breast carcinogenesis: expression of HIF-1alpha, GLUT1, and CAIX. Virchows Archiv : an international journal of pathology, Vol.457, No.1, pp. 53-61, ISSN 1432-2307

Chen, G.S.; Yu, H.S.; Lan, C.C.E.; Chow, K.C.; Lin, T.Y.; Kok, L.F.; Lu, M.P.; Liu, C.H. & Wu, M.T. (2006). CXC chemokine receptor CXCR4 expression enhances tumorigenesis and angiogenesis of basal cell carcinoma. British Journal of Dermatology, Vol. 154, No. 5, pp. 910-918, ISSN 1365-2133

Chen, S.T.;Pan, T.L.;Juan, H.F.;Chen, T.Y.;Lin, Y.S. & Huang, C.M. (2008). Breast tumor microenvironment: proteomics highlights the treatments targeting secretome. J Proteome Res, Vol.7, No.4, pp. 1379-1387, ISSN 1535-3893

Chen, X.;Sood, S.;Yang, C.S.;Li, N. & Sun, Z. (2006). Five-lipoxygenase pathway of arachidonic acid metabolism in carcino-genesis and cancer chemoprevention. Curr Cancer Drug Targets, Vol.6, No.7, pp. 613-622, ISSN 1873-5576

Christian, S.;Winkler, R.;Helfrich, I.;Boos, A.M.;Besemfelder, E.;Schadendorf, D. & Augustin, H.G. (2008). Endosialin (Tem1) is a marker of tumor-associated myofibroblasts and tumor vessel-associated mural cells. The American journal of pathology, Vol.172, No.2, pp. 486-494, ISSN 0002-9440

Colotta, F.; Allavena, P.; Sica, A.; Garlanda, C. & Mantovani, A. (2009). Cancer-related inflammation, the seventh hallmark of cancer: links to genetic instability. Carcinogenesis, Vol. 30, No. 7, pp. 1073-1081, 1460-2180 (Electronic)

Colotta, F.;Allavena, P.;Sica, A.;Garlanda, C. & Mantovani, A. (2009). Cancer-related inflammation, the seventh hallmark of cancer: links to genetic instability. Carcinogenesis, Vol.30, No.7, pp. 1073-1081, ISSN 1460-2180

Coussens, L.M. & Werb, Z. (2002). Inflammation and cancer. Nature, Vol. 420, No. pp. 860-867,

Croitoru-Lamoury, J.; Guillemin, G.J.; Boussin, F.D.; Mognetti, B.; Gigout, L.I.; Cheret, A.; Vaslin, B.; Le Grand, R.; Brew, B.J. & Dormont, D. (2003). Expression of chemokines and their receptors in human and simian astrocytes: evidence for a central role of TNF alpha and IFN gamma in CXCR4 and CCR5 modulation. Glia, Vol. 41, No. pp. 354-370,

Crowther, M.; Brown, N.J.; Bishop, E.T. & Lewis, C.E. (2001). Microenvironmental influence
    on macrophage regulation of angiogenesis in wounds and malignant tumors.
    Journal of Leukocyte Biology, Vol. 70, No. 4, pp. 478-490,

Cucoranu, I.;Clempus, R.;Dikalova, A.;Phelan, P.J.;Ariyan, S.;Dikalov, S. & Sorescu, D.
    (2005). NAD(P)H oxidase 4 mediates transforming growth factor-beta1-induced
    differentiation of cardiac fibroblasts into myofibroblasts. Circulation research,
    Vol.97, No.9, pp. 900-907, ISSN 1524-4571

Cukierman, E. (2004). A visual-quantitative analysis of fibroblastic stromagenesis in breast
    cancer progression. Journal of mammary gland biology and neoplasia, Vol.9, No.4,
    pp. 311-324, ISSN 1083-3021

Cukierman, E. (2009). Stromagenesis. Encyclopedia of Cancer. M. Schwab.
    Heidelberg/Germany, Springer. 4: 2843-2845.

Cukierman, E. & Bassi, D.E. (2010). Physico-mechanical aspects of extracellular matrix
    influences on tumorigenic behaviors. Seminars in cancer biology, Vol.20, No.3, pp.
    139-145, ISSN 1096-3650 (

Cukierman, E. & Khan, D.R. (2010). The benefits and challenges associated with the use of
    drug delivery systems in cancer therapy. Biochem Pharmacol, Vol.80, No.5, pp.
    762-770, ISSN 1873-2968

Del Casar, J.M.;Gonzalez, L.O.;Alvarez, E.;Junquera, S.;Marin, L.;Gonzalez, L.;Bongera,
    M.;Vazquez, J. & Vizoso, F.J. (2009). Comparative analysis and clinical value of the
    expression of metalloproteases and their inhibitors by intratumor stromal
    fibroblasts and those at the invasive front of breast carcinomas. Breast cancer
    research and treatment, Vol.116, No.1, pp. 39-52, ISSN 1573-7217

Desmouliere, A.;Chaponnier, C. & Gabbiani, G. (2005). Tissue repair, contraction, and the
    myofibroblast. Wound Repair Regen, Vol.13, No.1, pp. 7-12, ISSN 1067-1927

Desmouliere, A.;Guyot, C. & Gabbiani, G. (2004). The stroma reaction myofibroblast: a key
    player in the control of tumor cell behavior. Int J Dev Biol, Vol.48, No.5-6, pp. 509-
    517, ISSN 0214-6282

Discher, D.E.;Janmey, P. & Wang, Y.L. (2005). Tissue cells feel and respond to the stiffness of
    their substrate. Science, Vol.310, No.5751, pp. 1139-1143, ISSN 1095-9203

Egeblad, M.;Nakasone, E.S. & Werb, Z. (2010). Tumors as organs: complex tissues that
    interface with the entire organism. Dev Cell, Vol.18, No.6, pp. 884-901, ISSN 1878-
    1551

Elaraj, D.M.;Weinreich, D.M.;Varghese, S.;Puhlmann, M.;Hewitt, S.M.;Carroll,
    N.M.;Feldman, E.D.;Turner, E.M. & Alexander, H.R. (2006). The role of interleukin
    1 in growth and metastasis of human cancer xenografts. Clinical cancer research :
    an official journal of the American Association for Cancer Research, Vol.12, No.4,
    pp. 1088-1096, ISSN 1078-0432

Ellsworth, D.L.;Ellsworth, R.E.;Love, B.;Deyarmin, B.;Lubert, S.M.;Mittal, V. & Shriver, C.D.
    (2004). Genomic patterns of allelic imbalance in disease free tissue adjacent to
    primary breast carcinomas. Breast cancer research and treatment, Vol.88, No.2, pp.
    131-139, ISSN 0167-6806

Erez, N.;Truitt, M.;Olson, P.;Arron, S.T. & Hanahan, D. (2010). Cancer-Associated
    Fibroblasts Are Activated in Incipient Neoplasia to Orchestrate Tumor-Promoting

Inflammation in an NF-kappaB-Dependent Manner. Cancer cell, Vol.17, No.2, pp. 135-147, ISSN 1878-3686

Erkan, M.;Michalski, C.W.;Rieder, S.;Reiser-Erkan, C.;Abiatari, I.;Kolb, A.;Giese, N.A.;Esposito, I.;Friess, H. & Kleeff, J. (2008). The Activated Stroma Index Is a Novel and Independent Prognostic Marker in Pancreatic Ductal Adenocarcinoma. Clin Gastroenterol Hepatol, Vol.6, No.10, pp. 1155-1161, ISSN 1542-7714 (Electronic)

Fidler, I.J. (2002). Critical determinants of metastasis. Seminars in cancer biology, Vol. 12, No. 2, pp. 89-96, ISSN 1044-579X

Flanagan, K.; Glover, R.T.; H_rig, H.; Yang, W. & Kaufman, H.L. (2004). Local delivery of recombinant vaccinia virus expressing secondary lymphoid chemokine (SLC) results in a CD4 T-cell dependent antitumor response. Vaccine, Vol. 22, No. 21-22, pp. 2894-2903, 0264-410X

Franco-Barraza, J.; Valdivia-Silva, J.E.; Zamudio-Meza, H.; Castillo, A.; Garcia-Zepeda, E.A.; Benitez-Bribiesca, L. & Meza, I. (2010). Actin cytoskeleton participation in the onset of IL-1beta induction of an invasive mesenchymal-like phenotype in epithelial MCF-7 cells. Archives of medical research, Vol. 41, No. 3, pp. 170-181, 1873-5487 (Electronic)

Franco, O.E.;Shaw, A.K.;Strand, D.W. & Hayward, S.W. (2010). Cancer associated fibroblasts in cancer pathogenesis. Seminars in cell & developmental biology, Vol.21, No.1, pp. 33-39, ISSN 1096-3634

Freund, A.; Chauveau, C.; Brouillet, J.; Lucas, A.; Lacroix, M.; Licznar, A.; Vignon, F. & Lazennec, G. (2003). IL-8 expression and its possible relationship with estrogen-receptor-negative status of breast cancer cells. Oncogene, Vol. 22, No. pp. 256 - 265,

Freund, A.; Jolivel, V.; Durand, S.; Kersual, N.; Chalbos, D.; Chavey, C.; Vignon, F. & Lazennec, G. (2004). Mechanisms underlying differential expression of interleukin-8 in breast cancer cells. Oncogene, Vol. 23, No. pp. 6105 - 6114,

Fujimoto, K.; Imaizumi, T.; Yoshida, H.; Takanashi, S.; Okumura, K. & Satoh, K. (2001). Interferon-gamma Stimulates Fractalkine Expression in Human Bronchial Epithelial Cells and Regulates Mononuclear Cell Adherence. Am. J. Respir. Cell Mol. Biol., Vol. 25, No. 2, pp. 233-238,

Garg, A.K. & Aggarwal, B.B. (2002). Reactive oxygen intermediates in TNF signalling. Molecular Immunology, Vol. 39, No. 9, pp. 509-517, 0161-5890

Goicoechea, S.M.;Bednarski, B.;Stack, C.;Cowan, D.W.;Volmar, K.;Thorne, L.;Cukierman, E.;Rustgi, A.K.;Brentnall, T.;Hwang, R.F.;McCulloch, C.A.;Yeh, J.J.;Bentrem, D.J.;Hochwald, S.N.;Hingorani, S.R.;Kim, H.J. & Otey, C.A. (2010). Isoform-specific upregulation of palladin in human and murine pancreas tumors. PloS one, Vol.5, No.4, pp. e10347, ISSN 1932-6203

Goldberg, J.E. & Schwertfeger, K.L. (2010). Proinflammatory cytokines in breast cancer: mechanisms of action and potential targets for therapeutics. Current drug targets, Vol.11, No.9, pp. 1133-1146, ISSN 1873-5592

Goldstein, R.H.;Reagan, M.R.;Anderson, K.;Kaplan, D.L. & Rosenblatt, M. (2010). Human bone marrow-derived MSCs can home to orthotopic breast cancer tumors and promote bone metastasis. Cancer research, Vol.70, No.24, pp. 10044-10050, ISSN 1538-7445

Gross, N. & Meier, R. (2009). Chemokines in neuroectodermal cancers: The crucial growth signal from the soil. Seminars in cancer biology, Vol. 19, No. 2, pp. 103-110, ISSN 1044-579X

Gudjonsson, T.;Ronnov-Jessen, L.;Villadsen, R.;Rank, F.;Bissell, M.J. & Petersen, O.W. (2002). Normal and tumor-derived myoepithelial cells differ in their ability to interact with luminal breast epithelial cells for polarity and basement membrane deposition. Journal of cell science, Vol.115, No.Pt 1, pp. 39-50, ISSN 0021-9533

Guleng, B.;Tateishi, K.;Ohta, M.;Kanai, F.;Jazag, A.;Ijichi, H.;Tanaka, Y.;Washida, M.;Morikane, K.;Fukushima, Y.;Yamori, T.;Tsuruo, T.;Kawabe, T.;Miyagishi, M.;Taira, K.;Sata, M. & Omata, M. (2005). Blockade of the stromal cell-derived factor-1/CXCR4 axis attenuates in vivo tumor growth by inhibiting angiogenesis in a vascular endothelial growth factor-independent manner. Cancer research, Vol.65, No.13, pp. 5864-5871, ISSN 0008-5472

Gupta, V.;Bassi, D.E.;Simons, J.D.;Al-Saleem, T.I.;Devarajan, K.;Uzzo, R.G. & Cukierman, E. (2011). Elevated expression of stromal palladin predicts poor clinical outcome in renal cell carcinoma. PloS one, Vol. 6, No.6, pp. e21494, ISSN

Guttery, D.S.;Hancox, R.A.;Mulligan, K.T.;Hughes, S.;Lambe, S.M.;Pringle, J.H.;Walker, R.A.;Jones, J.L. & Shaw, J.A. (2010). Association of invasion-promoting tenascin-C additional domains with breast cancers in young women. Breast Cancer Res, Vol.12, No.4, pp. R57, ISSN 1465-542X

Hadden, J.W. (1999). The immunology and immunotherapy of breast cancer: an update. International journal of immunopharmacology, Vol. 21, No. pp. 79-101,

Half, E.; Tang, X.M.; Gwyn, K.; Sahin, A.; Wathen, K. & Sinicrope, F.A. (2002). Cyclooxygenase-2 Expression in Human Breast Cancers and Adjacent Ductal Carcinoma in Situ. Cancer research, Vol. 62, No. 6, pp. 1676-1681,

He, X.;Fang, L.;Wang, J.;Yi, Y.;Zhang, S. & Xie, X. (2008). Bryostatin-5 blocks stromal cell-derived factor-1 induced chemotaxis via desensitization and down-regulation of cell surface CXCR4 receptors. Cancer research, Vol.68, No.21, pp. 8678-8686, ISSN 1538-7445

Hinz, B. (2010). The myofibroblast: paradigm for a mechanically active cell. Journal of biomechanics, Vol.43, No.1, pp. 146-155, ISSN 1873-2380

Holliday, C.;Rummel, S.;Hooke, J.A.;Shriver, C.D.;Ellsworth, D.L. & Ellsworth, R.E. (2009). Genomic instability in the breast microenvironment? A critical evaluation of the evidence. Expert review of molecular diagnostics, Vol.9, No.7, pp. 667-678, ISSN 1744-8352

Hsiao, Y.H.; Chou, M.C.; Fowler, C.; Mason, J.T. & Man, Y. (2010). Breast cancer heterogeneity: mechanisms, proofs, and implications. Journal of cancer, Vol. 1, No. pp. 6-13,

Hu, M. & Polyak, K. (2008). Molecular characterisation of the tumor microenvironment in breast cancer. European journal of cancer, Vol.44, No.18, pp. 2760-2765, ISSN 1879-0852

Hu, M.;Peluffo, G.;Chen, H.;Gelman, R.;Schnitt, S. & Polyak, K. (2009). Role of COX-2 in epithelial-stromal cell interactions and progression of ductal carcinoma in situ of the breast. Proceedings of the National Academy of Sciences of the United States of America, Vol.106, No.9, pp. 3372-3377, ISSN 1091-6490

Hu, M.;Yao, J.;Carroll, D.K.;Weremowicz, S.;Chen, H.;Carrasco, D.;Richardson, A.;Violette, S.;Nikolskaya, T.;Nikolsky, Y.;Bauerlein, E.L.;Hahn, W.C.;Gelman, R.S.;Allred, C.;Bissell, M.J.;Schnitt, S. & Polyak, K. (2008). Regulation of in situ to invasive breast carcinoma transition. Cancer cell, Vol.13, No.5, pp. 394-406, ISSN 1878-3686

Huber, M.A.;Kraut, N.;Park, J.E.;Schubert, R.D.;Rettig, W.J.;Peter, R.U. & Garin-Chesa, P. (2003). Fibroblast activation protein: differential expression and serine protease activity in reactive stromal fibroblasts of melanocytic skin tumors. The Journal of investigative dermatology, Vol.120, No.2, pp. 182-188, ISSN 0022-202X

Iliopoulos, D.;Hirsch, H.A. & Struhl, K. (2009). An epigenetic switch involving NF-kappaB, Lin28, Let-7 MicroRNA, and IL6 links inflammation to cell transformation. Cell, Vol.139, No.4, pp. 693-706, ISSN 1097-4172

Ishii, G.;Sangai, T.;Oda, T.;Aoyagi, Y.;Hasebe, T.;Kanomata, N.;Endoh, Y.;Okumura, C.;Okuhara, Y.;Magae, J.;Emura, M.;Ochiya, T. & Ochiai, A. (2003). Bone-marrow-derived myofibroblasts contribute to the cancer-induced stromal reaction. Biochem Biophys Res Commun, Vol.309, No.1, pp. 232-240, ISSN 0006-291X

Jemal, A.; Bray, F.; Center, M.M.; Ferlay, J.; Ward, E. & Forman, D. (2011). Global cancer statistics. CA: A Cancer Journal for Clinicians, Vol. 61, No. 2, pp. 69-90, ISSN 1542-4863

Jiang, B.H.; Rue, E.; Wang, G.; Roe, R. & Semenza, G.L. (1996). Dimerization, DNA binding, and transactivation properties of hypoxia-inducible factor 1. J Biol Chem, Vol. 271:, No. pp. 17771-17778,

Jin, L.; Yuan, R.Q.; Fuchs, A.; Yao, Y.; Joseph, A.; Schwall, R.; Schnitt, S.J.; Guida, A.; Hastings, H.M.; Andres, J.; Turkel, G.; Polverini, P.J.; Goldberg, I.D. & Rosen, E.M. (1997). Expression of interleukin-1? in human breast carcinoma. Cancer, Vol. 80, No. 3, pp. 421-434, 1097-0142

Jodele, S.;Blavier, L.;Yoon, J.M. & DeClerck, Y.A. (2006). Modifying the soil to affect the seed: role of stromal-derived matrix metalloproteinases in cancer progression. Cancer metastasis reviews, Vol.25, No.1, pp. 35-43, ISSN 0167-7659

Johnson-Holiday, C.; Singh, S.; Johnson, E.; Singh, U. & Lillard, J.W. (2007). CCR9- CCL25 interaction mediates breast cancer cell survival via Akt activation. Journal of immunology, Vol. 178, No. pp. 49.22,

Johnson, H.L. (2010). A rare presentation of metastatic breast cancer in a woman with apparent cholangiocarcinoma. Journal of the american academy of physician assistants, Vol. 23, No. 3, pp. 32-36,

Joyce, J.A. & Pollard, J.W. (2009). Microenvironmental regulation of metastasis. Nature reviews. Cancer, Vol. 9, No. 4, pp. 239-252, ISSN 1474-175X

Kalluri, R. & Weinberg, R.A. (2009). The basics of epithelial-mesenchymal transition. The Journal of clinical investigation, Vol.119, No.6, pp. 1420-1428, ISSN 1558-8238

Kalluri, R. & Zeisberg, M. (2006). Fibroblasts in cancer. Nature reviews. Cancer, Vol.6, No.5, pp. 392-401, ISSN 1474-175X

Kanoh, K.; Shimura, T.; Tsutsumi, S.; Suzuki, H.; Kashiwabara, K.; Nakajima, T. & Kuwano, H. (2001). Significance of contracted cholecystitis lesions as high risk for gallbladder carcinogenesis. Cancer letters, Vol. 169, No. 1, pp. 7-14, 0304-3835

Karczewska, A.; Nawrocki, S.; Br?borowicz, D.; Filas, V. & Mackiewicz, A. (2000). Expression of interleukin-6, interleukin-6 receptor, and glycoprotein 130 correlates with good prognoses for patients with breast carcinoma. Cancer, Vol. 88, No. 9, pp. 2061-2071, 1097-0142

Karnoub, A.E. & Weinberg, R.A. (2006). Chemokine networks and breast cancer metastasis. Breast disease, Vol. 26, No. pp. 75-85,

Kaspar, M.;Zardi, L. & Neri, D. (2006). Fibronectin as target for tumor therapy. International journal of cancer. Journal international du cancer, Vol.118, No.6, pp. 1331-1339, ISSN 0020-7136

Katoh, H.;Hosono, K.;Ito, Y.;Suzuki, T.;Ogawa, Y.;Kubo, H.;Kamata, H.;Mishima, T.;Tamaki, H.;Sakagami, H.;Sugimoto, Y.;Narumiya, S.;Watanabe, M. & Majima, M. (2010). COX-2 and prostaglandin EP3/EP4 signaling regulate the tumor stromal proangiogenic microenvironment via CXCL12-CXCR4 chemokine systems. The American journal of pathology, Vol.176, No.3, pp. 1469-1483, ISSN 1525-2191

Keeley, E.C.; Mehrad, B.; Strieter, R.M.; George, F.V.W. & George, K. (2010). CXC Chemokines in Cancer Angiogenesis and Metastases. In: CXC Chemokines in Cancer Angiogenesis and MetastasesBook. pp. 91-111. Academic Press, ISBN 0065-230X

Kilgore, T.; Grewal, A.; Bechtold, M.; Miick, R.; Diaz-Arias, A.; Ibdah, J. & Bragg, J. (2007). Breast Cancer Metastasis To The Colon: A Case Report And Review Of The Literature. The Internet Journal of Gastroenterology, Vol. 6, No. 1, pp. on-line, ISSN 1528-8323

Kirschmann, D.A.; Seftor, E.A.; Nieva, D.R.C.; Mariano, E.A. & Hendrix, M.J.C. (1999). Differentially expressed genes associated with the metastatic phenotype in breast cancer. Breast cancer research and treatment, Vol. 55, No. 2, pp. 125-134, 0167-6806

Koizumi, K.; Hojo, S.; Akashi, T.; Yasumoto, K. & Saiki, I. (2007). Chemokine receptors in cancer metastasis and cancer cell-derived chemokines in host immune response. Cancer science, Vol. 98, No. pp. 1652-1658,

Komori, A.; Yatsunami, J.; Suganuma, M.; Okabe, S.; Abe, S.; Sakai, A.; Sasaki, K. & Fujiki, H. (1993). Tumor Necrosis Factor Acts as a Tumor Promoter in BALB/3T3 Cell Transformation. Cancer research, Vol. 53, No. 9, pp. 1982-1985,

Kraman, M.;Bambrough, P.J.;Arnold, J.N.;Roberts, E.W.;Magiera, L.;Jones, J.O.;Gopinathan, A.;Tuveson, D.A. & Fearon, D.T. (2010). Suppression of antitumor immunity by stromal cells expressing fibroblast activation protein-alpha. Science, Vol.330, No.6005, pp. 827-830, ISSN 1095-9203

Kundu, N. & Fulton, A.M. (2002). Selective Cyclooxygenase (COX)-1 or COX-2 Inhibitors Control Metastatic Disease in a Murine Model of Breast Cancer. Cancer research, Vol. 62, No. 8, pp. 2343-2346,

Kunz-Schughart, L.A. & Knuechel, R. (2002a). Tumor-associated fibroblasts (part II): Functional impact on tumor tissue. Histol Histopathol, Vol.17, No.2, pp. 623-637, ISSN 0213-3911

Kunz-Schughart, L.A. & Knuechel, R. (2002b). Tumor-associated fibroblasts (part I): Active stromal participants in tumor development and progression? Histol Histopathol, Vol.17, No.2, pp. 599-621, ISSN 0213-3911

Kuperwasser, C.;Chavarria, T.;Wu, M.;Magrane, G.;Gray, J.W.;Carey, L.;Richardson, A. & Weinberg, R.A. (2004). Reconstruction of functionally normal and malignant human breast tissues in mice. Proceedings of the National Academy of Sciences of the United States of America, Vol.101, No.14, pp. 4966-4971, ISSN 0027-8424

Kurebayashi, J. (2000). Regulation of interleukin-6 secretion from breast cancer cells and its clinical implications. Breast cancer, Vol. 7, No. 2, pp. 124-129,

Kurose, K.; Gilley, K.; Matsumoto, S.; Watson, P.H.; Zhou, X.-P. & Eng, C. (2002). Frequent somatic mutations in PTEN and TP53 are mutually exclusive in the stroma of breast carcinomas. Nat Genet, Vol. 32, No. 3, pp. 355-357, ISSN 1061-4036

Kurose, K.; Hoshaw-Woodard, S.; Adeyinka, A.; Lemeshow, S.; Watson, P.H. & Eng, C. (2001). Genetic model of multi-step breast carcinogenesis involving the epithelium and stroma: clues to tumor—microenvironment interactions. Human molecular genetics, Vol. 10, No. 18, pp. 1907-1913, ISSN 1460-2083

Landi, S.; Moreno, V.; Gioia-Patricola, L.; Guino, E.; Navarro, M.; de Oca, J.; Capella, G.; Canzian, F. & Group, f.t.B.C.C.S. (2003). Association of Common Polymorphisms in Inflammatory Genes Interleukin (IL)6, IL8, Tumor Necrosis Factor âÒ, NFKB1, and Peroxisome Proliferator-activated Receptor â? with Colorectal Cancer. Cancer research, Vol. 63, No. 13, pp. 3560-3566,

Langhans, T. (1879). Pulsirende cavernoese Geschwulst der Miltz mit metastatischen Knoten in der Leber. Virchows Archiv, Vol.75, pp. 273-291, ISSN (N/A)

Lavergne, E.; Combadiere, B.; Bonduelle, O.; Iga, M.; Gao, J.L.; Maho, M.; Boissonnas, A.; Murphy, P.M.; Debre, P. & Combadiere, C. (2003). Fractalkine mediates natural killer-dependent antitumor responses in vivo. Cancer research, Vol. 63, No. pp. 7468-7474,

LeBeau, A.M.;Brennen, W.N.;Aggarwal, S. & Denmeade, S.R. (2009). Targeting the cancer stroma with a fibroblast activation protein-activated promelittin protoxin. Molecular cancer therapeutics, Vol.8, No.5, pp. 1378-1386, ISSN 1538-8514

Lee, H.O.M., S.R.; Franco-Barraza, J.; Valinaou, M.; Cukierman, E. & Cheng, J.D. (2011). Fap-overexpressing fibroblasts produce an extracellular matrix that enhances invasive velocity and directionality of pancreatic cancer cells. BMC Cancer, ISSN Vol. 13, No.11, pp. 245, ISSN

Leek, R.D.; Landers, R.; Fox, S.B.; Ng, F.; Harris, A.L. & Lewis, C.E. (1998). Association of tumor necrosis factor alpha and its receptors with thymidine phosphorylase expression in invasive breast carcinoma. British journal of cancer, Vol. 77, No. 12, pp. 2246-2251,

Letsch, A.; Keilholz, U.; Schadendorf, D.; Assfalg, G.; Asemissen, A.M.; Thiel, E. & Scheibenbogen, C. (2004). Functional CCR9 Expression Is Associated with Small Intestinal Metastasis. J Investig Dermatol, Vol. 122, No. 3, pp. 685-690, ISSN 0022-202X

Levental, K.R.;Yu, H.;Kass, L.;Lakins, J.N.;Egeblad, M.;Erler, J.T.;Fong, S.F.;Csiszar, K.;Giaccia, A.;Weninger, W.;Yamauchi, M.;Gasser, D.L. & Weaver, V.M. (2009).

Matrix crosslinking forces tumor progression by enhancing integrin signaling. Cell, Vol.139, No.5, pp. 891-906, ISSN 1097-4172

Li, H.;Fan, X. & Houghton, J. (2007). Tumor microenvironment: the role of the tumor stroma in cancer. J Cell Biochem, Vol.101, No.4, pp. 805-815, ISSN 0730-2312

Li, Y.M.; Pan, Y.; Wei, Y.; Cheng, X.; Zhou, B.P.; Tan, M.; Zhou, X.; Xia, W.; Hortobagyi, G.N.; Yu, D. & Hung, M.-C. (2004). Upregulation of CXCR4 is essential for HER2-mediated tumor metastasis. Cancer cell, Vol. 6, No. 5, pp. 459-469, 1535-6108

Liang, Z.; Wu, T.; Lou, H.; Yu, X.; Taichman, R.S.; Lau, S.K.; Nie, S.; Umbreit, J. & Shim, H. (2004). Inhibition of Breast Cancer Metastasis by Selective Synthetic Polypeptide against CXCR4. Cancer research, Vol. 64, No. 12, pp. 4302-4308,

Liu, W.; Reinmuth, N.; Stoeltzing, O.; Parikh, A.A.; Tellez, C.; Williams, S.; Jung, Y.D.; Fan, F.; Takeda, A.; Akagi, M.; Bar-Eli, M.; Gallick, G.E. & Ellis, L.M. (2003). Cyclooxygenase-2 Is Up-Regulated by Interleukin-1â? in Human Colorectal Cancer Cells via Multiple Signaling Pathways. Cancer research, Vol. 63, No. 13, pp. 3632-3636,

Lochter, A. & Bissell, M.J. (1995). Involvement of extracellular matrix constituents in breast cancer. Seminars in cancer biology, Vol.6, No.3, pp. 165-173, ISSN 1044-579X

Loeffler, M.;Kruger, J.A.;Niethammer, A.G. & Reisfeld, R.A. (2006). Targeting tumor-associated fibroblasts improves cancer chemotherapy by increasing intratumoral drug uptake. The Journal of clinical investigation, Vol.116, No.7, pp. 1955-1962, ISSN 0021-9738

Lu, X. & Kang, Y. (2007). Organotropism of breast cancer metastasis. Journal of mammary gland biology and neoplasia, Vol. 12, No. 2-3, pp. 153-162, ISSN 1083-3021

Luster, A.D. (1998). Chemokines - Chemotactic Cytokines That Mediate Inflammation. New England Journal of Medicine, Vol. 338, No. 7, pp. 436-445,

MacDonald, I.C.; Groom, A.C. & Chambers, A.F. (2002). Cancer spread and micrometastasis development: quantitative approaches for in vivo models. Bioessays, Vol. 24, No. pp. 885-893,

Madhusudan, S.;Foster, M.;Muthuramalingam, S.R.;Braybrooke, J.P.;Wilner, S.;Kaur, K.;Han, C.;Hoare, S.;Balkwill, F.;Talbot, D.C.;Ganesan, T.S. & Harris, A.L. (2004). A phase II study of etanercept (Enbrel), a tumor necrosis factor alpha inhibitor in patients with metastatic breast cancer. Clinical cancer research : an official journal of the American Association for Cancer Research, Vol.10, No.19, pp. 6528-6534, ISSN 1078-0432

Maquart, F.X.;Pasco, S.;Ramont, L.;Hornebeck, W. & Monboisse, J.C. (2004). An introduction to matrikines: extracellular matrix-derived peptides which regulate cell activity. Implication in tumor invasion. Critical reviews in oncology/hematology, Vol.49, No.3, pp. 199-202, ISSN 1040-8428

Mathew, S.;Scanlan, M.J.;Mohan Raj, B.K.;Murty, V.V.;Garin-Chesa, P.;Old, L.J.;Rettig, W.J. & Chaganti, R.S. (1995). The gene for fibroblast activation protein alpha (FAP), a putative cell surface-bound serine protease expressed in cancer stroma and wound healing, maps to chromosome band 2q23. Genomics, Vol.25, No.1, pp. 335-337, ISSN 0888-7543

Matsumiya, T.; Imaizumi, T.; Fujimoto, K.; Cui, X.; Shibata, T.; Tamo, W.; Kumagai, M.; Tanji, K.; Yoshida, H.; Kimura, H. & Satoh, K. (2001). Soluble Interleukin-6 Receptor [alpha] Inhibits the Cytokine-Induced Fractalkine/CX3CL1 Expression in Human Vascular Endothelial Cells in Culture. Experimental Cell Research, Vol. 269, No. 1, pp. 35-41, 0014-4827

Matsumoto, E.;Yoshida, T.;Kawarada, Y. & Sakakura, T. (1999). Expression of fibronectin isoforms in human breast tissue: production of extra domain A+/extra domain B+ by cancer cells and extra domain A+ by stromal cells. Jpn J Cancer Res, Vol.90, No.3, pp. 320-325, ISSN 0910-5050

McAllister, S.S. & Weinberg, R.A. (2010). Tumor-host interactions: a far-reaching relationship. Journal of clinical oncology : official journal of the American Society of Clinical Oncology, Vol.28, No.26, pp. 4022-4028, ISSN 1527-7755

Mersmann, M.;Schmidt, A.;Rippmann, J.F.;Wuest, T.;Brocks, B.;Rettig, W.J.;Garin-Chesa, P.;Pfizenmaier, K. & Moosmayer, D. (2001). Human antibody derivatives against the fibroblast activation protein for tumor stroma targeting of carcinomas. International journal of cancer. Journal international du cancer, Vol.92, No.2, pp. 240-248, ISSN 0020-7136

Miller, L.J.; Kurtzman, S.H.; Wang, Y.; Anderson, K.H.; Lindquist, R.R. & Kreutzer, D.L. (1998). Expression of interleukin-8 receptors on tumor cells and vascular endothelial cells in human breast cancer tissue. Anticancer research, Vol. 18, No. 1A, pp. 77-88, ISSN 0250-7005

Mimeault, M. & Batra, S.K. (2007). Interplay of distinct growth factors during epithelial mesenchymal transition of cancer progenitor cells and molecular targeting as novel cancer therapies. Annals of oncology : official journal of the European Society for Medical Oncology / ESMO, Vol.18, No.10, pp. 1605-1619, ISSN 1569-8041

Mintz, B. & Illmensee, K. (1975). Normal genetically mosaic mice produced from malignant teratocarcinoma cells. Proceedings of the National Academy of Sciences of the United States of America, Vol.72, No.9, pp. 3585-3589, ISSN 0027-8424

Mishra, P.; Banerjee, D. & Ben-Baruch, A. (2011). Chemokines at the crossroads of tumor-fibroblast interactions that promote malignancy. J Leukoc Biol, Vol. 89, No. 1, pp. 31-39, 1938-3673 (Electronic)

Moinfar, F.; Man, Y.G.; Arnould, L.; Bratthauer, G.L.; Ratschek, M. & Tavassoli, F.A. (2000). Concurrent and Independent Genetic Alterations in the Stromal and Epithelial Cells of Mammary Carcinoma: Implications for Tumorigenesis. Cancer research, Vol. 60, No. 9, pp. 2562-2566, ISSN: 1538-7445

Moser, B. & Loetscher, P. (2001). Lymphocyte traffic control by chemokines. Nat Immunol, Vol. 2, No. 2, pp. 123-128, ISSN 1529-2908

Moser, B. & Willimann, K. (2004). Chemokines: role in inflammation and immune surveillance. Annals of the Rheumatic Diseases, Vol. 63, No. suppl 2, pp. ii84-ii89, ISSN 1468-2060

Mourad, P.D.; Farrell, L.; Stamps, L.D.; Chicoine, M.R. & Silbergeld, D.L. (2005). Why are systemic glioblastoma metastases rare? Systemic and cerebral growth of mouse glioblastoma. Surgical neurology, Vol. 63, No. 6, pp. 511-519, ISSN 0090-3019

Mueller, M.M. & Fusenig, N.E. (2002). Tumor-stroma interactions directing phenotype and progression of epithelial skin tumor cells. Differentiation, Vol.70, No.9-10, pp. 486-497, ISSN 1538-7445

Muller, A.; Homey, B.; Soto, H.; Ge, N.; Catron, D.; Buchanan, M.E.; McClanahan, T.; Murphy, E.; Yuan, W.; Wagner, S.N.; Barrera, J.L.; Mohar, A.; Verastegui, E. & Zlotnik, A. (2001). Involvement of chemokine receptors in breast cancer metastasis. Nature medicine, Vol. 410, No. pp. 50-56,

Nanki, T.; Imai, T.; Nagasaka, K.; Urasaki, Y.; Nonomura, Y.; Taniguchi, K.; Hayashida, K.; Hasegawa, J.; Yoshie, O. & Miyasaka, N. (2002). Migration of CX3CR1-positive T cells producing type 1 cytokines and cytotoxic molecules into the synovium of patients with rheumatoid arthritis. Arthritis & Rheumatism, Vol. 46, No. 11, pp. 2878-2883, 1529-0131

Nevo, I.; Sagi-Assif, O.; Meshel, T.; Geminder, H.; Goldberg-Bittman, L.; Ben-Menachem, S.; Shalmon, B.; Goldberg, I.; Ben-Baruch, A. & Witz, I.P. (2004). The tumor microenvironment: CXCR4 is associated with distinct protein expression patterns in neuroblastoma cells. Immunology Letters, Vol. 92, No. pp. 163-169,

O'Sullivan, C. & Lewis, C.E. (1994). Tumor-associated leucocytes: Friends or foes in breast carcinoma. The Journal of pathology, Vol. 172, No. 3, pp. 229-235, 1096-9896

Offersen, B.V.; Knap, M.M.; Marcussen, N.; Horsman, M.R.; Hamilton-Dutoit, S. & Overgaard, J. (2002). Intense inflammation in bladder carcinoma is associated with angiogenesis and indicates good prognosis. British journal of cancer, Vol. 87, No. 12, pp. 1422-1430,

Okada, N.; Gao, J.-Q.; Sasaki, A.; Niwa, M.; Okada, Y.; Nakayama, T.; Yoshie, O.; Mizuguchi, H.; Hayakawa, T.; Fujita, T.; Yamamoto, A.; Tsutsumi, Y.; Mayumi, T. & Nakagawa, S. (2004). Anti-tumor activity of chemokine is affected by both kinds of tumors and the activation state of the host's immune system: implications for chemokine-based cancer immunotherapy. Biochemical and Biophysical Research Communications, Vol. 317, No. 1, pp. 68-76, 0006-291X

Okamoto, M.; Kawamata, H.; Kawai, K. & Oyasu, R. (1995). Enhancement of Transformation in Vitro of a Nontumorigenic Rat Urothelial Cell Line by Interleukin 6. Cancer research, Vol. 55, No. 20, pp. 4581-4585,

Orimo, A.; Gupta, P.B.; Sgroi, D.C.; Arenzana-Seisdedos, F.; Delaunay, T.; Naeem, R.; Carey, V.J.; Richardson, A.L. & Weinberg, R.A. (2005). Stromal Fibroblasts Present in Invasive Human Breast Carcinomas Promote Tumor Growth and Angiogenesis through Elevated SDF-1/CXCL12 Secretion. Cell, Vol. 121, No. 3, pp. 335-348, ISSN 0092-8674

Orimo, A.;Gupta, P.B.;Sgroi, D.C.;Arenzana-Seisdedos, F.;Delaunay, T.;Naeem, R.;Carey, V.J.;Richardson, A.L. & Weinberg, R.A. (2005). Stromal fibroblasts present in invasive human breast carcinomas promote tumor growth and angiogenesis through elevated SDF-1/CXCL12 secretion. Cell, Vol.121, No.3, pp. 335-348, ISSN 0092-8674

Ou, D.L.; Chen, C.L.; Lin, S.B.; Hsu, C.H. & L.I. Lin, L.I. (2006). Chemokine receptor expression profiles in nasopharyngeal carcinoma and their association with metastasis and radiotherapy. Journal of pathology, Vol. 210, No. pp. 363-373,

Paget, S. (1889). The distribution of secondary growths in cancer of the breast Lancet, Vol.133, pp. 571-573, ISSN

Pantschenko, A.G.;Pushkar, I.;Anderson, K.H.;Wang, Y.;Miller, L.J.;Kurtzman, S.H.;Barrows, G.&Kreutzer, D.L. (2003). The interleukin-1 family of cytokines and receptors in human breast cancer: implications for tumor progression. International journal of oncology, Vol.23, No.2, pp. 269-284, ISSN 1019-6439

Papageorgis, P.;Lambert, A.W.;Ozturk, S.;Gao, F.;Pan, H.;Manne, U.;Alekseyev, Y.O.;Thiagalingam, A.;Abdolmaleky, H.M.;Lenburg, M. & Thiagalingam, S. (2010). Smad signaling is required to maintain epigenetic silencing during breast cancer progression. Cancer research, Vol.70, No.3, pp. 968-978, ISSN 1538-7445

Petersen, O.W.;Nielsen, H.L.;Gudjonsson, T.;Villadsen, R.;Rank, F.;Niebuhr, E.;Bissell, M.J. & Ronnov-Jessen, L. (2003). Epithelial to mesenchymal transition in human breast cancer can provide a nonmalignant stroma. The American journal of pathology, Vol.162, No.2, pp. 391-402, ISSN 0002-9440

Polyak, K. & Kalluri, R. (2010). The role of the microenvironment in mammary gland development and cancer. Cold Spring Harb Perspect Biol, Vol.2, No.11, pp. a003244, ISSN 1943-0264

Postovit, L.M.;Margaryan, N.V.;Seftor, E.A.;Kirschmann, D.A.;Lipavsky, A.;Wheaton, W.W.;Abbott, D.E.;Seftor, R.E. & Hendrix, M.J. (2008). Human embryonic stem cell microenvironment suppresses the tumorigenic phenotype of aggressive cancer cells. Proceedings of the National Academy of Sciences of the United States of America, Vol.105, No.11, pp. 4329-4334, ISSN 1091-6490

Powell, D.W.;Mifflin, R.C.;Valentich, J.D.;Crowe, S.E.;Saada, J.I. & West, A.B. (1999). Myofibroblasts. I. Paracrine cells important in health and disease. The American journal of physiology, Vol.277, No.1 Pt 1, pp. C1-9, ISSN 0002-9513

Provenzano, P.P.;Eliceiri, K.W.;Campbell, J.M.;Inman, D.R.;White, J.G. & Keely, P.J. (2006). Collagen reorganization at the tumor-stromal interface facilitates local invasion. BMC Med, Vol.4, No.1, pp. 38, ISSN 1741-7015

Quiros, R.M.;Valianou, M.;Kwon, Y.;Brown, K.M.;Godwin, A.K. & Cukierman, E. (2008). Ovarian normal and tumor-associated fibroblasts retain in vivo stromal characteristics in a 3-D matrix-dependent manner. Gynecologic Oncology, Vol.110, No.1, pp. 99-109, ISSN 0090-8258

Radisky, D.C.;Levy, D.D.;Littlepage, L.E.;Liu, H.;Nelson, C.M.;Fata, J.E.;Leake, D.;Godden, E.L.;Albertson, D.G.;Nieto, M.A.;Werb, Z. & Bissell, M.J. (2005). Rac1b and reactive oxygen species mediate MMP-3-induced EMT and genomic instability. Nature, Vol.436, No.7047, pp. 123-127, ISSN 1476-4687

Radisky, E.S. & Radisky, D.C. (2007). Stromal induction of breast cancer: inflammation and invasion. Reviews in endocrine & metabolic disorders, Vol.8, No.3, pp. 279-287, ISSN 1389-9155

Rajagopalan, H.; Nowak, M.A.; Vogelstein, B. & Lengauer, C. (2003). The significance of unstable chromosomes in colorectal cancer. Nature reviews. Cancer, Vol. 3, No. 9, pp. 695-701, ISSN 1474-175X

Rasanen, K. & Vaheri, A. (2010). Activation of fibroblasts in cancer stroma. Exp Cell Res, Vol.316, No.17, pp. 2713-2722, ISSN 1090-2422

Reardon, D.A.;Akabani, G.;Coleman, R.E.;Friedman, A.H.;Friedman, H.S.;Herndon, J.E., 2nd;McLendon, R.E.;Pegram, C.N.;Provenzale, J.M.;Quinn, J.A.;Rich, J.N.;Vredenburgh, J.J.;Desjardins, A.;Gururangan, S.;Badruddoja, M.;Dowell, J.M.;Wong, T.Z.;Zhao, X.G.;Zalutsky, M.R. & Bigner, D.D. (2006). Salvage radioimmunotherapy with murine iodine-131-labeled antitenascin monoclonal antibody 81C6 for patients with recurrent primary and metastatic malignant brain tumors: phase II study results. Journal of clinical oncology : official journal of the American Society of Clinical Oncology, Vol.24, No.1, pp. 115-122, ISSN 1527-7755

Robert, N.;Krekow, L.;Stokoe, C.;Clawson, A.;Iglesias, J. & O'Shaughnessy, J. (2011). Adjuvant dose-dense doxorubicin plus cyclophosphamide followed by dose-dense nab-paclitaxel is safe in women with early-stage breast cancer: a pilot study. Breast cancer research and treatment, Vol.125, No.1, pp. 115-120, ISSN 1573-7217

Robinson, S.C.; Scott, K.A.; Wilson, J.L.; Thompson, R.G.; Proudfoot, A.E.I. & Balkwill, F.R. (2003). A Chemokine Receptor Antagonist Inhibits Experimental Breast Tumor Growth. Cancer research, Vol. 63, No. 23, pp. 8360-8365,

Rocic, P. & Lucchesi, P.A. (2005). NAD(P)H oxidases and TGF-beta-induced cardiac fibroblast differentiation: Nox-4 gets Smad. Circulation research, Vol.97, No.9, pp. 850-852, ISSN 1524-4571

Ronnov-Jessen, L. & Bissell, M.J. (2009). Breast cancer by proxy: can the microenvironment be both the cause and consequence? Trends Mol Med, Vol.15, No.1, pp. 5-13, ISSN 1471-4914

Ronty, M.J.;Leivonen, S.K.;Hinz, B.;Rachlin, A.;Otey, C.A.;Kahari, V.M. & Carpen, O.M. (2006). Isoform-specific regulation of the actin-organizing protein palladin during TGF-beta1-induced myofibroblast differentiation. The Journal of investigative dermatology, Vol.126, No.11, pp. 2387-2396, ISSN 1523-1747

Ruffini, P.A.; Morandi, P.; Cabioglu, N.; Altundag, K. & Cristofanilli, M. (2007). Manipulating the chemokine-chemokine receptor network to treat cancer. Cancer, Vol. 109, No. pp. 2392-2404,

Ryan, D.G.;Taliana, L.;Sun, L.;Wei, Z.G.;Masur, S.K. & Lavker, R.M. (2003). Involvement of S100A4 in stromal fibroblasts of the regenerating cornea. Invest Ophthalmol Vis Sci, Vol.44, No.10, pp. 4255-4262, ISSN 0146-0404

Saisho, S.; Takashima, S.; Ohsumi, S.; Saeki, S.; Aogi, K.; Saeki, T.; Mandai, K.; Iwata, S. & Takeda, T. (2005). Two Cases with Long-Term Disease-Free Survival after Resection and Radiotherapy for Solitary Brain Metastasis from Breast Cancer with Extensive Nodal Metastases. Breast cancer, Vol. 12, No. pp. 221-225, ISSN 1880-4233

Sallusto, F.; Mackay, C.R. & Lanzavecchia, A. (2000). The role of chemokine receptors in primary, effector, and memory immune responses. Annual review of immunology, Vol. 18, No. pp. 593-620,

Santos, A.M.;Jung, J.;Aziz, N.;Kissil, J.L. & Pure, E. (2009). Targeting fibroblast activation protein inhibits tumor stromagenesis and growth in mice. The Journal of clinical investigation, Vol.119, No.12, pp. 3613-3625, ISSN 1558-8238

Schimanski, C.C.; Galle, P.R. & Moehler, M. (2008). Chemokine receptor CXCR4- prognostic factor for gastrointestinal tumors. World journal of gastroenterology, Vol. 14, No. pp. 4721-4724,

Schmid, E.;Osborn, M.;Rungger-Brandle, E.;Gabbiani, G.;Weber, K. & Franke, W.W. (1982). Distribution of vimentin and desmin filaments in smooth muscle tissue of mammalian and avian aorta. Exp Cell Res, Vol.137, No.2, pp. 329-340, ISSN 0014-4827

Schonbeck, U.;Mach, F. & Libby, P. (1998). Generation of biologically active IL-1 beta by matrix metalloproteinases: a novel caspase-1-independent pathway of IL-1 beta processing. Journal of immunology, Vol.161, No.7, pp. 3340-3346, ISSN 0022-1767

Schwarz, M.; Wahl, M.; Resch, K. & Radeke, H.H. (2002). IFN? induces functional chemokine receptor expression in human mesangial cells. Clinical & Experimental Immunology, Vol. 128, No. 2, pp. 285-294, 1365-2249

Seaton, A.; Maxwell, P.J.; Hill, A.; Gallagher, R.; Pettigrew, J.; Wilson, R.H. & Waugh, D.J.J. (2009). Inhibition of constitutive and cxc-chemokine-induced NF-[kappa]B activity potentiates ansamycin-based HSP90-inhibitor cytotoxicity in castrate-resistant prostate cancer cells. British journal of cancer, Vol. 101, No. 9, pp. 1620-1629, 0007-0920

Semenza, G.L. & Wang, G.L. (1992). A nuclear factor induced by hypoxia via de novo protein synthesis binds to the human erythropoietin gene enhancer at a site required for transcriptional activation. Mol. Cell. Biol., Vol. 12, No. 12, pp. 5447-5454,

Shao, Z.M.;Nguyen, M. & Barsky, S.H. (2000). Human breast carcinoma desmoplasia is PDGF initiated. Oncogene, Vol.19, No.38, pp. 4337-4345, ISSN 0950-9232

Shields, J.D.; Fleury, M.E.; Yong, C.; Tomei, A.A.; Randolph, G.J. & Swartz, M.A. (2007). Autologous chemotaxis as a mechanism of tumor cell homing to lymphatics via interstitial flow and autocrine CCR7 signalling. Cancer cell, Vol. 11, No. pp. 526-538,

Shulby, S.A.; Dolloff, N.G.; Stearns, M.E.; Meucci, O. & Fatatis, A. (2004). CX3CR1-fractalkine expression regulates cellular mechanisms involved in adhesion, migration, and survival of human prostate cancer cells. Cancer research, Vol. 64, No. pp. 4693-4698,

Silzle, T.;Randolph, G.J.;Kreutz, M. & Kunz-Schughart, L.A. (2004). The fibroblast: sentinel cell and local immune modulator in tumor tissue. International journal of cancer. Journal international du cancer, Vol.108, No.2, pp. 173-180, ISSN 0020-7136

Singer, C.F.;Kronsteiner, N.;Marton, E.;Kubista, M.;Cullen, K.J.;Hirtenlehner, K.;Seifert, M. & Kubista, E. (2002). MMP-2 and MMP-9 expression in breast cancer-derived human fibroblasts is differentially regulated by stromal-epithelial interactions. Breast cancer research and treatment, Vol.72, No.1, pp. 69-77, ISSN 0167-6806

Singh, S.; Singh, U.P.; Grizzle, W.E. & J.W. Lillard, J.W.J. (2004). CXCL12-CXCR4 interactions modulate prostate cancer cell migration, metalloproteinase expression and invasion. Laboratory investigation, Vol. 84, No. pp. 1666-1676,

Soria, G. & Ben-Baruch, A. (2008). The inflammatory chemokines CCL2 and CCL5 in breast cancer. Cancer letters, Vol. 267, No. 2, pp. 271-285, 0304-3835

Soto, A.M. & Sonnenschein, C. (2004). The somatic mutation theory of cancer: growing problems with the paradigm? Bioessays, Vol.26, No.10, pp. 1097-1107, ISSN 0265-9247

Strieter, R.M.; Burdick, M.D.; Mestas, J.; Gomperts, B.; Keane, M.P. & Belperio, J.A. (2006). Cancer CXC chemokine networks and tumor angiogenesis. European journal of cancer (Oxford, England : 1990), Vol. 42, No. 6, pp. 768-778, ISSN 0959-8049

Struyf, S.; Salogni, L.; Burdick, M.D.; Vandercappellen, J.; Gouwy, M.; Noppen, S.; Proost, P.; Opdenakker, G.; Parmentier, M.; Gerard, C.; Sozzani, S.; Strieter, R.M. & Van Damme, J. (2011). Angiostatic and chemotactic activities of the CXC chemokine CXCL4L1 (platelet factor-4 variant) are mediated by CXCR3. Blood, Vol. 117, No. 2, pp. 480-488, ISSN 1528-0020

Sugimoto, H.;Mundel, T.M.;Kieran, M.W. & Kalluri, R. (2006). Identification of fibroblast heterogeneity in the tumor microenvironment. Cancer biology & therapy, Vol.5, No.12, pp. 1640-1646, ISSN 1538-4047

Sullivan, N.J.;Sasser, A.K.;Axel, A.E.;Vesuna, F.;Raman, V.;Ramirez, N.;Oberyszyn, T.M. & Hall, B.M. (2009). Interleukin-6 induces an epithelial-mesenchymal transition phenotype in human breast cancer cells. Oncogene, Vol.28, No.33, pp. 2940-2947, ISSN 1476-5594

Tai, I.T. & Tang, M.J. (2008). SPARC in cancer biology: its role in cancer progression and potential for therapy. Drug Resist Updat, Vol.11, No.6, pp. 231-246, ISSN 1532-2084

Takahashi, N.;Haba, A.;Matsuno, F. & Seon, B.K. (2001). Antiangiogenic therapy of established tumors in human skin/severe combined immunodeficiency mouse chimeras by anti-endoglin (CD105) monoclonal antibodies, and synergy between anti-endoglin antibody and cyclophosphamide. Cancer research, Vol.61, No.21, pp. 7846-7854, ISSN 0008-5472

Takanami, I. (2003). Overexpression of CCR7 mRNA in nonsmall cell lung cancer: correlation with lymph node metastasis. International journal of cancer, Vol. 105, No. pp. 186-189,

Tarin, D. & Croft, C.B. (1969). Ultrastructural features of wound healing in mouse skin. J Anat, Vol.105, No.Pt 1, pp. 189-190, ISSN 0021-8782

Taylor, M.A.;Parvani, J.G. & Schiemann, W.P. (2010). The pathophysiology of epithelial-mesenchymal transition induced by transforming growth factor-beta in normal and malignant mammary epithelial cells. Journal of mammary gland biology and neoplasia, Vol.15, No.2, pp. 169-190, ISSN 1573-7039

Tenney, R.M. & Discher, D.E. (2009). Stem cells, microenvironment mechanics, and growth factor activation. Curr Opin Cell Biol, Vol.21, No.5, pp. 630-635, ISSN 1879-0410

Tesarov_, P.; Kvasnika, J.; Umlaufov, A.; Homolkov, H.; Jirsa, M. & Tesar, V. (2000). Soluble TNF and IL-2 receptors in patients with breast cancer. Medical science monitor, Vol. 6, No. 4, pp. 661-664,

Thomasset, N.;Lochter, A.;Sympson, C.J.;Lund, L.R.;Williams, D.R.;Behrendtsen, O.;Werb, Z. & Bissell, M.J. (1998). Expression of autoactivated stromelysin-1 in mammary glands of transgenic mice leads to a reactive stroma during early development. The American journal of pathology, Vol.153, No.2, pp. 457-467, ISSN 0002-9440

Tlsty, T.D. (2001). Stromal cells can contribute oncogenic signals. Seminars in cancer biology, Vol. 11, No. 2, pp. 97-104, 1044-579X

Tlsty, T.D. & Hein, P.W. (2001). Know thy neighbor: stromal cells can contribute oncogenic signals. Current Opinion in Genetics & Development, Vol. 11, No. 1, pp. 54-59, 0959-437X

Tomasek, J.J.;Gabbiani, G.;Hinz, B.;Chaponnier, C. & Brown, R.A. (2002). Myofibroblasts and mechano-regulation of connective tissue remodelling. Nature reviews. Molecular cell biology, Vol.3, No.5, pp. 349-363, ISSN 1471-0072

Toullec, A.;Gerald, D.;Despouy, G.;Bourachot, B.;Cardon, M.;Lefort, S.;Richardson, M.;Rigaill, G.;Parrini, M.C.;Lucchesi, C.;Bellanger, D.;Stern, M.H.;Dubois, T.;Sastre-Garau, X.;Delattre, O.;Vincent-Salomon, A. & Mechta-Grigoriou, F. (2010). Oxidative stress promotes myofibroblast differentiation and tumor spreading. EMBO molecular medicine, Vol.2, No.6, pp. 211-230, ISSN 1757-4684

Valdivia-Silva, J.E.; Franco-Barraza, J.; Silva, A.L.; Pont, G.D.; Soldevila, G.; Meza, I. & Garcia-Zepeda, E.A. (2009). Effect of pro-inflammatory cytokine stimulation on human breast cancer: implications of chemokine receptor expression in cancer metastasis. Cancer letters, Vol. 283, No. 2, pp. 176-185, 1872-7980 (Electronic)

van Diest, P.J. & Baak, J.P. (1991). The morphometric prognostic index is the strongest prognosticator in premenopausal lymph node-negative and lymph node-positive breast cancer patients. Human pathology, Vol. 22, No. pp. 326-330,

Vishnu, P. & Roy, V. (2010). nab-paclitaxel: a novel formulation of taxane for treatment of breast cancer. Womens Health (Lond Engl), Vol.6, No.4, pp. 495-506, ISSN 1745-5065

Volk, L.D.;Flister, M.J.;Chihade, D.;Desai, N.;Trieu, V. & Ran, S. (2011). Synergy of Nab-paclitaxel and Bevacizumab in Eradicating Large Orthotopic Breast Tumors and Preexisting Metastases. Neoplasia, Vol.13, No.4, pp. 327-338, ISSN 1476-5586

Voorzanger, N.; Touitou, R.; Garcia, E.; Delecluse, H.-J.; Rousset, F.o.; Joab, I.n.; Favrot, M.C. & Blay, J.-Y. (1996). Interleukin (IL)-10 and IL-6 Are Produced in Vivo by Non-Hodgkin's Lymphoma Cells and Act as Cooperative Growth Factors. Cancer research, Vol. 56, No. 23, pp. 5499-5505,

Walker, R.A. & Dearing, S.J. (1992). Transforming growth factor beta 1 in ductal carcinoma in situ and invasive carcinomas of the breast. European journal of cancer, Vol.28, No.2-3, pp. 641-644, ISSN 0959-8049

Walker, R.A.;Dearing, S.J. & Gallacher, B. (1994). Relationship of transforming growth factor beta 1 to extracellular matrix and stromal infiltrates in invasive breast carcinoma. British journal of cancer, Vol.69, No.6, pp. 1160-1165, ISSN 0007-0920

Wang, J.; Xi, L.; Gooding, W.; Godfrey, T.E. & Ferris, R.L. (2005). Chemokine receptors 6 and 7 identify a metastatic expression pattern in squamous cell carcinoma of the head and neck. Advances in otorhinolaryngology, Vol. 62, No. pp. 121-133,

Wipff, P.J. & Hinz, B. (2008). Integrins and the activation of latent transforming growth factor beta1 - an intimate relationship. European journal of cell biology, Vol.87, No.8-9, pp. 601-615, ISSN 0171-9335

Wipff, P.J.;Rifkin, D.B.;Meister, J.J. & Hinz, B. (2007). Myofibroblast contraction activates latent TGF-beta1 from the extracellular matrix. The Journal of cell biology, Vol.179, No.6, pp. 1311-1323, ISSN 1540-8140

Wong, Y.C. & Tam, N.N. (2002). Dedifferentiation of stromal smooth muscle as a factor in prostate carcinogenesis. Differentiation, Vol.70, No.9-10, pp. 633-645, ISSN 0301-4681

Woodworth, C.D.; McMullin, E.; Iglesias, M. & Plowman, G.D. (1995). Interleukin 1 alpha and tumor necrosis factor alpha stimulate autocrine amphiregulin expression and proliferation of human papillomavirus-immortalized and carcinoma-derived cervical epithelial cells. Proceedings of the National Academy of Sciences, Vol. 92, No. 7, pp. 2840-2844,

Wu, Y.;Deng, J.;Rychahou, P.G.;Qiu, S.;Evers, B.M. & Zhou, B.P. (2009). Stabilization of snail by NF-kappaB is required for inflammation-induced cell migration and invasion. Cancer cell, Vol.15, No.5, pp. 416-428, ISSN 1878-3686

Xouri, G. & Christian, S. (2010). Origin and function of tumor stroma fibroblasts. Seminars in cell & developmental biology, Vol.21, No.1, pp. 40-46, ISSN 1096-3634

Xu, S.-G.; Yan, P.-J. & Shao, Z.-M. (2010). Differential proteomic analysis of a highly metastatic variant of human breast cancer cells using two-dimensional differential gel electrophoresis. Journal of Cancer Research and Clinical Oncology, Vol. 136, No. 10, pp. 1545-1556, 0171-5216

Yaal-Hahoshen, N.; Shina, S.; Leider-Trejo, L.; Barnea, I.; Shabtai, E.L.; Azenshtein, E.; Greenberg, I.; Keydar, I. & Ben-Baruch, A. (2006). The chemokine CCL5 as a potential prognostic factor predicting disease progression in stage II breast cancer patients. Clinical cancer research, Vol. 12, No. pp. 4474- 4480,

Yang, L.;Pang, Y. & Moses, H.L. (2010). TGF-beta and immune cells: an important regulatory axis in the tumor microenvironment and progression. Trends in immunology, Vol.31, No.6, pp. 220-227, ISSN 1471-4981

Zeisberg, E.M.;Potenta, S.;Xie, L.;Zeisberg, M. & Kalluri, R. (2007). Discovery of endothelial to mesenchymal transition as a source for carcinoma-associated fibroblasts. Cancer research, Vol.67, No.21, pp. 10123-10128, ISSN 1538-7445

Zhou, W.; Guo, S. & Gonzalez-Perez, R.R. (2011). Leptin pro-angiogenic signature in breast cancer is linked to IL-1 signalling. British journal of cancer, Vol. 104, No. 1, pp. 128-137, 0007-0920

Zlotnik, A. (2006). Chemokines and cancer. International journal of cancer, Vol. 119, No. 9, pp. 2026-2029,

Zlotnik, A. (2008). New insights on the role of CXCR4 in cancer metastasis. The Journal of pathology, Vol. 215, No. 3, pp. 211-213, ISSN 1096-9896

8

The Role of Fibrin(ogen) in Transendothelial Cell Migration During Breast Cancer Metastasis

Patricia J. Simpson-Haidaris[1], Brian J. Rybarczyk[2] and Abha Sahni[3]
[1]Department of Medicine, University of Rochester School of Medicine and Dentistry,
[2]Department of Biology, University of North Carolina at Chapel Hill,
[3]Aab Cardiovascular Research Institute, University of Rochester
School of Medicine and Dentistry,
USA

1. Introduction

Despite all the modern advances in treatment for breast cancer, metastatic disease remains the hurdle to surmount in curing breast cancer or, at least, in significantly reducing morbidity and mortality to improve long-term survival and quality of life. For over a century, inflammation and thrombosis have been linked to metastatic cancer (Boccaccio & Medico, 2006). In addition to being known for describing the factors leading to venous thromboembolism (alterations in blood flow, vascular endothelial injury, and hypercoagulability) as Virchow's triad, in 1863 Virchow noted a connection between chronic inflammation and cancer based on the recruitment of leukocytes to cancerous lesions (reviewed in (Balkwill & Mantovani, 2001)) (**Fig. 1**).

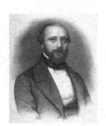

Trousseau's Syndrome

Described malignancy-associated hypercoagulable states and venous thromboembolism in cancer.

Hemostatic Factors

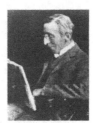

Rudolf Virchow
1863

Stephen Paget
1889

Inflammation in Cancer

Hypothesized that cancer originated at sites of chronic inflammation denoted by leukocyte infiltration.

Inflammatory cells, cytokines and chemokines

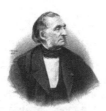

Armand Trousseau
1865

Seed and Soil Hypothesis

Suggested metastasis depends on cross-talk between cancer cells ('seeds') and microenvironment ('soil') of specific organs.

Extracellular matrix constituents, supporting cell populations

Fig. 1. The three faces of cancer metastasis. (Portraits obtained from public domain).

Rudolf Virchow, Armand Trousseau and Stephen Paget each provided valuable insight into the pathophysiology of invasive carcinomas—these theories still hold today to explain molecular mechanisms of cancer metastasis. Hypercoagulability is often diagnosed before identification of a coexisting malignancy, and is associated with increased thromboembolic risk (Sorensen et al., 2000). Armand Trousseau (Trousseau, 1865) (**Fig. 1**) identified and described the association between cancer and clot formation in 1865 and, shortly thereafter, self-identified these findings as a consequence of gastric cancer from which he later succumbed (Varki, 2007). Trousseau's Syndrome is associated with hypercoagulability and thromboembolic events in adenocarcinomas (Starakis et al., 2010). Another important contribution that has lead to better understanding of the mechanisms of cancer metastasis was provided by Stephen Paget in 1889 (Paget, 1889) when he propose the seed and soil concept of cancer metastasis (**Fig. 1**). By examining countless autopsy specimen from breast cancer patients, Paget determined that cancer cells, the "seed", had a preference to metastasize to distinct organs of the body based on favorable interactions with the stromal microenvironment, the "soil". As reviewed by Langley and Fiddler (Langley & Fidler, 2011), it is clear that cancer therapy is targeted to either the "seed" through chemotherapy with cytotoxic drugs or the "soil" by manipulating stromal contributions favorable to metastatic growth such as inhibiting angiogenesis.

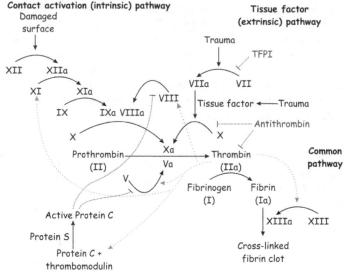

Fig. 2. Schematic view of intrinsic and extrinsic coagulation pathways.

Red lines denote pathway inhibitors of coagulation and green lines denote thrombin activation of hemostatic factors. (Reproduced from public domain image).

Appropriate activation of the clotting cascade is fundamental to arrest bleeding in response to vascular injury. The immediate response, known as primary hemostasis, involves vasoconstriction of blood vessels and activation and aggregation of platelets to form a plug at the site of vascular injury. Activated platelets release a panoply of stored constituents including: chemokines (IL-8) and growth factors such as platelet derived growth factor (PDGF), vascular endothelial growth factor (VEGF), fibroblast growth factor (FGF)-2 and transforming growth factor (TGF)-β; adhesive glycoproteins, including fibrinogen (Fg), fibronectin and von Willebrand factor; and lipid mediators such as lysophosphatidic acid, platelet-activating factor, leukotriene B_4, and thromboxanes. During secondary hemostasis, coagulation is activated either through the extrinsic pathway via tissue factor (TF)-Factor VII (FVII)/activated FVII (FVIIa) or the intrinsic pathway through Factor XII/FXIIa (**Fig. 2**). These pathways converge at the formation of the tenase complex that activates FX to FXa leading to thrombin activation. Thrombin cleaves soluble plasma Fg into fibrin monomers that form the insoluble fibrin clot after fibrin monomer polymerization and covalent crosslinking and stabilization by activated FXIII (FXIIIa). The fibrin clot provides a provisional matrix upon which injured endothelial cells adhere, proliferate and migrate to restore an intact endothelium lining blood vessels. Furthermore, fibrin and Fg provide a reservoir for sequestration of growth factors including FGF-2 (Sahni et al., 1998; Sahni et al., 1999), VEGF (Sahni & Francis, 2000), and TGF-β (Schachtrup et al., 2010), as well as an adhesive substrate for recruitment of leukocytes and stromal fibroblasts to aid in wound repair (Rybarczyk et al., 2003; Ugarova & Yakubenko, 2001). Normal wound repair is self-limiting as the provisional fibrin matrix is dissolved by various proteases, *e.g.*, plasmin, upon resolution of the vascular injury, reduction of inflammation and restoration of normal function (**Fig. 2**).

In the 1980s, however, Dvorak likened cancer progression to "wounds that never heal" in which Fg and fibrin also play prominent roles (Dvorak, 1986), and as reviewed by Coussens and Werb (Coussens & Werb, 2002). Several key steps in normal wound repair are also manifested during cancer progression (**Fig. 3**). As discussed above, a heighten state of coagulation occurs immediately after wound injury, and the release of chemokines and cytokines from activated platelets to recruit and activate proinflammatory cell types to the wound site amplify the inflammatory response system wide.

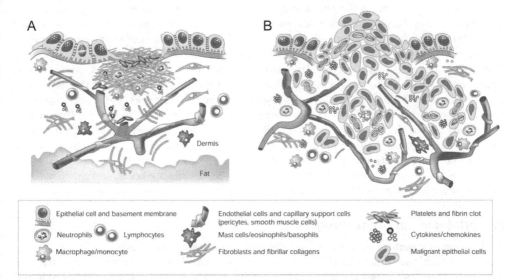

Fig. 3. Normal wound repair is depicted in panel A and mechanisms of wound repair left unchecked in cancer are depicted in Panel B. (Figure reprinted from (Coussens & Werb, 2002) with permission from Nature Publishing Group).

Systemic inflammation is best characterized by the innate acute phase response to injury or infection whereby the synthesis of a host of plasma proteins by the liver is altered to immediately respond to disruptions of homeostasis (Baumann & Gauldie, 1994). Of note, C-reactive protein and Fg are two positive (upregulated) acute phase proteins whose expression is also elevated in malignancies (Jones et al., 2006; Yamaguchi et al., 1998; Yigit et al., 2008). Coagulation and deposition of a provisional fibrin matrix occurs within minutes of vascular injury, and changes in expression of adhesion molecules on the surface of activated endothelium leads to the rolling and slowing of circulating leukocytes, firm attachment and the processes of diapedesis, *i.e.*, transmigration across the endothelial cell barrier into interstitial spaces. Neutrophils are the first proinflammatory cells to appear in the wound space where they release molecules to kill invading microorganisms and promote recruitment of stromal cells such as fibroblasts and endothelial cells to the wound space. Locally deposited growth factors promote cell proliferation and migration leading to the formation of granulation tissue over several days to a few weeks, which is the result of fibroblasts/myofibroblasts depositing extracellular matrix constituents (*e.g.*, collagens) and endothelial cells forming new blood vessels to facilitate would closure. In the case of cutaneous wounds, re-epithelialization begins to close the wound, the provisional fibrin matrix is dissolved, and infiltrating monocytes/macrophages clean up wound debris in preparation for matrix remodelling, deposition of a complete basement membrane (*e.g.*, laminin) and, over weeks to months, gradual restoration of the tensile strength of the tissue (Coussens & Werb, 2002). In contrast, the orderly array of signaling components that turn on and off cell migration, cell proliferation, and angiogenesis during wound repair goes array during cancer such that cell growth is unchecked, mechanisms of apoptosis are overridden and the stromal compartment is dramatically altered to perpetuate angiogenesis, tumor growth and cell migration to promote metastasis (**Fig. 3**).

Metastatic disease remains the prevailing reason for treatment failure and death from solid tumors including breast cancers. Only recently have three major areas of research outside the realm of the primary tumor cells themselves been considered viable for development of new therapeutic strategies to prevent the initiation, progression and metastasis of tumors. These include hemostatic factors, the tumor stromal microenvironment, and chronic inflammation. The blood coagulation protein Fg and its insoluble counterpart, fibrin, play central roles in inflammation, venous thromboembolism, and as components of the extracellular matrix. The goals of this chapter are three-fold: first, to review the current understanding of the roles of Fg and/or fibrin {commonly referred to as fibrin(ogen)} in cancer progression in general; second, to provide evidence that fibrin(ogen) likely plays a critical role in the metastatic spread of breast cancer; and third, to propose new therapies for treatment and future avenues of research to elucidate the molecular mechanisms that promote the phenotypic switch of breast epithelial cells to a metastatic cell phenotype.

2. Fibrin(ogen) in cancer progression

2.1 Hemostatic factors and vascular cells promote tumor metastasis

Molecules and cells linked to the prothrombotic state of Trousseau's syndrome that also facilitate cancer metastasis including thrombin, TF, selectins, platelets, endothelial cells and fibrin (Varki, 2007). It is well known that thrombin contributes to the severity of cancer progression by promoting tumor angiogenesis, cancer cell proliferation and metastasis by mechanisms other than just thrombin generation of fibrin (Nierodzik & Karpatkin, 2006).

Cell-associated TF expression by cancer cells correlates with disease severity and poor prognosis {reviewed in (Palumbo & Degen, 2007)}. Although tumor cell-associated TF expression is not required for the growth of primary tumors, it is necessary for their metastatic spread (Palumbo et al., 2007). Similarly, FXIII and Fg are important for the metastatic spread of tumor cells through both the circulation and lymphatic systems but not primary tumor growth (Palumbo et al., 2008; Palumbo & Degen, 2001; Palumbo & Degen, 2007; Palumbo et al., 2000; Palumbo et al., 2002; Palumbo et al., 2007; Palumbo et al., 2005). Moreover, FXIII, Fg and platelets are important substrates or cell targets for thrombin action demonstrating the critical role played by the hemostatic system in promoting cancer metastasis. Degen and colleagues suggest that tumor cell-associated TF mediates thrombin generation to support the early survival of micrometastases by at least two mechanisms: 1) the formation of platelet-fibrin microthrombi to protect newly formed micrometastases from natural killer (NK) cell-mediated cytotoxicity, and 2) by promoting mechanical stability of tumor cell emboli within vascular beds at distant metastatic sites (Palumbo et al., 2008; Palumbo & Degen, 2001; Palumbo & Degen, 2007; Palumbo et al., 2000; Palumbo et al., 2002; Palumbo et al., 2007; Palumbo et al., 2005).

2.2 Chronic inflammation is associated with cancer initiation and progression

Systemic inflammation is clearly linked with adverse prognosis in patients with cancer, and is characterized by elevated expression of pro-inflammatory mediators including interleukin (IL)-6 (Gao et al., 2007; Knupfer & Preiss, 2007). IL-6 is the major cytokine responsible for upregulation of specific plasma proteins in the liver during an acute phase response (Baumann & Gauldie, 1994), and also in chronic inflammation (Barton, 2001; Lin & Karin, 2007; Neurath & Finotto, 2011). IL-6 induces expression of target genes, including Fg, by activation of Stat3 (Duan & Simpson-Haidaris, 2003); Stat3 is often constitutively active in breast cancer, and tumor growth can become dependent on Stat3 signaling (Pensa et al., 2009). Both IL-6 and Fg levels are elevated in patients with advanced lung cancer (Yamaguchi et al., 1998). In breast cancer patients, serum IL-6 correlates with increasing numbers of involved sites, liver metastasis, and disease progression (Knupfer & Preiss, 2007; Salgado et al., 2003). In 2002, Drix et al demonstrated that IL-6, VEGF and D-dimer levels are elevated in patients with progressive breast cancer; these markers correlate positively with disease severity, and serum IL-6 is an independent prognostic factor in patients with metastatic disease (Dirix et al., 2002). Elevated levels of Fg, D-dimers, IL-6, VEGF and soluble P-selectin, an indicator of platelet activation, were also found in the plasma of breast cancer patients by Caine et al, who furthered demonstrated that IL-6 induces dose-dependent release of VEGF from platelets in vitro (Caine et al., 2004). Steinbrecher et al demonstrated a direct link between fibrin(ogen), elevated IL-6 levels and the development of inflammation-driven cancer using a mouse model of colitis-associated cancer (Steinbrecher et al., 2010). IL-6 serves as a marker to predict which patients will respond poorly to anti-endocrine chemotherapy (Zhang & Adachi, 1999), as a marker of tumor staging and a predictor of micrometastases (Ravishankaran & Karunanithi, 2011). IL-6 also induces VEGF expression (Cohen et al., 1996) and invasion and migration of breast cancer cells (Walter et al., 2009). Furthermore, overexpression of Her2 in breast cancer cells upregulates IL-6 leading to Stat3 activation and altered gene expression resulting in an autocrine feedback loop promoting cell survival (Hartman et al., 2011). Together, these reports substantiate the importance of fibrin(ogen) and inflammation in cancer metastasis.

2.3 Fibrin(ogen) functions as a bridging molecule in cell-cell interactions during coagulation and inflammatory cell trafficking

Excessive fibrin deposition is accompanied by local expression of proinflammatory mediators, vascular leakage, and inflammatory cell recruitment and activation, leading to amplification of the inflammatory response (Clark, 1996; Simpson-Haidaris & Rybarczyk, 2001; van Hinsbergh et al., 2001). Specific structural features of fibrin(ogen) modulate the functions of a variety of different cell types including endothelial, epithelial, leukocytes, platelets and fibroblasts (**Fig. 4**). Cell receptors that bind to fibrin(ogen) include: β3 integrins (αIIbβ3 and αvβ3) (Bennett et al., 2009); β2 integrins (CD11a/CD18 and CD11b/CD18) (Altieri et al., 1993; Flick et al., 2004; Lishko et al., 2004; Loike et al., 1991; Ugarova et al., 2003; Yakovlev et al., 2005); and β1 integrin, α5β1 (Asakura et al., 1997; Suehiro et al., 1997). Nonintegrin adhesion molecules that bind to fibrin(ogen) include intercellular adhesion molecule (ICAM)-1 (Languino et al., 1993; Pluskota & D'Souza, 2000), vascular endothelial (VE)-cadherin (Bach et al., 1998b) and heparan sulfate proteoglycans (HSPG) (Odrljin et al., 1996a; Odrljin et al., 1996b). Fibrin(ogen) also modulates a number of signaling molecules important in innate immunity. Fg-bound FGF-2 induces expression of uPA, uPA receptor and PAI-1, and fibrin(ogen) induce IL-8, MCP-1 or IL-1β expression in endothelial cells (Guo et al., 2004; Harley & Powell, 1999; Kuhns et al., 2001; Lee et al., 2001; Qi & Kreutzer, 1995; Ramsby & Kreutzer, 1994; Sahni et al., 2004). Fg and fibrin activate NF-κB and AP-1 (Guo et al., 2004; Sitrin et al., 1998), transcription factors critical for propagation of inflammation.

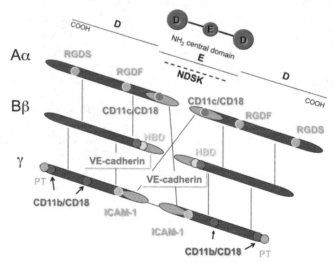

Fig. 4. Fibrin(ogen) enzyme and CNBr cleavage fragments and cell recognition domains.

Fg Aα, Bβ and γ chains are held together by 29 pairs of disulfide bonds (approximated by the vertical lines) with the N-termini of all six chains held together in the central domain. Electron microscopy studies indicate that the dimeric Fg molecule appears as a trinodular structure as depicted by the red ball and stick cartoon. Thrombin release of fibrinopeptides, FPA and FPB, from Aα and Bβ N-termini, respectively, produces soluble fibrin leading to fibrin polymerization into an insoluble gel stabilized by FXIIIA-mediated crosslinks between γ-γ and α-γ chains. Lines below the ball and stick cartoon denote N-terminal plasmin cleavage fragment E and C-terminal fragments D. N-terminal disulfide knot (NDSK) (dashed line) is the minimal sequence of the central domain after CNBr cleavage and is structurally similar to plasmin E fragment. Residues on Fg for receptor-cell binding domains are: CD11c/CD18, $A\alpha^{17-19}$; integrin RGDF, $A\alpha^{95-98}$ and RGDS, $A\alpha^{572-575}$; ICAM-1, $\gamma^{117-133}$; CD11b/CD18, $\gamma^{190-202}$, $\gamma^{228-253}$ and $\gamma^{390-396}$; platelet (PT) binding, $\gamma^{400-411}$. The heparin binding domain (HBD) at β^{15-42} overlaps the VE-cadherin binding site. The first fibrin degradation products (FDPs) released by plasmin cleavage are the β^{15-42} domain and the C-terminal 2/3rd of the $A\alpha$ chain, termed αC, which contain several cell binding domains.

2.4 Fibrin(ogen) in the stromal microenvironment in breast cancer

The tumor microenvironment is a complex entity composed not only of extracellular matrix (ECM) constituents including: i) growth factors; ii) cytokines and chemokines; iii) proteases; and iv) matrix glycoproteins, glycosaminoglycans and proteoglycans—but also diverse cell populations that influence the behavior of cancer cells including: v) immune cells such as lymphocytes, NK cells, dendritic cells, macrophages and neutrophils; vi) stromal fibroblasts/myofibroblasts, adipocytes and stem cells; and vii) cells of the vasculature including endothelial cells, pericytes and smooth muscle cells (reviewed in (Andre et al., 2010; Anton & Glod, 2009; De Wever et al., 2008; Deryugina & Quigley, 2006; Tlsty & Coussens, 2006; Ulisse et al., 2009)). Although activated inflammatory cells in the tumor microenvironment play important roles in cancer initiation, progression, angiogenesis and metastasis, they are not the most numerous. Cancer-associated fibroblasts, similar to myofibroblasts of healing wounds, are the most abundant stromal cells in the tumor microenvironment (Tlsty & Coussens, 2006), and contribute significantly to chronic inflammation by production of chemokines, cytokines, and pro-angiogenic factors and deposition of matrix constituents that support new blood vessel formation required for tumor growth, cell migration and metastasis (De Wever et al., 2008). Solid tumors need to develop their own blood supply for nutrient delivery and removal of toxic waste. Angiogenesis, the formation of new blood vessels from existing vasculature, requires activation of proteases leading to degradation of the basement membrane, endothelial cell sprouting and pericyte attachment for vessel stabilization. Cancer-associated fibroblasts play an important role in synchronizing these events (De Wever et al., 2008). Furthermore, the topography of the ECM mediates vascular development and regulates the speed at which cells migrate during angiogenesis (Bauer et al., 2009). Vascular endothelial cells play a pivotal role in regulating leukocyte recruitment during inflammation (McGettrick et al., 2007). In most cases, cancers exploit pro-inflammatory mediators and recruited inflammatory cells to benefit their own survival (Lorusso & Ruegg, 2008) (also as reviewed in (Simpson-Haidaris et al., 2010)).

Fg and fibrin deposition is found within the stroma of most solid tumors (Simpson-Haidaris & Rybarczyk, 2001), and elevated levels of plasma Fg and fibrin degradation products (FDPs) correlate positively with lymph node involvement and metastatic spread of colorectal, ovarian, lung and breast cancers (Sahni et al., 2009; Varki, 2007). Fibrin deposition at the tumor-normal host cell interface as well as in the stroma of primary tumors is well documented, and is thought to protect tumors from infiltrating inflammatory cells by acting as a barrier thereby preventing inflammatory reactions directed towards the tumor cells (reviewed in (Simpson-Haidaris & Rybarczyk, 2001)). The presence of D-dimer, a fibrin degradation product indicative of pathological fibrin formation and dissolution, correlates with poor prognosis in most solid tumors including colon, prostate, lung and breast (Batschauer et al., 2010; Kilic et al., 2008; Knowlson et al., 2010). However, in some malignancies, including breast, evidence demonstrating deposition of fibrin within the primary tumor is lacking (reviewed in (Simpson-Haidaris & Rybarczyk, 2001)). Instead, abundant Fg deposition occurs in breast tumor stroma in the absence of thrombin generation (Costantini et al., 1991).

2.5 Cancer cells, including breast, synthesize and secrete fibrinogen

The origin of tumor-associated fibrin(ogen) and fibrin(ogen) degradation products has historically been thought to be from exudation of plasma Fg due to the increased vascular permeability and subsequent procoagulant or fibrinolytic activity at the tumor site (Rybarczyk & Simpson-Haidaris, 2000). However, because Fg deposition in the stroma, but not fibrin formation, is considered a hallmark of breast cancer (Costantini et al., 1991), we hypothesized that breast cancer cells were capable of endogenous synthesis and secretion of Fg. We demonstrated that human MCF-7 cells are capable of synthesizing Fg chains, although assembly of intact Fg is defective due to degradation of the Bβ chain (Rybarczyk & Simpson-Haidaris, 2000). In addition, we have shown that lung, prostate and breast cancer epithelial cells synthesize and secrete Fg that enhances FGF-2-mediated cell proliferation, assembles into the ECM and binds to cancer cell surface receptors (Rybarczyk & Simpson-Haidaris, 2000; Sahni et al., 2008; Simpson-Haidaris, 1997; Simpson-Haidaris & Rybarczyk, 2001). Others have shown Fg production in cervical (Lee et al., 1996) and intestinal (Molmenti et al., 1993) cancer cell lines. Expression array profiling studies confirmed that Fg genes are expressed in breast (Pentecost et al., 2005) and lung carcinomas (Tan et al., 2005) from patients. Thus, Fg synthesized by cancer cells promotes growth of the primary tumor and supports tumor-associated angiogenesis characterized by localized VEGF production and leaky vessels (Dvorak, 2006). The importance of VEGF in promoting tumor vascular permeability, angiogenesis and leakage of plasma Fg into the perivascular space to induce tumor stroma desmoplasia is well known. However, whether *tumor-associated fibrin(ogen)* contributes to permeability of tumor vessels and breast cancer metastasis is unknown.

2.6 Fibrinogen is an extracellular matrix protein

Although Fg is known for its hemostatic role, we showed that Fg, not fibrin, is a component of the insoluble fibrillar ECM of fibroblasts, alveolar epithelial cells, endothelial cells and breast epithelial cells (Guadiz et al., 1997; Pereira et al., 2002; Sahni et al., 2009; Simpson-Haidaris et al., 2010; Simpson-Haidaris & Sahni, 2010). Upon assembly into matrix fibrils, Fg undergoes conformational changes exposing the cryptic β^{15-42} epitope in the absence of thrombin cleavage or covalent crosslinking (Guadiz et al., 1997; Simpson-Haidaris & Sahni, 2010). When Fg is pre-established in the ECM of adventitial fibroblasts prior to wounding, increased cell proliferation and migration enhance wound closure (Rybarczyk et al., 2003), which is dependent on *de novo* protein synthesis (Pereira & Simpson-Haidaris, 2001) but independent of added growth factors, PDGF and FGF-2 (Rybarczyk et al., 2003). However, assembly of Fg into mature matrix fibrils of breast epithelial cells appears to correlate negatively with the increasing invasive potential of the cell (**Fig. 5**). We also determined whether the cryptic HBD in soluble Fg (Odrljin et al., 1996b) was accessible in matrix Fg using a specific MoAb (T2G1) (Kudryk et al., 1984). Whereas the T2G1 epitope (β^{15-21}) within β^{15-42} is not accessible for antibody binding in soluble Fg or Fg immobilized to a surface, the results indicated that $\beta^{15\text{-}21}$ is exposed on Fg assembled into matrix fibrils (Guadiz et al., 1997; Rybarczyk et al., 2003). Together these data suggest that matrix Fg possesses "fibrin-like" properties in the absence of fibrin polymerization and that Fg deposition rapidly changes the topology of the ECM to provide a surface for cell migration and matrix remodeling during wound repair. However, the mechanisms by which $\beta^{15\text{-}42}$ modulates cell-cell or cell-matrix adhesion are not well understood.

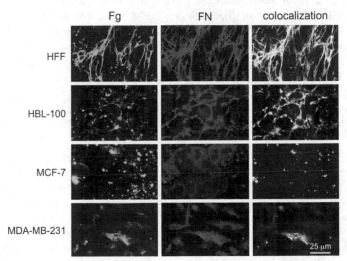

Fig. 5. Plasma fibrinogen assembles into mature matrix fibrils of nonmalinant cells (HFF and HBL-100) but poorly assembles in the matrix of malignant breast cancer cells (MCF-7 and MDA-MB-231). Primary human fibroblasts (HFF), a nonmalignant human breast cancer cell line (HBL-100) and two human breast cancer cell lines (MCF-7 and MDA-MB-231) were grown on gelatin-coated glass coverslips and treated with Fg conjugated to Oregon Green™ (30 µg/ml) for 24 hr. The cells were washed, fixed, stained with anti-fibronectin (FN) polyclonal antibodies followed by rhodamine-goat anti-rabbit secondary antibodies, and visualized by epifluorescence microscopy. Green fluorescence is Fg-specific and red fluorescence denotes FN staining. Colocalization of Fg and FN results in yellow fluorescence. The loss of FN in the more invasive cell lines (MCF-7 and MDA-MB-231) is likely an explanation for purified plasma Fg binding to the surface of cells but failure to assembly into mature matrix fibrils, as we have shown that assembly of Fg into an elaborate fibrillar ECM depends on the assembly of FN fibrils as well (Pereira et al., 2002).

3. Role of Fibrin(ogen) in breast cancer metastasis

3.1 Importance of Fg peptide $\beta^{15\text{-}42}$ in Fg-endothelial cell interactions

Fibrin(ogen) $\beta^{15\text{-}42}$ sequences support a diverse array of biological functions mediated by fibrin(ogen). Although the primary structure of fibrinopeptide B (FPB) is poorly conserved across species, the fibrin $\beta^{15\text{-}42}$ domain is highly conserved, implying evolutionary conservation of function (Courtney et al., 1994). The $\beta^{15\text{-}42}$ region constitutes a cryptic domain in soluble Fg that is exposed in fibrin after thrombin cleavage (Odrljin et al., 1996b). Both the HBD and overlapping binding site for VE-cadherin are localized to $\beta^{15\text{-}42}$. VE-cadherin mediates homophilic cell-cell adhesion critical for the maintenance of barrier integrity of the endothelium. Disruption of VE-cadherin-mediated endothelial barrier function leads to altered vascular permeability found in a number of diseases including ischemia-reperfusion (IR) injury, inflammation, angiogenesis, and cancer growth and metastasis (discussed in (Sahni et al., 2009)). Exposure of β^{15-42} and binding by VE-cadherin is also required for endothelial capillary tube formation in fibrin gels (Bach et al., 1998a; Chalupowicz et al., 1995); portions of the third extracellular domain (EC3) of VE-cadherin constitute a fibrin β^{15-42} receptor (Bach et al., 1998b; Yakovlev & Medved, 2009). Newly exposed β chain residues, β15-GHRP-18, play a critical role in fibrin monomer aggregation during polymerization and clot formation during secondary hemostasis (Mosesson, 2005). Furthermore, exposure of the β^{15-42} domain mediates heparin-dependent fibrin binding to endothelial cell surfaces (Odrljin et al., 1996a); promotes endothelial cell adhesion and spreading (Bunce et al., 1992); promotes the release of endothelial cell-specific markers of endothelial activation (Ribes et al., 1989); and stimulates proliferation of endothelial cells, fibroblasts and cancer cells (Rybarczyk et al., 2003; Sahni et al., 2008; Sporn et al., 1995).

3.2 Fibrin β^{15-42} protects the myocardium from Ischemic-Reperfusion (IR) injury

A synthetic peptide of fibrin residues β^{15-42} has been implicated as a potential therapeutic agent to reduce tissue damage and scarring after a heart attack (Hirschfield & Pepys, 2003; Petzelbauer et al., 2005b; Roesner et al., 2007; Zacharowski et al., 2006; Zacharowski et al., 2007). Peptide β^{15-42} works by inhibiting leukocyte migration across the endothelium into heart tissue, which prevents excessive inflammation and tissue damage. Peptide β^{15-42}-mediated reduction of tissue injury depends on its ability to bind to VE-cadherin. Peptide β^{15-42} competes with FDP (*e.g.*, the plasmin E domain of fibrin as depicted in **Fig. 4**) for binding to VE-cadherin to prevent transendothelial cell migration (TEM) of leukocytes during myocardial IR injury (Petzelbauer et al., 2005b; Roesner et al., 2007; Zacharowski et al., 2006; Zacharowski et al., 2007). These published reports demonstrate the physiologic efficacy of fibrin β^{15-42} for treating IR injury. *However, the molecular mechanisms induced by fibrin(ogen) β^{15-42} binding to VE-cadherin to mediate enhanced paracellular permeability and whether fibrinogen-induced cancer metastasis involves binding interactions with fibrin(ogen) β^{15-42} have not been previously studied.*

3.3 Fibrin(ogen) β^{15-42} induces endothelial barrier permeability via VE-cadherin binding interactions

In a recent report (Sahni et al., 2009), we sought to determine whether fibrin(ogen) β^{15-42} binding to VE-cadherin induced endothelial cell permeability, and whether fibrinogen-induced cancer metastasis involves binding interactions between VE-cadherin and fibrin(ogen) β^{15-42}. Using transwell insert culture systems, we showed that Fg β^{15-42} and VE-cadherin binding interactions promote endothelial cell barrier permeability (Sahni et al., 2009) (**Fig. 6**). Peptides containing or missing residues β15-17 critical for β^{15-42} binding to VE-cadherin (Gorlatov & Medved, 2002) and neutralizing antibodies that bind to Fg β15-21 (T2G1) and VE-cadherin (BV9) (**Fig. 7A**) were used to induce or inhibit permeability. Fg induced dose-dependent permeability of human umbilical vein endothelial cells (HUVEC) and microvascular endothelial cells (HMEC-1) (**Fig. 6**), but not epithelial cell barriers (as shown in Fig. 1 in ref (Sahni et al., 2009)), which could be inhibited by neutralizing antibodies against β15-21 (T2G1) and VE-cadherin (BV9) and synthetic peptides (not shown).

However, the neutralizing antibodies (T2G1 and BV9) did not completely inhibit Fg-induced permeability (**Fig. 7B**), suggesting that additional cell recognition domains on Fg participate in fibrin(ogen)-induced vascular permeability.

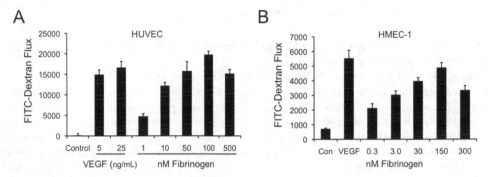

Fig. 6. Fg-induced EC permeability involves Fg β^{15-42} and VE-cadherin. Cells were grown to confluency on Millicell™ 24-well cell culture inserts. Panel 6A, HUVEC were left untreated (control) or treated for 15 min with increasing concentrations of Fg or VEGF as indicated. Panel 6B, HUVEC were treated with 30 nM of Fg plus 1 mg/ml FITC-Dextran for the times indicated. The FITC-Dextran flux to the bottom chamber was measured by fluorometry and the data presented as the mean relative FITC-Dextran Flux ± SEM. Data points were derived from 3 or more independent experiments with the total number of replicates per condition ranging from 6-13. (Reprinted from (Sahni et al., 2009) with permission). P-values can be found in ref (Sahni et al., 2009).

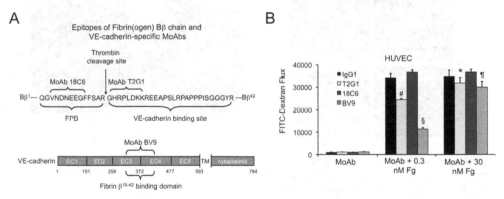

Fig. 7. Fg-induced EC permeability involves Fg β^{15-42} sequences and VE-cadherin. Panel 7A, schematics of the aminoterminus of the fibrin(ogen) Bβ chain and the domain structure of VE-cadherin are depicted. The arrow denotes the thrombin cleavage site for release of FPB. The 18C6 epitope maps to FPB, the T2G1 epitope maps to β^{15-21} and the VE-cadherin binding site on fibrin maps to β^{15-42}. The epitope of the VE-cadherin-specific monoclonal antibody BV9 maps to the third and fourth extracellular domains (EC3-EC4). The fibrin β^{15-42} binding site on VE cadherin maps to EC3 near the EC3-EC4 junction. TM, transmembrane domain. Panel 7B, all monoclonal antibodies used are IgG$_1$ isotype murine antibodies and

nonimmune IgG$_1$ was used for the control. Monoclonal antibodies were used at 3 nM in the absence of Fg, or with 0.3 nM or 30 nM Fg for 45 min. The data were plotted as the mean ± SEM of relative FITC-Dextran Flux and were obtained from three independent experiments with a total sample size of 6-9 per condition. (Reprinted from (Sahni et al., 2009) with permission). P-values can be found in ref (Sahni et al., 2009).

3.4 VE-cadherin binding domain of Fg (β^{15-42}) enhances transendothelial migration of malignant breast epithelial cells

Because plasma Fg promotes metastasis of some types of cancer and Fg β^{15-42} sequences promote endothelial cell permeability, we hypothesized Fg β^{15-42} sequences would play a role in promoting TEM of breast cancer cells. To test this hypothesis, breast cancer cells were labeled with a fluorescence cell-tracking dye (DiI) before they were mixed with increasing concentrations Fg. Breast cancer cells and Fg were allowed to pre-incubate for 15 minutes prior to addition to the upper chamber of a barrier monolayer of endothelial cells. After 45 minutes incubation, the relative number of breast cancer cells migrating to the underside of the transwell insert membrane were quantified by relative fluorescence and

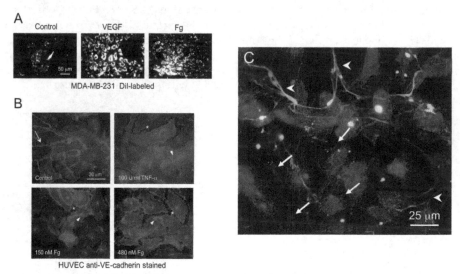

Fig. 8. Fg enhances TEM of malignant breast epithelial cells (Panel A), induces gap formation between adjacent endothelial cells (Panel B, asterisks), promotes intracellular relocalization (Panel B, arrowheads) of VE-cadherin at membrane cell-cell junctions (Panel B, Control, arrow), assembles into ECM (Panel C, arrowhead), and shows punctate, cell surface receptor-like binding between adjacent endothelial cells (Panel C, arrows). Cells in Panels A and B were treated as described in Section 3.3. In Panel C, endothelial cells were treated for 24 hours with purified plasma Fg conjugated to Oregon Green. Cells were fixed, permeabilized and stained with anti-FGF-2 (red fluoresence). After staining, the coverslip was mounted upside down on a microscope slide so that the basolateral aspect (bottom of cells) and the subendothelial ECM appear as the "top" of the cells. Matrix Fg and receptor bound Fg are shown in green fluorescence. Cover Figure ref (Sahni et al., 2009).

visualized by microscopy. VEGF was used as a positive control to induce endothelial cell permeability and TEM of breast cancer cells. The results indicated that TEM of both MCF-7 and MDA-MB-231 cells was increased in a Fg-concentration-dependent manner (see Fig. 3a of ref (Sahni et al., 2009)) and as visualized by immunofluorescence microscopy showing MDA-MB-231 cells adhered to the bottom side of the transwell filter (**Fig. 8A**).

To determine whether VE-cadherin and/or Fg β[15-42] were involved in Fg-enhanced TEM of MDA-MB-231 cells, the assay was repeated in the presence of the neutralizing and control antibodies (as shown in Fig. 3c of ref (Sahni et al., 2009)). To determine whether Fg promoted gap formation between cells, confluent HUVEC were treated with 150 or 480 nM Fg or 100 Units/ml TNF-α, a known inducer of endothelial permeability and gap formation, for 30 minutes then cells were fixed, permeabilized and immunostained with an anti-VE-cadherin. Fg treatment induced gap formation between adjacent endothelial cells, and such treatment promoted the subcellular relocalization of VE-cadherin from the cell periphery as in control cells into the cytoplasm in Fg- and TNF-α-treated cells (**Fig. 8B**). Indirect evidence for Fg binding at endothelial cell-cell junctions was obtained by fluorescence microscopy. The data reveal that Fg binds to endothelial cell-cell junctions in a punctate pattern, consistent with cell surface receptor binding to the cell-cell adhesion receptor, VE-cadherin (**Fig. 8C, arrows**). Fg also assembles as part of the fibrillar subendothelial ECM (**Fig. 8C, arrowhead**). Taken together, the data in **Fig. 6-8** demonstrate that the VE-cadherin binding domain defined by residues 15-42 on the β-chain of human Fg induces permeability of endothelial but not epithelial cell barriers and enhances TEM of malignant breast cancer cells by a VE-cadherin-dependent mechanism. In contrast, the basal level of TEM of nonmalignant breast epithelial cells was not enhanced by Fg treatment (Sahni et al., 2009).

3.5 Fibrinogen potentiates endothelial cell permeability at low doses of VEGF

Both FGF-2 and VEGF bind to fibrin(ogen) at distinct sites with high affinity (Sahni & Francis, 2000; Sahni et al., 1998). Fg bound-FGF-2 potentiates endothelial cell proliferation over FGF-2 alone (Sahni et al., 2003; Sahni & Francis, 2004; Sahni et al., 2006; Sahni et al., 1999). Although Fg-bound VEGF remains active, it does not potentiate endothelial cell proliferation over VEGF alone (Sahni & Francis, 2000). Because Fg induces endothelial cell permeability through VE-cadherin binding interactions (Sahni et al., 2009) and VEGF binds to Fg (Sahni & Francis, 2000), we tested the hypothesis that Fg would potentiate VEGF-induced EC permeability (**Fig. 9**).

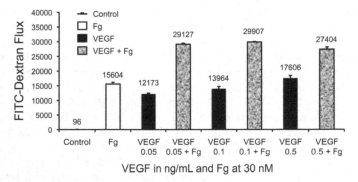

Fig. 9. Fg enhances permeability induced by low concentrations of VEGF.

The data indicate that 10 μg/ml (30 nM) Fg enhanced the flux of FITC-dextran to the bottom chamber of the transwell plate at low doses of VEGF (0.05 and 0.1 ng/ml); however, the additive effect on induction of endothelial cell permeability was lost at 0.5 ng/ml and higher concentrations of VEGF (**Fig. 9**). Fg-enhancement of VEGF-induced permeability is rapid and saturated within 5 min, whereas 5 ng/ml of VEGF is required to induce a similar amount of FITC-dextran flux as 30 nM Fg + 0.05 ng/ml, *i.e.*, 100-fold less VEGF. Studies by others suggest that low-dose VEGF mediates inflammation to promote cell survival of vascular and nonvascular cells such as those of the CNS, prior to induction of angiogenesis (Abumiya et al., 2005; Croll et al., 2004). Furthermore, VEGF colocalizes with exuded Fg at sites of edema in renal cell carcinoma (Verheul et al., 2010). Together with the aforementioned published data, our results suggest that Fg may regulate vascular permeability induced by low doses of VEGF without inducing EC proliferation—such a response would be conducive to fibrinogen induction of breast cancer cell TEM.

4. Summary, therapeutic strategies and future research to elucidate fibrin(ogen)-mediated mechanisms of breast cancer metastasis

4.1 Summary and therapeutic strategy using free peptide $\beta^{15\text{-}42}$ to inhibit breast cancer metastasis as depicted in Fig. 10, Steps 1-11

Regardless of the subtype of breast cancer, once the primary tumor becomes established (*Step 1*), it needs to develop its own blood supply for nutrient delivery and removal of toxic waste (*Step 2*). Breast cancer cells produce VEGF, which initiates permeability of nearby blood vessels allowing plasma Fg to leak into the tumor stroma promoting desmoplasia and deposition of a provisional fibrin(ogen) matrix in the tumor microenvironment (*Step 2*). Alternatively, endogenous synthesis of Fg by breast cancer cells could induce cancer progression. Thus, the innate immune response is activated to defend the host against this neoplastic insult. Release of IL-6 systemically leads to increased production of plasma Fg and fibrin formation resulting in exposure of $\beta^{15\text{-}42}$ and binding to VE-cadherin, a step critical for angiogenesis (Bach et al., 1998b; Martinez et al., 2001). Furthermore, VEGF binds to Fg and fibrin with high affinity (Sahni & Francis, 2000), which may be necessary for Fg to enhance VEGF-mediated endothelial cell permeability without potentiating endothelial cell proliferation. In contrast, VE-cadherin and VEGF receptor-2 form a signaling complex to promote endothelial cell proliferation (Carmeliet et al., 1999; Dejana, 2004; Esser et al., 1998). Fibrin(ogen) potentiates FGF-2- but not VEGF-induced proliferation of endothelial cells, angiogenesis and cancer cell growth (Rybarczyk & Simpson-Haidaris, 2000; Sahni & Francis, 2000; Sahni et al., 2006; Sahni et al., 2008; Sahni et al., 1999; Simpson-Haidaris, 1997; Simpson-Haidaris & Rybarczyk, 2001). Furthermore, fibrin(ogen) enhances cell migration and cancer invasion through tumor stroma, and TEM, *i.e.*, intravasation of breast cancer cells into the blood stream (*Step 3*) (Roche et al., 2003; Rybarczyk et al., 2003; Sahni et al., 2009). Fg and fibrin can bridge between cells of the same or different kinds (Kloczewiak et al., 1983; Languino et al., 1995; Languino et al., 1993; Saito et al., 2002; Sriramarao et al., 1996) and form aggregates or tumor emboli coated with fibrin(ogen) (*Step 4*). Because the host immune system does not recognize fibrin(ogen)-coated tumor emboli (Palumbo et al., 2005), immune-mediated destruction of tumor cells does not occur and these tumor emboli travel through the circulation to sites favorable for metastatic growth (*Steps 5 & 6*) such as lung. To establish metastatic growth, tumor emboli need to leave the circulation and enter lung tissue (*Steps 7 and 8*) where they find a receptive niche (*Step 9*) to begin the process again. Tumor cell proliferation and angiogenesis (*Step 10*) in lung results in metastatic disease (*Step 11*). We *hypothesize* that free peptide β^{15-42} will bind to VE-cadherin between endothelial cells to block endothelial cell binding to β^{15-42} on intact fibrin(ogen) found in the tumor stroma or tumor vessels, thereby inhibiting tumor-associated angiogenesis (*Step 2*), intravasation (*Step 3*), extravasation (*Step 8*), and angiogenesis at metastatic tumor sites (*Step 10*) (**as denoted by the lightening bolts at these steps in Fig. 10**).

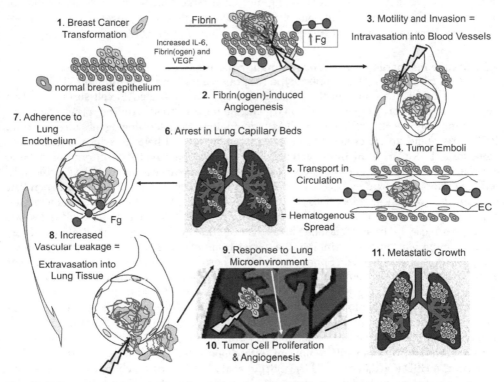

Fig. 10. Schematic summarizing role of fibrin(ogen) β^{15-42} in breast cancer metastasis and hypothesis development for employing free peptide β^{15-42} as a therapeutic strategy to treat metastatic breast cancers.

Successful demonstration of peptide β^{15-42} as an inhibitor of breast cancer metastasis and tumor-associated inflammation and angiogenesis *in vivo* would significantly impact breast cancer treatment in a timely manner. Peptide β^{15-42}, an endogenous fragment of fibrin, is already shown to be well tolerated in humans and effective in reducing damage to heart muscle after a heart attack in preclinical models of IR injury. However, until now, no one has proposed the use of peptide β^{15-42} as an inhibitor of breast cancer metastasis. A precedent and pipeline for production of viable therapeutics based on peptide β^{15-42} exists for treatment of damaged heart tissue, and Phase I and Phase II clinical trials are ongoing to test the safety and efficacy, respectively, of free β^{15-42} peptide for IR injury (Hallen et al., 2010; Petzelbauer et al., 2005a; Petzelbauer et al., 2005b; Roesner et al., 2007; Roesner et al., 2009; Wiedemann et al., 2010; Zacharowski et al., 2006). Therefore, the timeline for successful translational to a therapeutic agent to treat metastatic disease in breast cancer patients with different subtypes of the disease would be significantly shortened. Moreover, even if the primary tumor develops its own blood supply before adjuvant therapy with peptide $\beta^{15\text{-}42}$ is begun, we predict that free peptide $\beta^{15\text{-}42}$ will prevent subsequent steps required for metastatic spread and growth of breast cancers. Another advantage to this therapeutic strategy is that peptide $\beta^{15\text{-}42}$ functions outside the cell, precluding the need to deliver the peptide inside cells. Identifying molecular targets for therapeutic intervention of breast cancer metastasis, recruitment of inflammatory cells and angiogenesis will increase long-term disease-free survival and improve the quality of life for breast cancer patients.

4.2 Putative mechanisms whereby nonmalignant breast epithelial cells switch to a metastatic breast cancer cell phenotype responsive to fibrinogen induced TEM

A class of molecules found in the ECM, inside cells and attached to cell surfaces, called heparan sulfate proteoglycans (HSPG), contribute to breast cancer progression by promoting cancer cell proliferation, TEM, and tumor-associated angiogenesis (Koo et al., 2008). The ability to affect any one of these functions would help to reduce breast cancer metastasis; however, if all three of the functions could be targeted with one therapeutic approach, the morbidity and mortality due to metastatic breast cancer could be significantly reduced. Heparin is widely used as an anticoagulant, but it also inhibits HSPG-dependent mechanisms of cancer metastasis (Levy-Adam et al., 2005). However, anti-metastatic heparins that also inhibit blood coagulation are, therefore, not good candidates for widespread use to treat metastatic breast cancer due to bleeding complications. Thus, another molecular target to inhibit the prometastatic effects of HSPG but not inhibit coagulation is greatly needed. Spontaneous blood-borne and lymphatic metastasis of tumor emboli requires fibrin(ogen) (Palumbo et al., 2002). In addition to binding to VE-cadherin (Yakovlev et al., 2003), Fg $\beta^{15\text{-}42}$ also binds to heparin and HSPG on endothelial cells with high affinity (Odrljin et al., 1996a; Odrljin et al., 1996b); however, a role for HSPG in Fg-mediated breast cancer metastasis has not been studied. Fg binding to heparin and HSPG involves residues $\beta^{15\text{-}42}$, and $\beta^{15\text{-}42}$-dependent fibrin binding to EC surfaces can be inhibited with heparin and heparan sulfate but not with chondroitin sulfate, indicating that Fg-$\beta^{15\text{-}42}$ represents a HBD (Odrljin et al., 1996a; Odrljin et al., 1996b). The Fg HBD was later mapped to residues $\beta^{15\text{-}57}$, which includes the $\beta^{15\text{-}42}$ VE-cadherin binding domain (Yakovlev et al., 2003; Yakovlev & Medved, 2009). In our recent publication (Sahni et al., 2009), we unexpectedly discovered that Fg enhanced TEM of only malignant breast cancer cells (MCF-7 and MDA-MB-231) but not nonmalignant breast epithelial cells (MCF-10A), suggesting inherent differences in the ability of cancer vs. normal breast epithelial cells to interact with fibrin(ogen). Because TEM of nonmalignant epithelial cells (MCF-10A) could not be enhanced in the presence of Fg (Sahni et al., 2009), we hypothesize that loss of HSPG from the surface of premalignant breast epithelial cells serves as a molecular switch to induce a highly aggressive, metastatic breast cancer phenotype (Fig. 11A). We plan to investigate this hypothesis in future studies.

Another mechanism to regulate Fg-enhanced TEM of malignant breast cancer cells is a gain in function of cancer-associated Mucin-1 (MUC1), which is a membrane-associated mucin expressed at low levels on the apical surface of normal polarized epithelial cells. MUC1 is a tumor-associated glycoprotein aberrantly expressed in >90% of breast cancers (Singh & Bandyopadhyay, 2007), promotes cancer cell proliferation and metastasis, and is associated with poor survival (Hattrup & Gendler, 2006; Yuan et al., 2007). MUC1 is upregulated and hypoglycosylated in breast cancers. The polarized expression of MUC1 is lost on cancer cells such that it is expressed on the entire cell surface (Kondo et al., 1998; Moase et al., 2001; Wesseling et al., 1996; Yang et al., 2007). The MUC1 extracellular domain protrudes ~200 nm above the cell surface, whereas most cell surface receptors are ~35 nm long (Wesseling et al., 1996). When MUC1 is interspersed between adhesion molecules, it nonspecifically reduces cell-cell and cell-ECM interactions in vitro and in vivo, likely by steric hindrance caused by the extreme length and high density of the MUC1 at the cell surface (Wesseling et al., 1996) (**Fig. 11B**). MUC1 expression is found on MCF-7, MDA-MB-231, as well as other types of breast cancer cells, particularly on those isolated from patients with a highly aggressive subtype called inflammatory breast cancer (Alpaugh et al., 2002; Schroeder et al., 2003; Walsh et al., 1999); elevated expression of MUC1 contributes to lymphovascular tumor invasion of inflammatory breast cancer cells (Alpaugh et al., 2002).

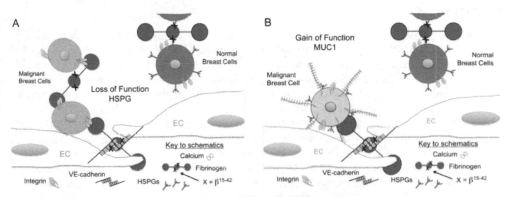

Fig. 11. Putative mechanisms whereby nonmalignant breast epithelial cells switch to a metastatic breast cancer cell phenotype responsive to fibrinogen-induced TEM. Panel A, schematic depicting loss of function due to release of cell-surface HSPG. Panel B, schematic depicting gain of function by overexpression of MUC1 leading to loss of polarity and cell-cell adhesion in breast epithelial cells.

We predict that Fg could bind to normal breast cell surface HSPG through Fg β^{15-42}, thus preventing Fg β^{15-42} binding to VE-cadherin extracellular domain 3 (EC3) and inhibition of TEM. Enhanced heparanase expression and enzymatic digestion of HSPG in human tumors correlates with metastatic potential, tumor vascularity, and reduced postoperative survival of cancer patients (Vlodavsky et al., 2008). Heparanase-induced loss of breast epithelial cell surface HSPG during conversion of non- or pre-malignant to malignant breast cancers would allow Fg β^{15-42} binding to VE-cadherin at cell-cell junctions to induce EC permeability. Fg would also bind to breast cancer cell integrins via binding sites on Fg C-terminal domains (**see Fig. 4**) then movement of VE-cadherin (induced by Fg binding to VE-cadherin as shown in **Fig. 8B**) in the endothelial cell membrane would induce paracellular transfer of Fg-bound breast cancer cells across the endothelial cell barrier to promote cancer metastasis. A precedent for this mechanism is already established; Fg binding to a counter adhesion molecule facilitates neutrophil TEM 20- to 30-fold (Languino et al., 1995). Overexpression of MUC1 could block accessibility of HSPG on breast cancer cells, which would also prevent Fg β^{15-42}–HSPG binding interactions leaving Fg β^{15-42} available for binding to VE-cadherin. Alternatively, loss of cell surface HSPG and elevated expression of MUC1 may contribute to Fg-enhanced TEM of malignant compared to nonmalignant breast epithelial cells. These possibilities will be addressed by future experiments.

5. Acknowledgements

We thank present and past members of the Simpson-Haidaris lab and our collaborators for all their contributions to elucidate the role of fibrin(ogen) in wound repair, endothelial cell biology and cancer progression. Our work has been supported by numerous grants from the National Institutes of Health NHLBI and NIAID, the Breast Cancer Research Program sponsored by the Department of Defense, the Komen Race for the Cure Foundation, and the American Heart Association.

6. References

Abumiya, T., Yokota, C., Kuge, Y. & Minematsu, K. (2005). Aggravation of hemorrhagic transformation by early intraarterial infusion of low-dose vascular endothelial growth factor after transient focal cerebral ischemia in rats. *Brain Res* 1049(1):95-103.

Alpaugh, M.L., Tomlinson, J.S., Kasraeian, S. & Barsky, S.H. (2002). Cooperative role of E-cadherin and sialyl-Lewis X/A-deficient MUC1 in the passive dissemination of tumor emboli in inflammatory breast carcinoma. *Oncogene* 21(22):3631-43.

Altieri, D.C., Plescia, J. & Plow, E.F. (1993). The structural motif glycine 190-valine 202 of the fibrinogen gamma chain interacts with CD11b/CD18 integrin (alpha M beta 2, Mac-1) and promotes leukocyte adhesion. *J Biol Chem* 268(3):1847-53.

Andre, F., Berrada, N. & Desmedt, C. (2010). Implication of tumor microenvironment in the resistance to chemotherapy in breast cancer patients. *Curr Opin Oncol* 22(6):547-51.

Anton, K. & Glod, J. (2009). Targeting the tumor stroma in cancer therapy. *Curr Pharm Biotechnol* 10(2):185-91.

Asakura, S., Niwa, K., Tomozawa, T., Jin, Y., Madoiwa, S., Sakata, Y., Sakai, T., Funayama, H., Soe, G., Forgerty, F., Hirata, H. & Matsuda, M. (1997). Fibroblasts spread on immobilized fibrin monomer by mobilizing a beta1-class integrin, together with a vitronectin receptor alphavbeta3 on their surface. *J Biol Chem* 272(13):8824-9.

Bach, T.L., Barsigian, C., Chalupowicz, D.G., Busler, D., Yaen, C.H., Grant, D.S. & Martinez, J. (1998a). VE-Cadherin mediates endothelial cell capillary tube formation in fibrin and collagen gels. *Exp Cell Res* 238(2):324-34.

Bach, T.L., Barsigian, C., Yaen, C.H. & Martinez, J. (1998b). Endothelial cell VE-cadherin functions as a receptor for the $\beta15$-42 sequence of fibrin. *J Biol Chem* 273(46):30719-28.

Balkwill, F. & Mantovani, A. (2001). Inflammation and cancer: back to Virchow? *Lancet* 357(9255):539-45.

Barton, B.E. (2001). IL-6-like cytokines and cancer cachexia: consequences of chronic inflammation. *Immunol Res* 23(1):41-58.

Batschauer, A.P., Figueiredo, C.P., Bueno, E.C., Ribeiro, M.A., Dusse, L.M., Fernandes, A.P., Gomes, K.B. & Carvalho, M.G. (2010). D-dimer as a possible prognostic marker of operable hormone receptor-negative breast cancer. *Ann Oncol* 21(6):1267-72.

Bauer, A.L., Jackson, T.L. & Jiang, Y. (2009). Topography of extracellular matrix mediates vascular morphogenesis and migration speeds in angiogenesis. *PLoS Comput Biol* 5(7):e1000445.

Baumann, H. & Gauldie, J. (1994). The acute phase response. *Immunol Today* 15(2):74-80.

Bennett, J.S., Berger, B.W. & Billings, P.C. (2009). The structure and function of platelet integrins. *J Thromb Haemost* 7 Suppl 1200-5.

Bunce, L.A., Sporn, L.A. & Francis, C.W. (1992). Endothelial cell spreading on fibrin requires fibrinopeptide B cleavage and amino acid residues 15-42 of the β chain. *J Clin Invest* 89(3):842-50.

Caine, G.J., Lip, G.Y., Stonelake, P.S., Ryan, P. & Blann, A.D. (2004). Platelet activation, coagulation and angiogenesis in breast and prostate carcinoma. *Thromb Haemost* 92(1):185-90.

Carmeliet, P., Lampugnani, M.G., Moons, L., Breviario, F., Compernolle, V., Bono, F., Balconi, G., Spagnuolo, R., Oostuyse, B., Dewerchin, M., Zanetti, A., Angellilo, A., Mattot, V., Nuyens, D., Lutgens, E., Clotman, F., de Ruiter, M.C., Gittenberger-de Groot, A., Poelmann, R., Lupu, F., Herbert, J.M., Collen, D. & Dejana, E. (1999). Targeted deficiency or cytosolic truncation of the VE-cadherin gene in mice impairs VEGF-mediated endothelial survival and angiogenesis. *Cell* 98(2):147-57.

Chalupowicz, D.G., Chowdhury, Z.A., Bach, T.L., Barsigian, C. & Martinez, J. (1995). Fibrin II induces endothelial cell capillary tube formation. *J Cell Biol* 130(1):207-15.

Clark, R.A.F. The molecular and cellular biology of wound repair. New York: Plenum Press 1996.

Cohen, T., Nahari, D., Cerem, L.W., Neufeld, G. & Levi, B.Z. (1996). Interleukin 6 induces the expression of vascular endothelial growth factor. *J Biol Chem* 271(2):736-41.

Costantini, V., Zacharski, L.R., Memoli, V.A., Kisiel, W., Kudryk, B.J. & Rousseau, S.M. (1991). Fibrinogen deposition without thrombin generation in primary human breast cancer tissue. *Cancer Res* 51(1):349-53.

Courtney, M.A., Bunce, L.A., Neroni, L.A. & Simpson-Haidaris, P.J. (1994). Cloning of the complete coding sequence of rat fibrinogen Bβ chain cDNA: interspecies conservation of fibrin β15-42 primary structure. *Blood Coagul Fibrinolysis* 5(4):487-96.

Coussens, L.M. & Werb, Z. (2002). Inflammation and cancer. *Nature* 420(6917):860-7.

Croll, S.D., Ransohoff, R.M., Cai, N., Zhang, Q., Martin, F.J., Wei, T., Kasselman, L.J., Kintner, J., Murphy, A.J., Yancopoulos, G.D. & Wiegand, S.J. (2004). VEGF-mediated inflammation precedes angiogenesis in adult brain. *Exp Neurol* 187(2):388-402.

De Wever, O., Demetter, P., Mareel, M. & Bracke, M. (2008). Stromal myofibroblasts are drivers of invasive cancer growth. *Int J Cancer* 123(10):2229-38.

Dejana, E. (2004). Endothelial cell-cell junctions: happy together. *Nat Rev Mol Cell Biol* 5(4):261-70.

Deryugina, E.I. & Quigley, J.P. (2006). Matrix metalloproteinases and tumor metastasis. *Cancer Metastasis Rev* 25(1):9-34.

Dirix, L.Y., Salgado, R., Weytjens, R., Colpaert, C., Benoy, I., Huget, P., van Dam, P., Prove, A., Lemmens, J. & Vermeulen, P. (2002). Plasma fibrin D-dimer levels correlate with tumour volume, progression rate and survival in patients with metastatic breast cancer. *Br J Cancer* 86(3):389-95.

Duan, H.O. & Simpson-Haidaris, P.J. (2003). Functional analysis of interleukin 6 response elements (IL-6REs) on the human gamma-fibrinogen promoter: binding of hepatic

Stat3 correlates negatively with transactivation potential of type II IL-6REs. *J Biol Chem* 278(42):41270-81.

Dvorak, H.F. (1986). Tumors: wounds that do not heal. Similarities between tumor stroma generation and wound healing. *N Engl J Med* 315(26):1650-9.

Dvorak, H.F. (2006). Discovery of vascular permeability factor (VPF). *Exp Cell Res*

Esser, S., Lampugnani, M.G., Corada, M., Dejana, E. & Risau, W. (1998). Vascular endothelial growth factor induces VE-cadherin tyrosine phosphorylation in endothelial cells. *J Cell Sci* 111(Pt 13):1853-65.

Flick, M.J., Du, X., Witte, D.P., Jirouskova, M., Soloviev, D.A., Busuttil, S.J., Plow, E.F. & Degen, J.L. (2004). Leukocyte engagement of fibrin(ogen) via the integrin receptor aMb2/Mac-1 is critical for host inflammatory response in vivo. *J Clin Invest* 113(11):1596-606.

Gao, S.P., Mark, K.G., Leslie, K., Pao, W., Motoi, N., Gerald, W.L., Travis, W.D., Bornmann, W., Veach, D., Clarkson, B. & Bromberg, J.F. (2007). Mutations in the EGFR kinase domain mediate STAT3 activation via IL-6 production in human lung adenocarcinomas. *J Clin Invest* 117(12):3846-56.

Gorlatov, S. & Medved, L. (2002). Interaction of fibrin(ogen) with the endothelial cell receptor VE-cadherin: mapping of the receptor-binding site in the NH_2-terminal portions of the fibrin β chains. *Biochemistry* 41(12):4107-16.

Guadiz, G., Sporn, L.A. & Simpson-Haidaris, P.J. (1997). Thrombin cleavage-independent deposition of fibrinogen in extracellular matrices. *Blood* 90(7):2644-53.

Guo, M., Sahni, S.K., Sahni, A. & Francis, C.W. (2004). Fibrinogen regulates the expression of inflammatory chemokines through NF-κB activation of endothelial cells. *Thromb Haemost* 92(4):858-66.

Hallen, J., Petzelbauer, P., Schwitter, J., Geudelin, B., Buser, P. & Atar, D. (2010). Impact of time to therapy and presence of collaterals on the efficacy of FX06 in acute ST elevation myocardial infarction: a substudy of the F.I.R.E., the Efficacy of FX06 in the prevention of myocardial reperfusion injury trial. *EuroIntervention* 5(8):946-52.

Harley, S.L. & Powell, J.T. (1999). Fibrinogen up-regulates the expression of monocyte chemoattractant protein 1 in human saphenous vein endothelial cells. *Biochem J* 341 (Pt 3):739-44.

Hartman, Z.C., Yang, X.Y., Glass, O., Lei, G., Osada, T., Dave, S.S., Morse, M.A., Clay, T.M. & Lyerly, H.K. (2011). HER2 overexpression elicits a proinflammatory IL-6 autocrine signaling loop that is critical for tumorigenesis. *Cancer Res* 71(13):4380-91.

Hattrup, C.L. & Gendler, S.J. (2006). MUC1 alters oncogenic events and transcription in human breast cancer cells. *Breast Cancer Res* 8(4):R37.

Hirschfield, G.M. & Pepys, M.B. (2003). C-reactive protein and cardiovascular disease: new insights from an old molecule. *QJM* 96(11):793-807.

Jones, J.M., McGonigle, N.C., McAnespie, M., Cran, G.W. & Graham, A.N. (2006). Plasma fibrinogen and serum C-reactive protein are associated with non-small cell lung cancer. *Lung Cancer* 53(1):97-101.

Kilic, M., Yoldas, O., Keskek, M., Ertan, T., Tez, M., Gocmen, E. & Koc, M. (2008). Prognostic value of plasma D-dimer levels in patients with colorectal cancer. *Colorectal Dis* 10(3):238-41.

Kloczewiak, M., Timmons, S. & Hawiger, J. (1983). Recognition site for the platelet receptor is present on the 15-residue carboxy-terminal fragment of the gamma chain of human fibrinogen and is not involved in the fibrin polymerization reaction. *Thromb Res* 29(2):249-55.

Knowlson, L., Bacchu, S., Paneesha, S., McManus, A., Randall, K. & Rose, P. (2010). Elevated D-dimers are also a marker of underlying malignancy and increased mortality in the absence of venous thromboembolism. *J Clin Pathol* 63(9):818-22.

Knupfer, H. & Preiss, R. (2007). Significance of interleukin-6 (IL-6) in breast cancer. *Breast Cancer Res Treat* 102(2):129-35.

Kondo, K., Kohno, N., Yokoyama, A. & Hiwada, K. (1998). Decreased MUC1 expression induces E-cadherin-mediated cell adhesion of breast cancer cell lines. *Cancer Res* 58(9):2014-9.

Koo, C.Y., Sen, Y.P., Bay, B.H. & Yip, G.W. (2008). Targeting heparan sulfate proteoglycans in breast cancer treatment. *Recent Patents Anticancer Drug Discov* 3(3):151-8.

Kudryk, B., Rohoza, A., Ahadi, M., Chin, J. & Wiebe, M.E. (1984). Specificity of a monoclonal antibody for the NH$_2$-terminal region of fibrin. *Mol Immunol* 21(1):89-94.

Kuhns, D.B., Nelson, E.L., Alvord, W.G. & Gallin, J.I. (2001). Fibrinogen induces IL-8 synthesis in human neutrophils stimulated with formyl-methionyl-leucyl-phenylalanine or leukotriene B(4). *J Immunol* 167(5):2869-78.

Langley, R.R. & Fidler, I.J. (2011). The seed and soil hypothesis revisited-The role of tumor-stroma interactions in metastasis to different organs. *Int J Cancer* 128(11):2527-35.

Languino, L.R., Duperray, A., Joganic, K.J., Fornaro, M., Thornton, G.B. & Altieri, D.C. (1995). Regulation of leukocyte-endothelium interaction and leukocyte transendothelial migration by intercellular adhesion molecule 1-fibrinogen recognition. *Proc Natl Acad Sci U S A* 92(5):1505-9.

Languino, L.R., Plescia, J., Duperray, A., Brian, A.A., Plow, E.F., Geltosky, J.E. & Altieri, D.C. (1993). Fibrinogen mediates leukocyte adhesion to vascular endothelium through an ICAM-1-dependent pathway. *Cell* 73(7):1423-34.

Lee, M.E., Kweon, S.M., Ha, K.S. & Nham, S.U. (2001). Fibrin stimulates microfilament reorganization and IL-1β production in human monocytic THP-1 cells. *Mol Cells* 11(1):13-20.

Lee, S.Y., Lee, K.P. & Lim, J.W. (1996). Identification and biosynthesis of fibrinogen in human uterine cervix carcinoma cells. *Thromb Haemostas* 75(3):466-70.

Levy-Adam, F., Abboud-Jarrous, G., Guerrini, M., Beccati, D., Vlodavsky, I. & Ilan, N. (2005). Identification and characterization of heparin/heparan sulfate binding domains of the endoglycosidase heparanase. *J Biol Chem* 280(21):20457-66.

Lin, W.W. & Karin, M. (2007). A cytokine-mediated link between innate immunity, inflammation, and cancer. *J Clin Invest* 117(5):1175-83.

Lishko, V.K., Podolnikova, N.P., Yakubenko, V.P., Yakovlev, S., Medved, L., Yadav, S.P. & Ugarova, T.P. (2004). Multiple binding sites in fibrinogen for integrin alphaMbeta2 (Mac-1). *J Biol Chem* 279(43):44897-906.

Loike, J.D., Sodeik, B., Cao, L., Leucona, S., Weitz, J.I., Detmers, P.A., Wright, S.D. & Silverstein, S.C. (1991). CD11c/CD18 on neutrophils recognizes a domain at the N terminus of the A alpha chain of fibrinogen. *Proc Natl Acad Sci U S A* 88(3):1044-8.

Lorusso, G. & Ruegg, C. (2008). The tumor microenvironment and its contribution to tumor evolution toward metastasis. *Histochem Cell Biol* 130(6):1091-103.

Martinez, J., Ferber, A., Bach, T.L. & Yaen, C.H. (2001). Interaction of fibrin with VE-cadherin. *Ann N Y Acad Sci* 936386-405.

McGettrick, H.M., Filer, A., Rainger, G.E., Buckley, C.D. & Nash, G.B. (2007). Modulation of endothelial responses by the stromal microenvironment: effects on leucocyte recruitment. *Biochem Soc Trans* 35(Pt 5):1161-2.

Moase, E.H., Qi, W., Ishida, T., Gabos, Z., Longenecker, B.M., Zimmermann, G.L., Ding, L., Krantz, M. & Allen, T.M. (2001). Anti-MUC-1 immunoliposomal doxorubicin in the treatment of murine models of metastatic breast cancer. *Biochim Biophys Acta* 1510(1-2):43-55.

Molmenti, E.P., Ziambaras, T. & Perlmutter, D.H. (1993). Evidence for an acute phase response in human intestinal epithelial cells. *J Biol Chem* 268(19):14116-24.

Mosesson, M.W. (2005). Fibrinogen and fibrin structure and functions. *J Thromb Haemost* 3(8):1894-904.

Neurath, M.F. & Finotto, S. (2011). IL-6 signaling in autoimmunity, chronic inflammation and inflammation-associated cancer. *Cytokine Growth Factor Rev* 22(2):83-9.

Nierodzik, M.L. & Karpatkin, S. (2006). Thrombin induces tumor growth, metastasis, and angiogenesis: Evidence for a thrombin-regulated dormant tumor phenotype. *Cancer Cell* 10(5):355-62.

Odrljin, T.M., Francis, C.W., Sporn, L.A., Bunce, L.A., Marder, V.J. & Simpson-Haidaris, P.J. (1996a). Heparin-binding domain of fibrin mediates its binding to endothelial cells. *Arterioscler Thromb Vasc Biol* 16(12):1544-51.

Odrljin, T.M., Shainoff, J.R., Lawrence, S.O. & Simpson-Haidaris, P.J. (1996b). Thrombin cleavage enhances exposure of a heparin binding domain in the N-terminus of the fibrin beta chain. *Blood* 88(6):2050-61.

Paget, S. (1889). The distribution of secondary growths in cancer of the breast. *Lancet* 1571-3.

Palumbo, J.S., Barney, K.A., Blevins, E.A., Shaw, M.A., Mishra, A., Flick, M.J., Kombrinck, K.W., Talmage, K.E., Souri, M., Ichinose, A. & Degen, J.L. (2008). Factor XIII transglutaminase supports hematogenous tumor cell metastasis through a mechanism dependent on natural killer cell function. *J Thromb Haemost* 6(5):812-9.

Palumbo, J.S. & Degen, J.L. (2001). Fibrinogen and tumor cell metastasis. *Haemostasis* 31(Suppl 1):11-5.

Palumbo, J.S. & Degen, J.L. (2007). Mechanisms linking tumor cell-associated procoagulant function to tumor metastasis. *Thromb Res* 120 Suppl 2S22-8.

Palumbo, J.S., Kombrinck, K.W., Drew, A.F., Grimes, T.S., Kiser, J.H., Degen, J.L. & Bugge, T.H. (2000). Fibrinogen is an important determinant of the metastatic potential of circulating tumor cells. *Blood* 96(10):3302-9.

Palumbo, J.S., Potter, J.M., Kaplan, L.S., Talmage, K., Jackson, D.G. & Degen, J.L. (2002). Spontaneous hematogenous and lymphatic metastasis, but not primary tumor growth or angiogenesis, is diminished in fibrinogen-deficient mice. *Cancer Res* 62(23):6966-72.

Palumbo, J.S., Talmage, K.E., Massari, J.V., La Jeunesse, C.M., Flick, M.J., Kombrinck, K.W., Hu, Z., Barney, K.A. & Degen, J.L. (2007). Tumor cell-associated tissue factor and circulating hemostatic factors cooperate to increase metastatic potential through natural killer cell-dependent and-independent mechanisms. *Blood* 110(1):133-41.

Palumbo, J.S., Talmage, K.E., Massari, J.V., La Jeunesse, C.M., Flick, M.J., Kombrinck, K.W., Jirouskova, M. & Degen, J.L. (2005). Platelets and fibrin(ogen) increase metastatic potential by impeding natural killer cell-mediated elimination of tumor cells. *Blood* 105(1):178-85.

Pensa, S., Watson, C.J. & Poli, V. (2009). Stat3 and the inflammation/acute phase response in involution and breast cancer. *J Mammary Gland Biol Neoplasia* 14(2):121-9.

Pentecost, B.T., Bradley, L.M., Gierthy, J.F., Ding, Y. & Fasco, M.J. (2005). Gene regulation in an MCF-7 cell line that naturally expresses an estrogen receptor unable to directly bind DNA. *Mol Cell Endocrinol* 238(1-2):9-25.

Pereira, M., Rybarczyk, B.J., Odrljin, T.M., Hocking, D.C., Sottile, J. & Simpson-Haidaris, P.J. (2002). The incorporation of fibrinogen into extracellular matrix is dependent on active assembly of a fibronectin matrix. *J Cell Sci* 115(3):609-17.

Pereira, M. & Simpson-Haidaris, P.J. (2001). Fibrinogen modulates gene expression in wounded fibroblasts. *Ann N Y Acad Sci* 936(1):438-43.

Petzelbauer, P., Zacharowski, P.A., Miyazaki, Y., Friedl, P., Wickenhauser, G., Castellino, F.J., Groger, M., Wolff, K. & Zacharowski, K. (2005a). The fibrin-derived peptide Bbeta15-42 protects the myocardium against ischemia-reperfusion injury. *Nat Med* 11(3):298-304.

Petzelbauer, P., Zacharowski, P.A., Miyazaki, Y., Friedl, P., Wickenhauser, G., Castellino, F.J., Groger, M., Wolff, K. & Zacharowski, K. (2005b). The fibrin-derived peptide Bβ15-42 protects the myocardium against ischemia-reperfusion injury. *Nat Med* 11(3):298-304.

Pluskota, E. & D'Souza, S.E. (2000). Fibrinogen interactions with ICAM-1 (CD54) regulate endothelial cell survival. *Eur J Biochem* 267(15):4693-704.

Qi, J. & Kreutzer, D.L. (1995). Fibrin activation of vascular endothelial cells. Induction of IL-8 expression. *J Immunol* 155(2):867-76.

Ramsby, M.L. & Kreutzer, D.L. (1994). Fibrin induction of interleukin-8 expression in corneal endothelial cells in vitro. *Invest Ophthalmol Vis Sci* 35(12):3980-90.

Ravishankaran, P. & Karunanithi, R. (2011). Clinical significance of preoperative serum interleukin-6 and C-reactive protein level in breast cancer patients. *World J Surg Oncol* 9(1):18.

Ribes, J.A., Ni, F., Wagner, D.D. & Francis, C.W. (1989). Mediation of fibrin-induced release of von Willebrand factor from cultured endothelial cells by the fibrin β chain. *J Clin Invest* 84(2):435-42.

Roche, Y., Pasquier, D., Rambeaud, J.J., Seigneurin, D. & Duperray, A. (2003). Fibrinogen mediates bladder cancer cell migration in an ICAM-1-dependent pathway. *Thromb Haemost* 89(6):1089-97.

Roesner, J.P., Petzelbauer, P., Koch, A., Mersmann, J., Zacharowski, P.A., Boehm, O., Reingruber, S., Pasteiner, W., Mascher, H.D., Wolzt, M., Barthuber, C., Noldge-Schomburg, G.E., Scheeren, T.W. & Zacharowski, K. (2007). The fibrin-derived peptide Bβ15-42 is cardioprotective in a pig model of myocardial ischemia-reperfusion injury. *Crit Care Med* (7):1730-5.

Roesner, J.P., Petzelbauer, P., Koch, A., Tran, N., Iber, T., Vagts, D.A., Scheeren, T.W., Vollmar, B., Noldge-Schomburg, G.E. & Zacharowski, K. (2009). Bbeta15-42 (FX06) reduces pulmonary, myocardial, liver, and small intestine damage in a pig model of hemorrhagic shock and reperfusion. *Crit Care Med* 37(2):598-605.

Rybarczyk, B.J., Lawrence, S.O. & Simpson-Haidaris, P.J. (2003). Matrix-fibrinogen enhances wound closure by increasing both cell proliferation and migration. *Blood* 102(12):4035-43.

Rybarczyk, B.J. & Simpson-Haidaris, P.J. (2000). Fibrinogen assembly, secretion, and deposition into extracellular matrix by MCF-7 human breast carcinoma cells. *Cancer Res* 60(7):2033-9.

Sahni, A., Altland, O.D. & Francis, C.W. (2003). FGF-2 but not FGF-1 binds fibrin and supports prolonged endothelial cell growth. *J Thromb Haemost* 1(6):1304-10.

Sahni, A., Arevalo, M.T., Sahni, S.K. & Simpson-Haidaris, P.J. (2009). The VE-cadherin binding domain of fibrinogen induces endothelial barrier permeability and enhances transendothelial migration of malignant breast epithelial cells. *Int J Cancer* 125(3):577-84.

Sahni, A. & Francis, C.W. (2000). Vascular endothelial growth factor binds to fibrinogen and fibrin and stimulates endothelial cell proliferation. *Blood* 96(12):3772-8.

Sahni, A. & Francis, C.W. (2004). Stimulation of endothelial cell proliferation by FGF-2 in the presence of fibrinogen requires $\alpha v \beta 3$. *Blood* 1043635-41.

Sahni, A., Khorana, A.A., Baggs, R.B., Peng, H. & Francis, C.W. (2006). FGF-2 binding to fibrin(ogen) is required for augmented angiogenesis. *Blood* 107(1):126-31.

Sahni, A., Odrljin, T. & Francis, C.W. (1998). Binding of basic fibroblast growth factor to fibrinogen and fibrin. *J Biol Chem* 273(13):7554-9.

Sahni, A., Sahni, S.K., Simpson-Haidaris, P.J. & Francis, C.W. (2004). Fibrinogen binding potentiates FGF-2 but not VEGF induced expression of u-PA, u-PAR, and PAI-1 in endothelial cells. *J Thromb Haemost* 2(9):1629-36.

Sahni, A., Simpson-Haidaris, P.J., Sahni, S.K., Vaday, G.G. & Francis, C.W. (2008). Fibrinogen synthesized by cancer cells augments the proliferative effect of FGF-2. *J Thromb Haemost* 6176-83.

Sahni, A., Sporn, L.A. & Francis, C.W. (1999). Potentiation of endothelial cell proliferation by fibrin(ogen)-bound fibroblast growth factor-2. *J Biol Chem* 274(21):14936-41.

Saito, M., Shima, C., Takagi, M., Ogino, M., Katori, M. & Majima, M. (2002). Enhanced exudation of fibrinogen into the perivascular space in acute inflammation triggered by neutrophil migration. *Inflamm Res* 51(7):324-31.

Salgado, R., Junius, S., Benoy, I., Van Dam, P., Vermeulen, P., Van Marck, E., Huget, P. & Dirix, L.Y. (2003). Circulating interleukin-6 predicts survival in patients with metastatic breast cancer. *Int J Cancer* 103(5):642-6.

Schachtrup, C., Ryu, J.K., Helmrick, M.J., Vagena, E., Galanakis, D.K., Degen, J.L., Margolis, R.U. & Akassoglou, K. (2010). Fibrinogen triggers astrocyte scar formation by promoting the availability of active TGF-beta after vascular damage. *J Neurosci* 30(17):5843-54.

Schroeder, J.A., Adriance, M.C., Thompson, M.C., Camenisch, T.D. & Gendler, S.J. (2003). MUC1 alters beta-catenin-dependent tumor formation and promotes cellular invasion. *Oncogene* 22(9):1324-32.

Simpson-Haidaris, P.J. (1997). Induction of fibrinogen biosynthesis and secretion from cultured pulmonary epithelial cells. *Blood* 89(3):873-82.

Simpson-Haidaris, P.J., Pollock, S.J., Ramon, S., Guo, N., Woeller, C.F., Feldon, S.E. & Phipps, R.P. (2010). Anticancer role of PPARgamma agonists in hematological malignancies found in the vasculature, marrow, and eyes. *PPAR Res* 2010814609.

Simpson-Haidaris, P.J. & Rybarczyk, B. (2001). Tumors and fibrinogen. The role of fibrinogen as an extracellular matrix protein. *Ann N Y Acad Sci* 936(1):406-25.

Simpson-Haidaris, P.J. & Sahni, A. (2010). Fibrin-specific beta(15-42) domain is exposed in cell-associated intact fibrinogen: Response to Weijers et al comment on the study by A. Sahni et al. *Int J Cancer* 127(12):2982-6.

Singh, R. & Bandyopadhyay, D. (2007). MUC1: a target molecule for cancer therapy. *Cancer Biol Ther* 6(4):481-6.

Sitrin, R.G., Pan, P.M., Srikanth, S. & Todd, R.F., 3rd. (1998). Fibrinogen activates NF-kappa B transcription factors in mononuclear phagocytes. *J Immunol* 161(3):1462-70.

Sorensen, H.T., Mellemkjaer, L., Olsen, J.H. & Baron, J.A. (2000). Prognosis of cancers associated with venous thromboembolism. *N Engl J Med* 343(25):1846-50.

Sporn, L.A., Bunce, L.A. & Francis, C.W. (1995). Cell proliferation on fibrin: modulation by fibrinopeptide cleavage. *Blood* 86(5):1802-10.

Sriramarao, P., Languino, L.R. & Altieri, D.C. (1996). Fibrinogen mediates leukocyte-endothelium bridging in vivo at low shear forces. *Blood* 88(9):3416-23.

Starakis, I., Koutras, A. & Mazokopakis, E.E. (2010). Drug-induced thromboembolic events in patients with malignancy. *Cardiovasc Hematol Disord Drug Targets* 10(2):94-102.

Steinbrecher, K.A., Horowitz, N.A., Blevins, E.A., Barney, K.A., Shaw, M.A., Harmel-Laws, E., Finkelman, F.D., Flick, M.J., Pinkerton, M.D., Talmage, K.E., Kombrinck, K.W., Witte, D.P. & Palumbo, J.S. (2010). Colitis-associated cancer is dependent on the interplay between the hemostatic and inflammatory systems and supported by integrin alpha(M)beta(2) engagement of fibrinogen. *Cancer Res* 70(7):2634-43.

Suehiro, K., Gailit, J. & Plow, E.F. (1997). Fibrinogen is a ligand for integrin a5b1 on endothelial cells. *J Biol Chem* 272(8):5360-6.

Tan, Y.J., Tham, P.Y., Chan, D.Z., Chou, C.F., Shen, S., Fielding, B.C., Tan, T.H., Lim, S.G. & Hong, W. (2005). The severe acute respiratory syndrome coronavirus 3a protein up-regulates expression of fibrinogen in lung epithelial cells. *J Virol* 79(15):10083-7.

Tlsty, T.D. & Coussens, L.M. (2006). Tumor stroma and regulation of cancer development. *Annu Rev Pathol* 1119-50.

Trousseau, A. (1865). Phlegmasia alba dolens. *In Clinique Medicale de l'Hotel-Dieu de Paris,* vol. 3, pp. 654–712. JB Bailliere.

Ugarova, T.P., Lishko, V.K., Podolnikova, N.P., Okumura, N., Merkulov, S.M., Yakubenko, V.P., Yee, V.C., Lord, S.T. & Haas, T.A. (2003). Sequence gamma 377-395(P2), but not gamma 190-202(P1), is the binding site for the alpha MI-domain of integrin alpha M beta 2 in the gamma C-domain of fibrinogen. *Biochemistry* 42(31):9365-73.

Ugarova, T.P. & Yakubenko, V.P. (2001). Recognition of fibrinogen by leukocyte integrins. *Ann N Y Acad Sci* 936(1):368-85.

Ulisse, S., Baldini, E., Sorrenti, S. & D'Armiento, M. (2009). The urokinase plasminogen activator system: a target for anti-cancer therapy. *Curr Cancer Drug Targets* 9(1):32-71.

van Hinsbergh, V.W., Collen, A. & Koolwijk, P. (2001). Role of fibrin matrix in angiogenesis. *Ann N Y Acad Sci* 936426-37.

Varki, A. (2007). Trousseau's syndrome: multiple definitions and multiple mechanisms. *Blood* 110(6):1723-9.

Verheul, H.M., van Erp, K., Homs, M.Y., Yoon, G.S., van der Groep, P., Rogers, C., Hansel, D.E., Netto, G.J. & Pili, R. (2010). The relationship of vascular endothelial growth factor and coagulation factor (fibrin and fibrinogen) expression in clear cell renal cell carcinoma. *Urology* 75(3):608-14.

Vlodavsky, I., Elkin, M., Abboud-Jarrous, G., Levi-Adam, F., Fuks, L., Shafat, I. & Ilan, N. (2008). Heparanase: one molecule with multiple functions in cancer progression. *Connect Tissue Res* 49(3):207-10.

Walsh, M.D., Luckie, S.M., Cummings, M.C., Antalis, T.M. & McGuckin, M.A. (1999). Heterogeneity of MUC1 expression by human breast carcinoma cell lines in vivo and in vitro. *Breast Cancer Res Treat* 58(3):255-66.

Walter, M., Liang, S., Ghosh, S., Hornsby, P.J. & Li, R. (2009). Interleukin 6 secreted from adipose stromal cells promotes migration and invasion of breast cancer cells. *Oncogene* 28(30):2745-55.

Wesseling, J., van der Valk, S.W. & Hilkens, J. (1996). A mechanism for inhibition of E-cadherin-mediated cell-cell adhesion by the membrane-associated mucin episialin/MUC1. *Mol Biol Cell* 7(4):565-77.

Wiedemann, D., Schneeberger, S., Friedl, P., Zacharowski, K., Wick, N., Boesch, F., Margreiter, R., Laufer, G., Petzelbauer, P. & Semsroth, S. (2010). The fibrin-derived peptide Bbeta(15-42) significantly attenuates ischemia-reperfusion injury in a cardiac transplant model. *Transplantation* 89(7):824-9.

Yakovlev, S., Gorlatov, S., Ingham, K. & Medved, L. (2003). Interaction of fibrin(ogen) with heparin: further characterization and localization of the heparin-binding site. *Biochemistry* 42(25):7709-16.

Yakovlev, S. & Medved, L. (2009). Interaction of fibrin(ogen) with the endothelial cell receptor VE-cadherin: Localization of the fibrin-binding site within the third extracellular VE-cadherin domain. *Biochemistry* 48(23):5171-9.

Yakovlev, S., Zhang, L., Ugarova, T. & Medved, L. (2005). Interaction of fibrin(ogen) with leukocyte receptor alpha M beta 2 (Mac-1): further characterization and identification of a novel binding region within the central domain of the fibrinogen gamma-module. *Biochemistry* 44(2):617-26.

Yamaguchi, T., Yamamoto, Y., Yokota, S., Nakagawa, M., Ito, M. & Ogura, T. (1998). Involvement of interleukin-6 in the elevation of plasma fibrinogen levels in lung cancer patients. *Jpn J Clin Oncol* 28(12):740-4.

Yang, E., Hu, X.F. & Xing, P.X. (2007). Advances of MUC1 as a target for breast cancer immunotherapy. *Histol Histopathol* 22(8):905-22.

Yigit, E., Gonullu, G., Yucel, I., Turgut, M., Erdem, D. & Cakar, B. (2008). Relation between hemostatic parameters and prognostic/predictive factors in breast cancer. *Eur J Intern Med* 19(8):602-7.

Yuan, Z., Wong, S., Borrelli, A. & Chung, M.A. (2007). Down-regulation of MUC1 in cancer cells inhibits cell migration by promoting E-cadherin/catenin complex formation. *Biochem Biophys Res Commun* 362(3):740-6.

Zacharowski, K., Zacharowski, P., Reingruber, S. & Petzelbauer, P. (2006). Fibrin(ogen) and its fragments in the pathophysiology and treatment of myocardial infarction. *J Mol Med* 84(6):469-77.

Zacharowski, K., Zacharowski, P.A., Friedl, P., Mastan, P., Koch, A., Boehm, O., Rother, R.P., Reingruber, S., Henning, R., Emeis, J.J. & Petzelbauer, P. (2007). The effects of the fibrin-derived peptide Bβ15-42 in acute and chronic rodent models of myocardial ischemia-reperfusion. *Shock* 27(6):631-7.

Zhang, G.J. & Adachi, I. (1999). Serum interleukin-6 levels correlate to tumor progression and prognosis in metastatic breast carcinoma. *Anticancer Res* 19(2B):1427-32.

9

Interleukin-6 in the Breast Tumor Microenvironment

Nicholas J. Sullivan
The Ohio State University, Columbus, Ohio
USA

1. Introduction

Greater than 200,000 new cases of breast cancer cases were diagnosed in 2010 in the United States, with approximately 40,000 women succumbing to the disease (www.cancer.gov). Globally, an estimated 1.38 million new cases of breast cancer were diagnosed in 2008, with greater than 450,000 women succumbing to the disease (Jemal *et al.*, 2011). Despite our improved understanding of breast carcinogenesis, breast cancer remains the second most commonly diagnosed cancer in women behind non-melanoma skin cancer and the second leading cause of death in women behind lung cancer. These epidemiological statistics highlight the overwhelming clinical dilemma of breast cancer and emphasize the need for novel therapeutic targets and prevention strategies. Countless studies in the fields of mammary gland development and breast cancer have led to an appreciation of a breast tumor microenvironment that actively contributes to the heterogeneous nature of breast cancer. The current review will focus on the impact of IL-6 and STAT3 activation in the breast tumor microenvironment and subsequently present rationale for targeting the IL-6/STAT3 signaling pathway in this setting. IL-6 is a quintessential pleiotropic cytokine produced by a diverse number of cell populations, most of which can localize to the breast tumor microenvironment. Excessive IL-6 has been demonstrated in primary breast tumors and breast cancer patient sera and is associated with poor clinical outcomes in breast cancer. These clinical associations are corroborated by emerging preclinical data revealing that IL-6 is a potent growth factor and promotes an epithelial-mesenchymal (EMT) phenotype in breast cancer cells to indicate that IL-6 in the breast tumor microenvironment is clinically relevant. Numerous clinical reports have now demonstrated the safety and efficacy of IL-6 signaling antagonists in multiple diseases, which supports future investigations of these therapies in breast cancer.

Estrogen receptor-alpha (ERα) is a latent cytoplasmic ligand-activated transcription factor utilized by clinicians to subclassify the heterogeneous disease of breast cancer. ERα-positive breast cancer incidence increases up to age 51, the mean age of menopause, and continues to increase until age 80. Conversely, ERα-negative breast cancer incidence plateaus and even slightly decreases at age 51, while demonstrating an increase prior to age 50 comparable to that of ERα-positive disease. This discrepancy between the two incidence rates at menopause produces an inflection in the incidence rate of all breast cancer cases which has been termed Clemmesen's hook (Anderson and Matsuno, 2006). Whereas the prevalence of

ERα-positive cells within terminal duct lobular units of the breast of healthy premenopausal women has been reported at 7%, this number is estimated at 42% in postmenopausal women (Shoker et al., 1999). In addition, approximately two-thirds of all breast cancers are diagnosed as ERα-positive, and 75% of postmenopausal breast cancers are ERα-positive (Macedo et al., 2009). Progesterone receptor (PR) and epidermal growth factor receptor 2 (EGFR2; HER2; or ErbB2), a receptor tyrosine kinase involved in cellular proliferation, have also acquired much clinical attention following reports of dismal survival rates in "triple negative" (ERα-negative/PR-negative/HER2 not overexpressed) breast cancer patients. Triple negative breast cancer represents approximately 15 to 20% of all breast cancer cases and can only be treated with standard chemotherapy as it lacks current adjuvant therapeutic targets. Such breast tumors are highly proliferative with a high mitotic index, increased necrosis, elevated apoptosis, and typically are of higher tumor grade. TP53 gene and p53 protein mutations as well as loss of the Rb tumor suppressor protein are common. Familial breast cancer patients with congenital BRCA1 mutations often present with triple negative breast cancer, as do relatively younger breast cancer patients and African American women. Currently, triple negative breast cancers are associated with a poor prognosis largely due to poor survival rates and early relapse. The fact that these breast tumors respond well if not completely to initial chemotherapy may seem counterintuitive, but enhanced invasiveness, consequent distant metastasis, and residual local recurrence eventually promote poor survival rates (Irvin and Carey, 2008).

Breast cancer most commonly metastasizes to bone, followed by lung, liver, and brain. Perhaps due to the heterogeneity across individual breast cancer cases, few prognostic molecular biomarkers have been demonstrated to accurately predict metastatic potential. One of the most important of these biomarkers is ERα, which is clinically exploited as a predictor of bone metastasis (Kominsky and Davidson, 2006). Whereas ERα-positive breast cancers have a strong tendency to metastasize to bone if at all (James et al., 2003), their ERα-negative counterparts favor visceral organs such as lung and liver (Hess et al., 2003). Primary mammary tumor cell dissemination has been quantified at 3 to 4 x 10^6 primary tumor cells in circulation per 24 hours per gram of tumor in a rat mammary carcinoma model, which exemplifies the inefficient nature of metastasis (Butler and Gullino, 1975). Although metastasis has been generally accepted as a relatively late event throughout cancer progression, recent work has revealed evidence of early primary tumor cell dissemination, thus refuting this paradigm (Klein, 2009). In particular, it has now been demonstrated that untransformed triple transgenic (doxycycline-inducible K-ras, MYC, and polyoma middle T antigen) mammary epithelial cells are capable of lung colonization when tail vein-injected into immunocompromised female mice on doxycycline. This work showed that untransformed "normal" mammary epithelial cells can colonize ectopic lung tissue, and upon oncogene activation, disseminated mammary epithelial cells within circulation or a foreign host microenvironment are capable of forming tumors at the ectopic site (Podsypanina et al., 2008). Additionally, reports of bone marrow cytokeratin-positive epithelial cells in up to 48% of breast cancer patients without overt metastases also offer support for early primary tumor cell dissemination. Decreased survival in patients with such cells was demonstrated in all studies (Braun et al., 2000; Diel et al., 1996; Gebauer et al., 2001; Pantel et al., 2003; Vannucchi et al., 1998). Furthermore, only 8% of these patients with bone marrow micrometastases exhibited cytokeratin-positive/Ki67-positive cells, suggesting that lack of overt bone metastasis may be due to disseminated tumor cell dormancy (Pantel et al., 2003).

2. The breast tumor microenvironment

A normal epithelial tissue can undergo hyperplasia and acquire tumorigenic properties that promote the development of a benign, non-invasive solid tumor known as carcinoma *in situ*. Normal epithelial tissues and non-invasive carcinoma *in situ* tumors are separated from a supportive stromal compartment by an intact basement membrane. Ultimately, carcinoma *in situ* can progress to a malignant, invasive carcinoma, the most common form of human cancer. The panoply of published investigations between the fields of mammary gland development and breast cancer has led to an appreciation for a supportive non-epithelial mammary stroma that mechanically and biologically restrains tumorigenesis. However, tumors of the breast and other epithelial tissues obviously overcome these growth restraints and exploit this stroma to sculpt a vastly divergent tumor stroma. Tumor stroma is generally divided into four main components: tumor vasculature, inflammatory leukocytes, extracellular matrix (ECM) and soluble growth factors, and fibroblasts. Malignant carcinoma cells and tumor stromal cells bi-directionally communicate with one another through paracrine signaling and intercellular contacts in a disorganized ECM to constitute a tumor microenvironment. Tumor-associated fibroblasts (TAF), the predominant stromal cell population within the tumor microenvironment, acquire and sustain an "activated" phenotype that promotes tumor progression (Rasanen and Vaheri, 2010). TAF are capable of enhancing breast tumor growth and metastasis by means of promoting angiogenesis (Orimo *et al.*, 2005), epithelial-mesenchymal transition (EMT) (Martin *et al.*, 2010; Radisky *et al.*, 2005), and progressive genetic instability (Kurose *et al.*, 2001; Moinfar *et al.*, 2000). In contrast, a normal mammary microenvironment can act in a dominant manner to inhibit tumor growth and "revert" the malignant phenotype of breast cancer cells (Kenny and Bissell, 2003). While resident breast tissue fibroblasts can inhabit breast tumors as TAF, breast tumors also recruit distant cell populations that engraft within the breast tumor microenvironment where they actively contribute as TAF. For example, mesenchymal stem cells (MSC), a bone marrow-derived stromal cell population, home to breast cancer cell xenograft tumors and persist as TAF (Spaeth *et al.*, 2009).

3. Cancer-associated inflammation

Although highly characterized for their protective capacity against infection, inflammatory leukocytes also reside within the tumor microenvironment. In fact, various immune cells are capable of eliminating transformed cells and thus preventing tumorigenesis in a process termed immunosurveillance (Dunn *et al.*, 2004). Whereas acute inflammation may prevent tumorigenesis by promoting an immune response directed against transformed cells, chronic inflammation promotes tumorigenesis. Rudolf Virchow is credited with making the seminal link between chronic inflammation and cancer by noting that human tumor biopsies were often infiltrated with inflammatory cells (Balkwill and Mantovani, 2001). Leukocytes can be detected in non-malignant tumors and carcinomas, including breast cancer (DeNardo and Coussens, 2007), which suggests an ongoing antitumor immune response. Despite the infiltration of leukocytes such as cytotoxic T-cells and NK-cells, the persistence of a tumor demonstrates immune evasion and highlights the local and systemic immune suppressive state of the tumor microenvironment and the tumor-bearing host, respectively.

4. Interleukin-6: A quintessential pleiotropic cytokine

Interleukin-6 (IL-6) is an inflammation-associated cytokine and major inducer of C-reactive protein (CRP) throughout the acute phase inflammatory response. *IL6* gene expression is nuclear factor-kappaB (NF-κB)-dependent (Chauhan *et al.*, 1996) and produces a 26 kDa IL-6 protein product. First characterized as a T-cell-derived factor that induced proliferation, differentiation, and immunoglobulin production in B-cells, IL-6 was originally named B-cell stimulating factor-2 (BSF-2). It was later thought to be a novel interferon (IFN-β2) due to studies demonstrating the ability of IL-6 to activate signal transducer and activator of transcription 3 (STAT3) (Kishimoto, 2006). Complementary DNA encoding the human IL-6 gene was subsequently cloned, and human IL-6 transgenic mice demonstrated a polyclonal IgG1 plasmacytosis phenotype (Suematsu *et al.*, 1989). Next, IL-6 knockout (IL-6-/-) mice were generated and characterized. IL-6-/- mice underwent normal development, but adult animals exhibited reduced numbers of peripheral T-cells and impaired antiviral cytotoxic T-cell activity (Kopf *et al.*, 1994). In addition, IL-6 is a critical factor during hematopoiesis and subsequent lymphocyte differentiation and activation. Multiple diverse cell populations including fibroblasts, T and B-cells, monocytes, macrophages, endothelial cells, keratinocytes, astrocytes, and smooth muscle cells all have the potential to produce constitutive or inducible IL-6 (Kishimoto, 2006).

Depending on cellular context, IL-6 can signal through multiple kinase-dependent proliferation and anti-apoptosis pathways including the mitogen-activated protein kinase (MAPK) pathway, the phosphatidylinositol-triphosphate kinase (PI-3K)/Akt pathway, and perhaps the most commonly evaluated in breast cancer, the Janus kinase (JAK)/signal transducer and activator of transcription-3 (STAT3) pathway (Hodge *et al.*, 2005). To do so, a plasma membrane-associated IL-6 receptor (IL-6R/CD126) homodimer first ligates two soluble IL-6 molecules, which leads to gp130 (CD130) homodimer ligation. Whereas IL-6R is only expressed on hepatocytes, osteoclasts, and most immune cells under normal physiological conditions, gp130 is a ubiquitous and promiscuous receptor involved in multiple cytokine signaling pathways (e.g., IL-11, leukemia inhibitory factor (LIF), oncostatin M (OSM), and ciliary neurotrophic factor (CNTF)) (Rose-John *et al.*, 2006). To initiate classical JAK/STAT3 signal transduction, JAK are recruited to the intracellular domain of the gp130 receptor where they bind and autophosphorylate. Subsequent gp130 phosphorylation via activated JAK offers docking sites for STAT3 and other receptor-associated proteins. Once bound to the intracellular domain of gp130, STAT3 is specifically phosphorylated (pSTAT3) by adjacent JAK on a C-terminal tyrosine residue (Y705), which grants its disengagement from the receptor. Dissociation of pSTAT3[Y705] from gp130 facilitates its homodimerization within the cytoplasm, and the pSTAT3[Y705] homodimer translocates to the nucleus. There, pSTAT3[Y705] binds to specific promoters whereby it initiates the transcription of multiple downstream target genes (Clevenger, 2004). Under normal physiological conditions, an inhibitory feedback loop maintains rapid and transient STAT3 activation. Following activation in normal cells, STAT3 induces suppressors of cytokine signaling (SOCS) and protein inhibitors of activated STATs (PIAS) expression. While SOCS-1 specifically inhibits JAK function, SOCS-3 binds the IL-6R complex to inhibit IL-6 signal transduction. PIAS-3 directly interacts with STAT3 to inhibit all STAT3 target gene expression (Kishimoto, 2006). In contrast, many human cancers, including breast cancer, exhibit constitutive STAT3 activity. Recent studies have demonstrated that unphosphorylated STAT3 (U-STAT3) accumulates in tumor cells with constitutively active

STAT3 where it forms a complex with NF-κB to activate a subset of NF-κB target genes (Yang and Stark, 2008).

Alternatively, IL-6 *trans*-signaling describes an IL-6 signaling pathway whereby an IL-6 soluble receptor (IL-6sR) binds IL-6 and subsequently ligates gp130 to stimulate STAT3 activation in cells that only express gp130. IL-6sR is naturally produced by either proteolytic cleavage of the membrane-bound IL-6R or alternative splicing of IL-6R mRNA (Rose-John *et al.*, 2006). Whereas IL-6 serum levels continue to increase with age, levels of serum IL-6sR rise until approximately age 70 at which time they gradually decline (Giuliani *et al.*, 2001). Furthermore, IL-6sR expression has been demonstrated in human breast cancer cell lines (Crichton *et al.*, 1996; Oh *et al.*, 1996; Singh *et al.*, 1995), suggesting that IL-6 *trans*-signaling mediates the effects of IL-6 in breast cancer cells. In contrast, an endogenous soluble gp130 (sgp130) specifically antagonizes IL-6 *trans*-signaling by exclusively ligating the IL-6/IL-6sR complex, thus having no effect on cells that express the membrane-bound IL-6R (Rose-John *et al.*, 2006) (Figure 1).

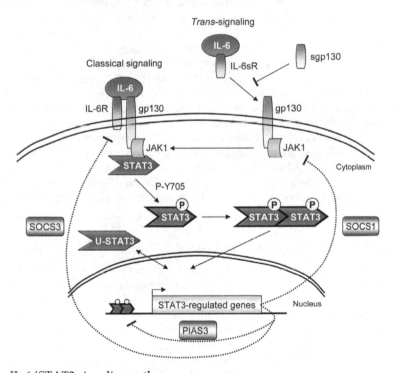

Fig. 1. The IL-6/STAT3 signaling pathway

5. Excessive IL-6 in human breast cancer

Aberrantly elevated IL-6 is associated with a poor prognosis in breast cancer (Bachelot *et al.*, 2003; Salgado *et al.*, 2003; Zhang and Adachi, 1999). Human breast tumors produce more IL-6 when compared to matched healthy breast tissue, and tumor IL-6 levels concurrently increase with tumor grade. In addition, increased serum IL-6 has been demonstrated in breast cancer patients compared to normal donors and correlates with advanced breast tumor stage (Kozlowski et al., 2003) and increased number of metastatic sites (Salgado et al., 2003). Furthermore, a single nucleotide polymorphism (SNP) exists at position -174 in the IL-6 gene promoter region, noted as IL-6 (-174 G>C), with the following allele frequency in a Caucasion population: 36% G/G, 44% G/C, and 18% C/C. An inflammatory stimulus such as Salmonella typhii vaccination induced higher serum IL-6 in those individuals with the G/G allele (Bennermo et al., 2004). Although the IL-6 (-174 G>C) SNP is not associated with increased risk of developing breast cancer (Gonzalez-Zuloeta Ladd et al., 2006; Litovkin et al., 2007; Yu et al., 2009b), it is significantly associated with disease-free and overall survival in breast cancer patients (DeMichele et al., 2003).

ERα is expressed in luminal subtype breast tumors (Perou et al., 2000) and therefore associated with improved patient survival (Buyse et al., 2006; Sorlie et al., 2001). A clear and well-characterized inverse correlation exists between breast cancer ERα status and IL-6. In fact, ERα directly binds to NF-κB, thus preventing transactivation of IL6 gene expression (Galien and Garcia, 1997), which demonstrates a direct mechanism for such a correlation. Furthermore, ERα-negative human breast tumors produce more IL-6 than tumors that express ERα (Chavey et al., 2007), and IL-6 serum levels are higher in ERα-negative breast cancer patients compared to ERα-positive patients (Jiang et al., 2000). Likewise, ERα-negative breast cancer cell lines produce autocrine IL-6 whereas ERα-positive breast cancer cell lines do not (Sasser et al., 2007). Therefore, this strongly suggests that ERα-negative breast cancer cells would exploit both paracrine (i.e., stromal cell-derived) and autocrine IL-6 signaling, whereas ERα-positive breast cancer cells could only utilize paracrine IL-6 signaling. In addition, ERα-negative breast cancer patients, whose tumors produce more IL-6 than those that express ERα (Chavey et al., 2007), showed no difference in survival between the G/G allele (higher inducible serum IL-6) and any C allele (lower inducible serum IL-6) at the IL-6 (-174 G>C) promoter SNP. In contrast, ERα-positive breast cancer patients with any C allele at the IL-6 (-174 G>C) promoter SNP demonstrated improved disease-free and overall survival compared to those with the G/G allele (DeMichele et al., 2003).

6. IL-6 promotes breast cancer cell growth

Stromal fibroblasts isolated from multiple types of tumors (i.e., TAF) or cancers (i.e., CAF) are now appreciated as influential players in cancer progression and metastasis (Orimo and Weinberg, 2006). CAF derived from multiple cancer types, including murine mammary cancers, exhibit an activated, proinflammatory phenotype with increased IL-6 production (Erez et al., 2010). Furthermore, work from our laboratory has demonstated that fibroblasts isolated from breast tissue and common sites of breast cancer metastasis such as bone and lung enhance the growth of breast cancer cells in an IL-6-dependent manner, and IL-6 is the major fibroblast-derived soluble factor that induced STAT3 activation in breast cancer cells (Sasser et al., 2007; Studebaker et al., 2008). MDA-MB-231 breast cancer cells are commonly utilized to model triple negative breast cancer and produce autocrine IL-6. MDA-MB-231 cells expressing a dominant negative isoform of gp130 lacked constitutively active STAT3 and exhibited impaired tumorigenicity in an orthotopic xenograft model (Selander et al., 2004), thus suggesting that IL-6 may drive tumor progression in this model. In addition, STAT3 is estimated to be constitutively activated in more than half of primary breast cancers due to IL-6 signaling (Berishaj et al., 2007).

Mesenchymal stem cells (MSC) are a bone marrow-derived fibroblast cell population that can be recruited to the breast tumor stroma, acquire a TAF phenotype, and produce high levels of IL-6. MSC enhance the growth of ERα-positive breast cancer cells, which do not express IL-6 or activated STAT3. In contrast, MSC have no effect on IL-6-producing ERα-negative breast cancer cells, which express constitutively activated STAT3. Moreover, ERα-positive breast cancer cells orthotopically co-injected with MSC or MSC conditioned medium and ERα-positive breast cancer cells that ectopically express IL-6 demonstrate enhanced xenograft tumor growth in the absence of exogenous 17β-estradiol (Sasser et al., 2007). Similar differential growth enhancement was demonstrated in vivo with ERα-positive and ERα-negative breast cancer cells co-injected with MSC, which also promoted metastasis (Karnoub et al., 2007). Interestingly, IL-6 has been reported to facilitate the recruitment of MSC to hypoxic breast tumor microenvironments (Rattigan et al., 2010). Likewise, IL-6 secreted from breast cancer cells has been shown to contribute to a recently characterized phenomenon termed "self-seeding" in which aggressive circulating tumor cells engraft within their original xenograft tumor (Kim et al., 2009). MSC have also been shown to mediate the self-renewal capacity of breast cancer stem cells, in part, through a reciprocal IL-6 loop (Liu et al., 2010). Taken together, preceding evidence strongly suggests that IL-6 promotes breast cancer cell growth by activating STAT3, which culminates with the upregulation of proliferative oncogenes such as c-Myc and cyclin D1 and and growth factors such as IL-6, hepatocyte growth factor (HGF), vascular endothelial growth factor (VEGF), and epidermal growth factor (EGF) (Yu et al., 2009a).

7. IL-6 promotes epithelial-mesenchymal transition in breast cancer cells

Normal polarized epithelial cells exhibit 'cobblestone' homophilic morphology and express E-cadherin, which is required for epithelial cell polarization, phenotype, and consequent homeostasis (Jeanes et al., 2008). E-cadherin is a key prognostic molecular biomarker clinically utilized to predict the metastatic propensity of breast cancer. Whereas very few studies have failed to demonstrate E-cadherin as an independent prognostic biomarker in breast cancer patients (Lipponen et al., 1994; Parker et al., 2001), the overwhelming majority of relevant studies have revealed E-cadherin as one of the strongest predictors of patient survival. Specifically, impaired E-cadherin expression in human breast tumors correlates with enhanced invasiveness, metastatic potential (Oka et al., 1993), and decreased breast cancer patient survival (Heimann and Hellman, 2000; Pedersen et al., 2002). While appropriate E-cadherin function is essential to the maintenance of epithelial cell morphology, phenotype, and homeostasis, regulation of E-cadherin expression is of equal importance. CDH1, the gene that encodes E-cadherin, is located on human chromosome 16q22.1 (Rakha et al., 2006) and is susceptible to inactivation by promoter hypermethylation, somatic mutation, or aberrant overexpression of repressive transcription factors including Twist, Snail, and Slug among others (Hirohashi, 1998). Likewise, E-cadherin loss of function can arise due to extracellular domain-specific proteolytic cleavage. Although uncommon, germline mutations of CDH1 predispose individuals to hereditary diffuse gastric cancer (HDGC) syndrome, and a proportion of these patients present with other cancers, including breast cancer (Guilford, 1999).

E-cadherin was initially termed uvomorulin in mice and L-CAM in chicks following its discovery as a 120 kDa calcium-dependent trypsin-labile cell surface glycoprotein required for intercellular adhesion in mouse blastomeres (Hyafil et al., 1981) and chick embryos

(Brackenbury *et al.*, 1981). It now represents the best studied member of the cadherin family of tissue-specific homophilic intercellular adhesion molecules. E-cadherin knockout studies have demonstrated early embryonic lethality due to impaired maintenance of epithelial polarity and failure to form an intact epithelium in E-cadherin$^{-/-}$ embryos (Larue *et al.*, 1994). E-cadherin is localized on the cell surface of epithelial cells, and each E-cadherin protein consists of an amino-terminal extracellular domain, a single-pass transmembrane segment, and a carboxy-terminal intracellular domain. Five calcium-binding repeated subunits comprise an extracellular domain that promotes homophilic interaction to ultimately form anti-parallel trans-E-cadherin dimers between adjacent cells (Guilford, 1999). The intracellular domain is comprised of a juxtamembrane p120-catenin binding subdomain and a C-terminal beta (β)-catenin binding subdomain. β-catenin, a potent transcription factor, binds E-cadherin and alpha (α)-catenin subsequently binds β-catenin. Although contentious (Weis and Nelson, 2006), it is generally acknowledged that α-catenin interacts with F-actin and thereby, facilitates the linkage of E-cadherin to the cytoskeleton. This E-cadherin-catenin-actin complex localizes to epithelial intercellular junctions called adherens junctions and is critical to epithelial cell adhesion, polarity, and morphology (Hartsock and Nelson, 2008). Furthermore, E-cadherin sequesters β-catenin at the cell surface as one means to inhibit β-catenin nuclear translocation and consequent expression of β-catenin responsive genes (Perez-Moreno *et al.*, 2003).

Another prominent role of E-cadherin is that of an invasion/metastasis suppressor protein. Upon loss of E-cadherin and subsequent dissociation of adherens junctions, epithelial cells acquire enhanced invasive capability (Behrens *et al.*, 1989). MDA-MB-231 cells, an ERα-negative breast cancer cell line, lack E-cadherin, whereas MCF-7 cells, an ERα-positive breast cancer cell line express high levels of E-cadherin (Kenny *et al.*, 2007), and MDA-MB-231 cells exhibit enhanced invasive capability compared to MCF-7 cells (Sommers *et al.*, 1991). Naturally, E-cadherin expression and consequent invasive capacity regulate the propensity of breast cancer metastasis. Multiple signaling pathways are activated following loss of E-cadherin protein, which promote transformed human breast epithelial cell metastasis in a xenograft model. Interestingly, Twist, a transcriptional repressor of *CDH1*, is induced upon loss of E-cadherin and is necessary for metastasis in this model. Furthermore, the E-cadherin binding partner, β-catenin, was shown to be necessary but not sufficient for the EMT phenotype induced following loss of E-cadherin (Onder *et al.*, 2008). Ectopic expression of murine E-cadherin in highly metastatic human MDA-MB-231 cells significantly reduced osteolytic bone metastases in a murine intracardiac dissemination model (Mbalaviele *et al.*, 1996). Likewise, aberrant cytoplasmic or diminished to negative E-cadherin immunostaining patterns are commonly detected in invasive poorly differentiated breast carcinomas compared to noninvasive well-differentiated breast carcinomas and are associated with increased probability of breast carcinoma metastasis (Oka *et al.*, 1993). The finding that distant metastases often express E-cadherin even in patients which exhibit primary breast carinomas which lack E-cadherin suggests that ultimate re-expression may be necessary for colonization of secondary tissues (Kowalski *et al.*, 2003; Saha *et al.*, 2007).

Loss of E-cadherin is a prerequisite for epithelial-mesenchymal transition (EMT), a highly conserved process which exemplifies the aberrant activation of an embryonic gene expression program during carcinoma progression. EMT is critical for multiple steps of developmental metazoan cellular morphogenesis as demonstrated in well-characterized

Drosophila and *Xenopus* models. Throughout embryonic development, EMT whereby epithelial cells give rise to more motile mesenchymal cells is essential for mesoderm and neural crest formation. Importantly, this is a transient process and mesenchymal-epithelial transition (MET) allows for cellular reversion (Yang and Weinberg, 2008).

Whereas EMT has been extensively studied for its essential role in embryogenesis, the concept of EMT-like cellular changes in human cancers has gained acceptance as a major mechanism to promote primary tumor cell invasion and subsequent tumor metastasis. A carcinoma cell must first detach from the primary tumor and invade through the basement membrane into the underlying tissue parenchyma to initiate the metastasic cascade. Although cancer-associated EMT was considered a controversial notion even in recent years (Tarin *et al.*, 2005), it has been demonstrated in multiple human carcinomas, including breast cancer (Cheng *et al.*, 2008; Heimann and Hellman, 2000; Moody *et al.*, 2005; Sarrio *et al.*, 2008), and is now recongnized as a putative mediator of tumor metastasis. An EMT phenotype including impaired E-cadherin expression with concominant induction of Vimentin, Alpha-smooth-muscle-actin, and/or N-cadherin is associated with the basal breast cancer subtype, suggesting that EMT may promote characteristic aggressiveness in these tumors and contribute to poor breast cancer patient survival (Sarrio *et al.*, 2008). Likewise, relatively noninvasive ERα-positive MCF-7 cells express E-cadherin, consistent with a characteristic epithelial phenotype, and are classified as luminal subtype, whereas highly invasive ERα-negative MDA-MB-231 cells lack E-cadherin and are classified as basal subtype (Blick *et al.*, 2008). Furthermore, ERα directly correlates with E-cadherin in primary human breast tumors (Ye *et al.*, 2010). While EMT may enhance carcinoma cell invasion and subsequent dissemination which would increase metastatic potential, it is not synonymous with metastasis in all models. For example, Lou, *et al.* demonstrated that EMT alone was insufficient for spontaneous murine mammary carcinoma metastasis (Lou *et al.*, 2008). Yet, Weinberg and colleagues described the promotion of metastasis with loss of E-cadherin and a consequent EMT phenotype in transformed human breast epithelial cells (Onder *et al.*, 2008).

Our laboratory has previously demonstrated that exogenous IL-6 exposure induced an EMT phenotype in a panel of human ERα-positive breast cancer cells, which included E-cadherin repression and concomitant induction of Vimentin, N-cadherin, Snail, and Twist. In addition, ectopic expression of IL-6 in ERα-positive MCF-7 breast cancer cells promoted an EMT phenotype and enhanced invasiveness. Likewise, MCF-7 cells with ectopic Twist expression exhibit an EMT phenotype (Mironchik *et al.*, 2005), autocrine IL-6 production, and constitutive STAT3 activation (Sullivan *et al.*, 2009).

8. Therapeutic targeting of the IL-6/STAT3 pathway

IL-6 levels are increased in human breast tumors and breast cancer patient sera, and excessive IL-6, both circulating and within the breast tumor microenvironment, is associated with poor clinical outcomes in breast cancer. STAT3, a critical downstream mediator of IL-6 signaling, is constitutively activated in more than half of human cancers and promotes the expression of proliferative, anti-apoptotic, immune suppressive, and pro-angiogenic target genes, which all potentiate carcinogenesis. Whereas the IL-6 signaling network has been targeted in numerous autoimmune diseases and cancers, this therapeutic strategy has yet to be clinically employed for breast cancer. Increased preclinical reports have revealed novel mechanisms underlying IL-6/STAT3 signaling in breast cancer cells such as enhanced growth, induction of EMT, multidrug resistance, and recruitment of peripheral fibroblasts. Taken together, accumulating preclinical and clinical data emphasize IL-6 as a highly attractive therapeutic target in breast cancer. It is therefore imperative that more work be done to evaluate current therapeutics and develop novel agents that target IL-6/STAT3 signaling in breast cancer models.

Multiple strategies could be utilized to target the IL-6/STAT3 pathway, but first and most obvious would be anti-IL-6 neutralizing antibodies. One such anti-IL-6 monoclonal antibody is Siltuximab (CNTO 328). The safety and efficacy of Situximab has been demonstrated in preclinical studies and phase I/II clinical trials of diverse human pathologies and malignancies including Castleman's disease (van Rhee *et al.*, 2010), multiple myeloma (Hunsucker *et al.*, 2011; Voorhees *et al.*, 2007), prostate cancer (Cavarretta *et al.*, 2007; Cavarretta *et al.*, 2008; Dorff *et al.*, 2010; Karkera *et al.*, 2011), renal cell carcinoma (Puchalski *et al.*, 2010; Rossi *et al.*, 2010), non-small cell lung cancer (Song *et al.*, 2010), and ovarian cancer (Guo *et al.*, 2010). Furthermore, IL-6R can be targeted with tocilizumab, an anti-IL-6R monoclonal antibody that has shown promising results in IL-6-driven autoimmune diseases (Tanaka et al., 2011) and was recently approved by the FDA for the treatment of rheumatoid arthritis. The promiscuous IL-6 coreceptor, gp130, also has an endogenous soluble form (sgp130) that exclusively inhibits IL-6 *trans*-signaling, thus preserving classical IL-6 signaling. Therapeutic sgp130 would potentially be more targeted toward breast cancer cells, which generally lack membrane-associated IL-6R and therefore utilize IL-6 trans-signaling through IL-6sR. Recombinant soluble gp130 (sgp130-Fc) has been shown to inhibit murine colon carcinogenesis (Becker *et al.*, 2004), suggesting that it may prove effective in breast cancer as well. Finally, a growing number of non-selective kinase inhibitors and recent focus on specific JAK and STAT3 inhibitor development will provide further insight into the roles of JAK and STAT3 in breast cancer.

9. Conclusions

Breast cancer is a heterogeneous disease and thus, highly variable across individual patients. This heterogenicity arises not only due to the diversity of genetic and molecular aberrations in primary breast cancer cells but also due to the diversity of cellular populations that inhabit the breast tumor microenvironment. Although IL-6 levels are higher in breast tumors and patient sera, the precise source of this IL-6 remains elusive. Importantly, many breast tumor stromal cells provide a paracrine source of IL-6 for breast cancer cells within the breast tumor microenvironment. In addition, certain clinical subtypes of breast cancers and research models, such as ERα-negative primary breast cancers and ERα-negative breast cancer cell lines, produce excessive IL-6 (Figure 2). Therefore, ERα-negative breast cancer cells may supply the tumor microenvironment with IL-6 by means of autocrine IL-6 production to exacerbate the poor prognosis associated with this clinical subtype. It will be critical to determine the specific cellular source of breast tumor-associated IL-6 to advance our understanding of this pleiotropic cytokine in breast cancer progression and metastasis. Moreover, this knowledge will facilitate the validation and subsequent clinical utility of current and novel targeted antagonists of the IL-6/STAT3 signaling network in breast cancer.

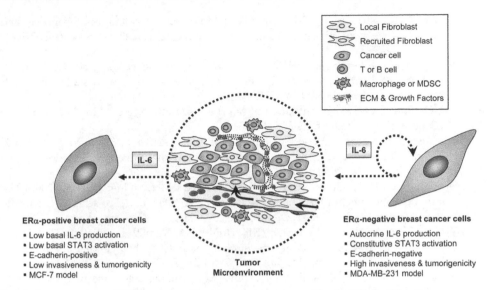

Fig. 2. Breast cancer cell ERα status dictates paracrine vs. autocrine IL-6 utilization.

10. References

Anderson WF, Matsuno R (2006) Breast cancer heterogeneity: a mixture of at least two main types? *J Natl Cancer Inst* 98:948-951.

Bachelot T, Ray-Coquard I, Menetrier-Caux C, Rastkha M, Duc Λ, Blay JY (2003) Prognostic value of serum levels of interleukin 6 and of serum and plasma levels of vascular endothelial growth factor in hormone-refractory metastatic breast cancer patients. *Br J Cancer* 88:1721-1726.

Balkwill F, Mantovani A (2001) Inflammation and cancer: back to Virchow? *Lancet* 357:539-545.

Becker C, Fantini MC, Schramm C, Lehr HA, Wirtz S, Nikolaev A, *et al.* (2004) TGF-beta suppresses tumor progression in colon cancer by inhibition of IL-6 trans-signaling. *Immunity* 21:491-501.

Behrens J, Mareel MM, Van Roy FM, Birchmeier W (1989) Dissecting tumor cell invasion: epithelial cells acquire invasive properties after the loss of uvomorulin-mediated cell-cell adhesion. *J Cell Biol* 108:2435-2447.

Bennermo M, Held C, Stemme S, Ericsson CG, Silveira A, Green F, *et al.* (2004) Genetic predisposition of the interleukin-6 response to inflammation: implications for a variety of major diseases? *Clin Chem* 50:2136-2140.

Berishaj M, Gao SP, Ahmed S, Leslie K, Al-Ahmadie H, Gerald WL, *et al.* (2007) Stat3 is tyrosine-phosphorylated through the interleukin-6/glycoprotein 130/Janus kinase pathway in breast cancer. *Breast Cancer Res* 9:R32.

Blick T, Widodo E, Hugo H, Waltham M, Lenburg ME, Neve RM, *et al.* (2008) Epithelial mesenchymal transition traits in human breast cancer cell lines. *Clin Exp Metastasis* 25:629-642.

Brackenbury R, Rutishauser U, Edelman GM (1981) Distinct calcium-independent and calcium-dependent adhesion systems of chicken embryo cells. *Proc Natl Acad Sci U S A* 78:387-391.

Braun S, Pantel K, Muller P, Janni W, Hepp F, Kentenich CR, *et al.* (2000) Cytokeratin-positive cells in the bone marrow and survival of patients with stage I, II, or III breast cancer. *N Engl J Med* 342:525-533.

Butler TP, Gullino PM (1975) Quantitation of cell shedding into efferent blood of mammary adenocarcinoma. *Cancer Res* 35:512-516.

Buyse M, Loi S, van't Veer L, Viale G, Delorenzi M, Glas AM, *et al.* (2006) Validation and clinical utility of a 70-gene prognostic signature for women with node-negative breast cancer. *J Natl Cancer Inst* 98:1183-1192.

Cavarretta IT, Neuwirt H, Untergasser G, Moser PL, Zaki MH, Steiner H, *et al.* (2007) The antiapoptotic effect of IL-6 autocrine loop in a cellular model of advanced prostate cancer is mediated by Mcl-1. *Oncogene* 26:2822-2832.

Cavarretta IT, Neuwirt H, Zaki MH, Steiner H, Hobisch A, Nemeth JA, *et al.* (2008) Mcl-1 is regulated by IL-6 and mediates the survival activity of the cytokine in a model of late stage prostate carcinoma. *Adv Exp Med Biol* 617:547-555.

Chauhan D, Uchiyama H, Akbarali Y, Urashima M, Yamamoto K, Libermann TA, *et al.* (1996) Multiple myeloma cell adhesion-induced interleukin-6 expression in bone marrow stromal cells involves activation of NF-kappa B. *Blood* 87:1104-1112.

Chavey C, Bibeau F, Gourgou-Bourgade S, Burlinchon S, Boissiere F, Laune D, *et al.* (2007) Oestrogen receptor negative breast cancers exhibit high cytokine content. *Breast Cancer Res* 9:R15.

Cheng GZ, Zhang WZ, Sun M, Wang Q, Coppola D, Mansour M, *et al.* (2008) Twist is transcriptionally induced by activation of STAT3 and mediates STAT3 oncogenic function. *J Biol Chem* 283:14665-14673.

Clevenger CV (2004) Roles and regulation of stat family transcription factors in human breast cancer. *Am J Pathol* 165:1449-1460.

Crichton MB, Nichols JE, Zhao Y, Bulun SE, Simpson ER (1996) Expression of transcripts of interleukin-6 and related cytokines by human breast tumors, breast cancer cells, and adipose stromal cells. *Mol Cell Endocrinol* 118:215-220.

DeMichele A, Martin AM, Mick R, Gor P, Wray L, Klein-Cabral M, *et al.* (2003) Interleukin-6 -174G-->C polymorphism is associated with improved outcome in high-risk breast cancer. *Cancer Res* 63:8051-8056.

DeNardo DG, Coussens LM (2007) Inflammation and breast cancer. Balancing immune response: crosstalk between adaptive and innate immune cells during breast cancer progression. *Breast Cancer Res* 9:212.

Diel IJ, Kaufmann M, Costa SD, Holle R, von Minckwitz G, Solomayer EF, *et al.* (1996) Micrometastatic breast cancer cells in bone marrow at primary surgery: prognostic value in comparison with nodal status. *J Natl Cancer Inst* 88:1652-1658.

Dorff TB, Goldman B, Pinski JK, Mack PC, Lara PN, Jr., Van Veldhuizen PJ, Jr., *et al.* (2010) Clinical and correlative results of SWOG S0354: a phase II trial of CNTO328 (siltuximab), a monoclonal antibody against interleukin-6, in chemotherapy-pretreated patients with castration-resistant prostate cancer. *Clin Cancer Res* 16:3028-3034.

Dunn GP, Old LJ, Schreiber RD (2004) The immunobiology of cancer immunosurveillance and immunoediting. *Immunity* 21:137-148.

Erez N, Truitt M, Olson P, Arron ST, Hanahan D (2010) Cancer-Associated Fibroblasts Are Activated in Incipient Neoplasia to Orchestrate Tumor-Promoting Inflammation in an NF-kappaB-Dependent Manner. *Cancer Cell* 17:135-147.

Galien R, Garcia T (1997) Estrogen receptor impairs interleukin-6 expression by preventing protein binding on the NF-kappaB site. *Nucleic Acids Res* 25:2424-2429.

Gebauer G, Fehm T, Merkle E, Beck EP, Lang N, Jager W (2001) Epithelial cells in bone marrow of breast cancer patients at time of primary surgery: clinical outcome during long-term follow-up. *J Clin Oncol* 19:3669-3674.

Giuliani N, Sansoni P, Girasole G, Vescovini R, Passeri G, Passeri M, et al. (2001) Serum interleukin-6, soluble interleukin-6 receptor and soluble gp130 exhibit different patterns of age- and menopause-related changes. *Exp Gerontol* 36:547-557.

Gonzalez-Zuloeta Ladd AM, Arias Vasquez A, Witteman J, Uitterlinden AG, Coebergh JW, Hofman A, et al. (2006) Interleukin 6 G-174 C polymorphism and breast cancer risk. *Eur J Epidemiol* 21:373-376.

Guilford P (1999) E-cadherin downregulation in cancer: fuel on the fire? *Mol Med Today* 5:172-177.

Guo Y, Nemeth J, O'Brien C, Susa M, Liu X, Zhang Z, et al. (2010) Effects of siltuximab on the IL-6-induced signaling pathway in ovarian cancer. *Clin Cancer Res* 16:5759-5769.

Hartsock A, Nelson WJ (2008) Adherens and tight junctions: structure, function and connections to the actin cytoskeleton. *Biochim Biophys Acta* 1778:660-669.

Heimann R, Hellman S (2000) Individual characterisation of the metastatic capacity of human breast carcinoma. *Eur J Cancer* 36:1631-1639.

Hess KR, Pusztai L, Buzdar AU, Hortobagyi GN (2003) Estrogen receptors and distinct patterns of breast cancer relapse. *Breast Cancer Res Treat* 78:105-118.

Hirohashi S (1998) Inactivation of the E-cadherin-mediated cell adhesion system in human cancers. *Am J Pathol* 153:333-339.

Hodge DR, Hurt EM, Farrar WL (2005) The role of IL-6 and STAT3 in inflammation and cancer. *Eur J Cancer* 41:2502-2512.

Hunsucker SA, Magarotto V, Kuhn DJ, Kornblau SM, Wang M, Weber DM, et al. (2011) Blockade of interleukin-6 signalling with siltuximab enhances melphalan cytotoxicity in preclinical models of multiple myeloma. *Br J Haematol* 152:579-592.

Hyafil F, Babinet C, Jacob F (1981) Cell-cell interactions in early embryogenesis: a molecular approach to the role of calcium. *Cell* 26:447-454.

Irvin WJ, Jr., Carey LA (2008) What is triple-negative breast cancer? *Eur J Cancer* 44:2799-2805.

James JJ, Evans AJ, Pinder SE, Gutteridge E, Cheung KL, Chan S, et al. (2003) Bone metastases from breast carcinoma: histopathological - radiological correlations and prognostic features. *Br J Cancer* 89:660-665.

Jeanes A, Gottardi CJ, Yap AS (2008) Cadherins and cancer: how does cadherin dysfunction promote tumor progression? *Oncogene* 27:6920-6929.

Jemal A, Bray F, Center MM, Ferlay J, Ward E, Forman D (2011) Global cancer statistics. *CA Cancer J Clin* 61:69-90.

Jiang XP, Yang DC, Elliott RL, Head JF (2000) Reduction in serum IL-6 after vacination of breast cancer patients with tumour-associated antigens is related to estrogen receptor status. *Cytokine* 12:458-465.

Karkera J, Steiner H, Li W, Skradski V, Moser PL, Riethdorf S, *et al.* (2011) The anti-interleukin-6 antibody siltuximab down-regulates genes implicated in tumorigenesis in prostate cancer patients from a phase I study. *Prostate.*

Karnoub AE, Dash AB, Vo AP, Sullivan A, Brooks MW, Bell GW, *et al.* (2007) Mesenchymal stem cells within tumour stroma promote breast cancer metastasis. *Nature* 449:557-563.

Kenny PA, Bissell MJ (2003) Tumor reversion: correction of malignant behavior by microenvironmental cues. *Int J Cancer* 107:688-695.

Kenny PA, Lee GY, Myers CA, Neve RM, Semeiks JR, Spellman PT, *et al.* (2007) The morphologies of breast cancer cell lines in three-dimensional assays correlate with their profiles of gene expression. *Mol Oncol* 1:84-96.

Kim MY, Oskarsson T, Acharyya S, Nguyen DX, Zhang XH, Norton L, *et al.* (2009) Tumor self-seeding by circulating cancer cells. *Cell* 139:1315-1326.

Kishimoto T (2006) Interleukin-6: discovery of a pleiotropic cytokine. *Arthritis Res Ther* 8 Suppl 2:S2.

Klein CA (2009) Parallel progression of primary tumours and metastases. *Nat Rev Cancer* 9:302-312.

Kominsky SL, Davidson NE (2006) A "bone" fide predictor of metastasis? Predicting breast cancer metastasis to bone. *J Clin Oncol* 24:2227-2229.

Kopf M, Baumann H, Freer G, Freudenberg M, Lamers M, Kishimoto T, *et al.* (1994) Impaired immune and acute-phase responses in interleukin-6-deficient mice. *Nature* 368:339-342.

Kowalski PJ, Rubin MA, Kleer CG (2003) E-cadherin expression in primary carcinomas of the breast and its distant metastases. *Breast Cancer Res* 5:R217-222.

Kozlowski L, Zakrzewska I, Tokajuk P, Wojtukiewicz MZ (2003) Concentration of interleukin-6 (IL-6), interleukin-8 (IL-8) and interleukin-10 (IL-10) in blood serum of breast cancer patients. *Rocz Akad Med Bialymst* 48:82-84.

Kurose K, Hoshaw-Woodard S, Adeyinka A, Lemeshow S, Watson PH, Eng C (2001) Genetic model of multi-step breast carcinogenesis involving the epithelium and stroma: clues to tumour-microenvironment interactions. *Hum Mol Genet* 10:1907-1913.

Larue L, Ohsugi M, Hirchenhain J, Kemler R (1994) E-cadherin null mutant embryos fail to form a trophectoderm epithelium. *Proc Natl Acad Sci U S A* 91:8263-8267.

Lipponen P, Saarelainen E, Ji H, Aaltomaa S, Syrjanen K (1994) Expression of E-cadherin (E-CD) as related to other prognostic factors and survival in breast cancer. *J Pathol* 174:101-109.

Litovkin KV, Domenyuk VP, Bubnov VV, Zaporozhan VN (2007) Interleukin-6 -174G/C polymorphism in breast cancer and uterine leiomyoma patients: a population-based case control study. *Exp Oncol* 29:295-298.

Liu S, Ginestier C, Ou SJ, Clouthier SG, Patel SH, Monville F, *et al.* (2010) Breast cancer stem cells are regulated by mesenchymal stem cells through cytokine networks. *Cancer Res* 71:614-624.

Lou Y, Preobrazhenska O, auf dem Keller U, Sutcliffe M, Barclay L, McDonald PC, et al. (2008) Epithelial-mesenchymal transition (EMT) is not sufficient for spontaneous murine breast cancer metastasis. Dev Dyn 237:2755-2768.

Macedo LF, Sabnis G, Brodie A (2009) Aromatase inhibitors and breast cancer. Ann N Y Acad Sci 1155:162-173.

Martin FT, Dwyer RM, Kelly J, Khan S, Murphy JM, Curran C, et al. (2010) Potential role of mesenchymal stem cells (MSCs) in the breast tumour microenvironment: stimulation of epithelial to mesenchymal transition (EMT). Breast Cancer Res Treat 124:317-326.

Mbalaviele G, Dunstan CR, Sasaki A, Williams PJ, Mundy GR, Yoneda T (1996) E-cadherin expression in human breast cancer cells suppresses the development of osteolytic bone metastases in an experimental metastasis model. Cancer Res 56:4063-4070.

Mironchik Y, Winnard PT, Jr., Vesuna F, Kato Y, Wildes F, Pathak AP, et al. (2005) Twist overexpression induces in vivo angiogenesis and correlates with chromosomal instability in breast cancer. Cancer Res 65:10801-10809.

Moinfar F, Man YG, Arnould L, Bratthauer GL, Ratschek M, Tavassoli FA (2000) Concurrent and independent genetic alterations in the stromal and epithelial cells of mammary carcinoma: implications for tumorigenesis. Cancer Res 60:2562-2566.

Moody SE, Perez D, Pan TC, Sarkisian CJ, Portocarrero CP, Sterner CJ, et al. (2005) The transcriptional repressor Snail promotes mammary tumor recurrence. Cancer Cell 8:197-209.

Oh JW, Revel M, Chebath J (1996) A soluble interleukin 6 receptor isolated from conditioned medium of human breast cancer cells is encoded by a differentially spliced mRNA. Cytokine 8:401-409.

Oka H, Shiozaki H, Kobayashi K, Inoue M, Tahara H, Kobayashi T, et al. (1993) Expression of E-cadherin cell adhesion molecules in human breast cancer tissues and its relationship to metastasis. Cancer Res 53:1696-1701.

Onder TT, Gupta PB, Mani SA, Yang J, Lander ES, Weinberg RA (2008) Loss of E-cadherin promotes metastasis via multiple downstream transcriptional pathways. Cancer Res 68:3645-3654.

Orimo A, Gupta PB, Sgroi DC, Arenzana-Seisdedos F, Delaunay T, Naeem R, et al. (2005) Stromal fibroblasts present in invasive human breast carcinomas promote tumor growth and angiogenesis through elevated SDF-1/CXCL12 secretion. Cell 121:335-348.

Orimo A, Weinberg RA (2006) Stromal fibroblasts in cancer: a novel tumor-promoting cell type. Cell Cycle 5:1597-1601.

Pantel K, Muller V, Auer M, Nusser N, Harbeck N, Braun S (2003) Detection and clinical implications of early systemic tumor cell dissemination in breast cancer. Clin Cancer Res 9:6326-6334.

Parker C, Rampaul RS, Pinder SE, Bell JA, Wencyk PM, Blamey RW, et al. (2001) E-cadherin as a prognostic indicator in primary breast cancer. Br J Cancer 85:1958-1963.

Pedersen KB, Nesland JM, Fodstad O, Maelandsmo GM (2002) Expression of S100A4, E-cadherin, alpha- and beta-catenin in breast cancer biopsies. Br J Cancer 87:1281-1286.

Perez-Moreno M, Jamora C, Fuchs E (2003) Sticky business: orchestrating cellular signals at adherens junctions. Cell 112:535-548.

Perou CM, Sorlie T, Eisen MB, van de Rijn M, Jeffrey SS, Rees CA, *et al.* (2000) Molecular portraits of human breast tumours. *Nature* 406:747-752.

Podsypanina K, Du YC, Jechlinger M, Beverly LJ, Hambardzumyan D, Varmus H (2008) Seeding and propagation of untransformed mouse mammary cells in the lung. *Science* 321:1841-1844.

Puchalski T, Prabhakar U, Jiao Q, Berns B, Davis HM (2010) Pharmacokinetic and pharmacodynamic modeling of an anti-interleukin-6 chimeric monoclonal antibody (siltuximab) in patients with metastatic renal cell carcinoma. *Clin Cancer Res* 16:1652-1661.

Radisky DC, Levy DD, Littlepage LE, Liu H, Nelson CM, Fata JE, *et al.* (2005) Rac1b and reactive oxygen species mediate MMP-3-induced EMT and genomic instability. *Nature* 436:123-127.

Rakha EA, Green AR, Powe DG, Roylance R, Ellis IO (2006) Chromosome 16 tumor-suppressor genes in breast cancer. *Genes Chromosomes Cancer* 45:527-535.

Rasanen K, Vaheri A (2010) Activation of fibroblasts in cancer stroma. *Exp Cell Res* 316:2713-2722.

Rattigan Y, Hsu JM, Mishra PJ, Glod J, Banerjee D (2010) Interleukin 6 mediated recruitment of mesenchymal stem cells to the hypoxic tumor milieu. *Exp Cell Res* 316:3417-3424.

Rose-John S, Scheller J, Elson G, Jones SA (2006) Interleukin-6 biology is coordinated by membrane-bound and soluble receptors: role in inflammation and cancer. *J Leukoc Biol* 80:227-236.

Rossi JF, Negrier S, James ND, Kocak I, Hawkins R, Davis H, *et al.* (2010) A phase I/II study of siltuximab (CNTO 328), an anti-interleukin-6 monoclonal antibody, in metastatic renal cell cancer. *Br J Cancer* 103:1154-1162.

Saha B, Chaiwun B, Imam SS, Tsao-Wei DD, Groshen S, Naritoku WY, *et al.* (2007) Overexpression of E-cadherin protein in metastatic breast cancer cells in bone. *Anticancer Res* 27:3903-3908.

Salgado R, Junius S, Benoy I, Van Dam P, Vermeulen P, Van Marck E, *et al.* (2003) Circulating interleukin-6 predicts survival in patients with metastatic breast cancer. *Int J Cancer* 103:642-646.

Sarrio D, Rodriguez-Pinilla SM, Hardisson D, Cano A, Moreno-Bueno G, Palacios J (2008) Epithelial-mesenchymal transition in breast cancer relates to the basal-like phenotype. *Cancer Res* 68:989-997.

Sasser AK, Sullivan NJ, Studebaker AW, Hendey LF, Axel AE, Hall BM (2007) Interleukin-6 is a potent growth factor for ER-alpha-positive human breast cancer. *Faseb J* 21:3763-3770.

Selander KS, Li L, Watson L, Merrell M, Dahmen H, Heinrich PC, *et al.* (2004) Inhibition of gp130 signaling in breast cancer blocks constitutive activation of Stat3 and inhibits in vivo malignancy. *Cancer Res* 64:6924-6933.

Shoker BS, Jarvis C, Clarke RB, Anderson E, Hewlett J, Davies MP, *et al.* (1999) Estrogen receptor-positive proliferating cells in the normal and precancerous breast. *Am J Pathol* 155:1811-1815.

Singh A, Purohit A, Wang DY, Duncan LJ, Ghilchik MW, Reed MJ (1995) IL-6sR: release from MCF-7 breast cancer cells and role in regulating peripheral oestrogen synthesis. *J Endocrinol* 147:R9-12.

Sommers CL, Thompson EW, Torri JA, Kemler R, Gelmann EP, Byers SW (1991) Cell adhesion molecule uvomorulin expression in human breast cancer cell lines: relationship to morphology and invasive capacities. *Cell Growth Differ* 2:365-372.

Song L, Rawal B, Nemeth JA, Haura EB (2010) JAK1 Activates STAT3 Activity in Non-Small-Cell Lung Cancer Cells and IL-6 Neutralizing Antibodies Can Suppress JAK1-STAT3 Signaling. *Mol Cancer Ther* 10:481-494.

Sorlie T, Perou CM, Tibshirani R, Aas T, Geisler S, Johnsen H, *et al.* (2001) Gene expression patterns of breast carcinomas distinguish tumor subclasses with clinical implications. *Proc Natl Acad Sci U S A* 98:10869-10874.

Spaeth EL, Dembinski JL, Sasser AK, Watson K, Klopp A, Hall B, *et al.* (2009) Mesenchymal stem cell transition to tumor-associated fibroblasts contributes to fibrovascular network expansion and tumor progression. *PLoS One* 4:e4992.

Studebaker AW, Storci G, Werbeck JL, Sansone P, Sasser AK, Tavolari S, *et al.* (2008) Fibroblasts isolated from common sites of breast cancer metastasis enhance cancer cell growth rates and invasiveness in an interleukin-6-dependent manner. *Cancer Res* 68:9087-9095.

Suematsu S, Matsuda T, Aozasa K, Akira S, Nakano N, Ohno S, *et al.* (1989) IgG1 plasmacytosis in interleukin 6 transgenic mice. *Proc Natl Acad Sci U S A* 86:7547-7551.

Sullivan NJ, Sasser AK, Axel AE, Vesuna F, Raman V, Ramirez N, *et al.* (2009) Interleukin-6 induces an epithelial-mesenchymal transition phenotype in human breast cancer cells. *Oncogene* 28:2940-2947.

Tanaka T, Narazaki M, Kishimoto T (2011) Anti-interleukin-6 receptor antibody, tocilizumab, for the treatment of autoimmune diseases. *FEBS Lett.*

Tarin D, Thompson EW, Newgreen DF (2005) The fallacy of epithelial mesenchymal transition in neoplasia. *Cancer Res* 65:5996-6000; discussion 6000-5991.

van Rhee F, Fayad L, Voorhees P, Furman R, Lonial S, Borghaei H, *et al.* (2010) Siltuximab, a novel anti-interleukin-6 monoclonal antibody, for Castleman's disease. *J Clin Oncol* 28:3701-3708.

Vannucchi AM, Bosi A, Glinz S, Pacini P, Linari S, Saccardi R, *et al.* (1998) Evaluation of breast tumour cell contamination in the bone marrow and leukapheresis collections by RT-PCR for cytokeratin-19 mRNA. *Br J Haematol* 103:610-617.

Voorhees PM, Chen Q, Kuhn DJ, Small GW, Hunsucker SA, Strader JS, *et al.* (2007) Inhibition of interleukin-6 signaling with CNTO 328 enhances the activity of bortezomib in preclinical models of multiple myeloma. *Clin Cancer Res* 13:6469-6478.

Weis WI, Nelson WJ (2006) Re-solving the cadherin-catenin-actin conundrum. *J Biol Chem* 281:35593-35597.

Yang J, Stark GR (2008) Roles of unphosphorylated STATs in signaling. *Cell Res* 18:443-451.

Yang J, Weinberg RA (2008) Epithelial-mesenchymal transition: at the crossroads of development and tumor metastasis. *Dev Cell* 14:818-829.

Ye Y, Xiao Y, Wang W, Yearsley K, Gao JX, Shetuni B, *et al.* (2010) ERalpha signaling through slug regulates E-cadherin and EMT. *Oncogene* 29:1451-1462.

Yu H, Pardoll D, Jove R (2009a) STATs in cancer inflammation and immunity: a leading role for STAT3. *Nat Rev Cancer* 9:798-809.

Yu KD, Di GH, Fan L, Chen AX, Yang C, Shao ZM (2009b) Lack of an association between a
    functional polymorphism in the interleukin-6 gene promoter and breast cancer risk:
    a meta-analysis involving 25,703 subjects. *Breast Cancer Res Treat* 122:483-488.
Zhang GJ, Adachi I (1999) Serum interleukin-6 levels correlate to tumor progression and
    prognosis in metastatic breast carcinoma. *Anticancer Res* 19:1427-1432.

10

Hyaluronan Associated Inflammation and Microenvironment Remodelling Influences Breast Cancer Progression

Caitlin Ward[1], Catalina Vasquez[1,2], Cornelia Tolg[1,3],
Patrick G. Telmer[1] and Eva Turley[1,4,5]
[1]London Regional Cancer Program, London Health Sciences Center,
Victoria Hospital, London ON
[2]Dept. of Medical Biophysics University of Western Ontario
[3]The Hospital for Sick Children, Toronto ON
[4]Dept. of Oncology, University of Western Ontario, London ON
[5]Dept. of Biochemistry, University of Western Ontario, London ON
Canada

1. Introduction

1.1 The breast microenvironment

The breast is an organ composed predominantly of glandular, fatty, and fibrous tissues. Glandular tissue is composed of ducts lined by luminal epithelial cells that secrete milk, and is surrounded by a layer of myoepithelial cells that contract to release milk. Myoepithelial cells produce proteases, growth factors and growth factor receptors that contribute to remodelling during breast tissue expansion. Each duct is enclosed by a laminin-rich basement membrane and embedded in extracellular matrix (ECM). Mammary gland ECM and is a mixture of fibrillar proteins such as collagens, laminins, fibronectin, and polysaccharides such as heparin sulphate, chondroitin sulphate and hyaluronan (HA). These collectively provide the mechanical and structural support required for maintaining mammary tissue architecture and for storage of the soluble regulatory molecules needed for tissue homeostasis, plasticity, and remodelling. ECM promotes both the differentiated, homeostatic integrity of mammary tissue and is also a key determinant in branching morphogenesis, response-to-injury and pathological processes such as neoplastic disease. The importance of the ECM in determining homeostatic vs. tumourigenic events was originally demonstrated three decades ago by Beatrice Mintz, who showed that marked embryonic carcinoma cells injected into blastocysts do not give rise to tumours but instead contribute to normal tissue architecture. The same cells injected into adult mice develop into tumours (Mintz and Illmensee, 1975). Components of the microenvironment that support tumour progression have since been identified. For example, chick embryos infected with Rous Sarcoma virus express the oncogene v-src in every cell but tumours develop only at sites of wounding due to the accumulation of TGF-β1 (Weigelt and Bissell, 2008).

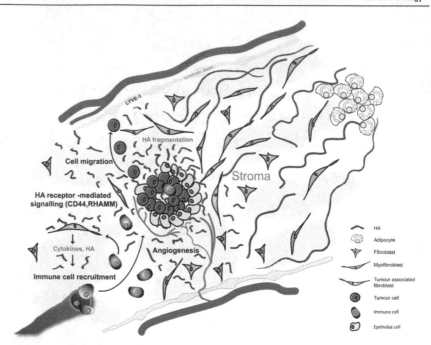

Fig. 1. Breast tumour microenvironment

Conversely, breast tumour cells can be reverted by blocking signalling through ECM receptors, including integrins (Turley *et al.*, 2008) and HA receptors such as RHAMM (Hall *et al.*, 1995). These and other studies have revealed a key role of ECM in initiating and sustaining breast cancer and introduced the novel concept that transformation can be a plastic rather than irreversible process. Specifically, increased HA accumulation in tumour cells or stroma is associated with poor outcome in Breast Cancer (BCA) (Tammi *et al.*, 2008). These studies predict that HA is an important component of ECM that determines a homeostatic vs. tumourigenesis "switch".

2. HA biology

2.1 Biochemical properties

HA belongs to the glycosaminoglycan group of polysaccharides composed of disaccharide units of a hexose linked to a hexosamine. It consists of repeating units of N-acetyl glucosamine and β-glucuronic acid (Fig. 2). The native polymer consists of up to 10^6 to 10^7 non-branching disaccharide units. The functions of HA within the ECM and cells depend upon its molecular weight, the type of cell, and the HA receptor(s) that target cells express. High molecular weight HA (e.g. >200 kDa) is a major biomechanical factor in ECM, which contributes to tissue hydration and elasticity by providing a template for the assembly of macromolecular complexes. A well known example is the "bottle brush" complex of aggrecan and link proteins, which provides the visco-elastic nature of synovial fluid. HA fragments provide signalling functions and are usually present during the ECM remodelling that is associated with morphogenesis or disease. Regulated synthesis and degradation are key factors in maintaining a delicate balance between structural (homeostatic) and signalling (wound and disease) functions of HA (Itano *et al.*, 2008, Jiang *et al.*, 2007, Veiseh and Turley, 2011). BCA cells are particularly adept at producing and responding to HA fragments. BCA cells produce increased levels of HA by increasing HA synthase expression, rapidly fragmenting HA as a result of increased Reactive Oxygen Species (ROS) production, and increasing hyaluronidase expression and release, and increasing expression and display of HA receptors to elevate the response to these fragments (Simpson and Lokeshwar, 2008, Toole and Slomiany, 2008, Veiseh and Turley, 2011).

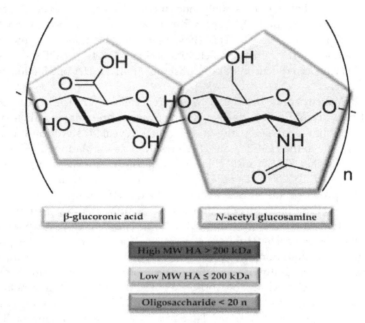

Fig. 2. HA structure and molecular weight ranges.

2.2 HA synthesis and tumourigenesis

HA is synthesized by three HAS isoforms, HAS1-3, which are located on different chromosomes but share from 57 to 80% sequence homology (Weigel *et al.*, 1997, Lokeshwar and Selzer, 2008, Stern, 2008). The mature enzymes are multi-pass integral proteins, which are primarily located in the plasma membrane and catalyze polymerization of HA from the uridine diphosphate (UDP) sugars uridine diphosphate glucuronic acid (UDP-Glc-UA) and uridine diphosphate N-acetylglucosamine (UDP-GlcNAC). Synthesis and secretion of HA occur concurrently, allowing for the rapid production and release of large polymers into the ECM (Weigel *et al.*, 1997). There is some evidence that HASs are resident in endosomes, ER and the perinuclear membrane although whether or not these produce intracellular HA is not yet clear (Karousou *et al.*, 2010, Vigetti *et al.*, 2010). HAS1 and 2 are widely expressed throughout the embryo while HAS3 expression is more restricted, for example, to developing tooth-forming neural crest cells and hair follicles. Genetic deletion of HAS2 is embryonic lethal in mice due to severe defects in cardiac tissue development, whereas targeted disruption of the HAS1 or 3 alleles results in fertile viable animals with only minor aberrations in tooth and follicle development (Weigel and DeAngelis, 2007). It is not fully understood why only HAS2 is absolutely required for organogenesis, but it has been suggested that it produces high molecular weight tissue HA while the other HASs produce the smaller HA sizes (Itano et al., 1999). There are differences in the mechanisms by which HAS isoform expression and enzyme activity are regulated that may be relevant to their functions and essential or non-essential roles in organogenesis (Tammi et al., 2008).

BCA cells use several mechanisms to rapidly control the synthesis and release of HA, thereby modifying their ECM, including substrate availability, gene expression, posttranslational control of enzyme activity, and differential response to cytokines and ECM signalling. The availability of UDP sugars can profoundly influence the yield of HAS enzymes (Kakizaki et al., 2004). This has been demonstrated by the use of 4-Methylumbelliferone (4-MU), which depletes intracellular levels of UDP-Glc-UA (Kakizaki et al., 2004) by serving as a glucuronidation substrate. It blocks HA production and reduces BCA tumourigenicty.

The genomic plasticity and instability of cancer cells often leads to chromosomal aberrations that can result in both de-regulation of gene expression and allele duplication. Chromatin breakpoint analysis using a BCA line revealed significant chromosomal rearrangements close to the HAS2 gene. These result in de-regulation of HAS2 expression and significantly higher HAS2 mRNA levels in transformed cells compared to normal breast cells (Unger et al., 2009). Detailed in vitro and in vivo studies of BCA lines and xenografts have provided numerous insights into the effects of genetically modifying HAS expression levels on HA concentration within the tumour and peri-tumoural stroma. Antisense inhibition of HAS2 in MDA-MB-231 BCA cells delays proliferation via a transient arrest of the cell cycle (Udabage et al., 2005). Knockdown of HAS expression also results in significant alterations in genes associated with HA metabolism. CD44 and HYAL1 expression are both down-regulated in response to antisense inhibition of HAS2. In vivo, MDA-MB-231 cells expressing antisense HAS2 do not form tumours in nude mice after 12 weeks, whereas the parental cell line readily establishes both primary and secondary tumours during this time. This clearly implicates tumour cell HA as a significant driver of BCA formation. Elevated HA accumulation within BCA peri-tumoural stroma is also a prognostic factor and appears to promote a microenvironment suitable for BCA growth. For example, HAS2-/- fibroblasts transplanted with BCA cells into the fat pads of NOD/SCID mice fail to recruit macrophages and promote angiogenesis to the same extent as HAS2+/+ fibroblasts. This defect results in decreased tumour volume (Kobayashi et al., 2010).

The expression of all three HASs is controlled by growth factors and cytokines. However, there appear to be subtle differences in the response of each isoform that depend upon the cell type. For example, PDGF and TGFβ induce HAS2 expression in fibroblasts but HAS1 or 3 expression in synoviocytes and keratinocytes, respectively (Karousou et al., 2010). H-Ras transformation increases only HAS2 expression in 3Y-1 tumour cells, while transformation with v-src or v-fos increases both HAS1 and HAS2 expression in the same cells (Itano et al., 2004). Posttranslational modification of HAS, including phosphorylation by PKC, PKA, and the ERK/ErbB2 MAPK pathways (Goentzel et al., 2006, Itano and Kimata, 2008) as well as mono-ubiquitination (Karousou et al., 2010) also affects HAS activity. HAS3 serine phosphorylation is enhanced upon treatment with a PKC activator (Goentzel et al., 2006). All three HAS isoforms expressed by SKOV3 ovarian cancer cell line are phosphorylated by

ERK1,2 in response to treatment with Heregulin (Bourguignon *et al.*, 2007) and mono-ubquitination of K190 on HAS2 rapidly inactivates this enzyme (Karousou *et al.*, 2010).

2.3 HA fragmentation and its role in tumourigenesis

In addition to HAS1-3 expression, the amount and polymer size of HA are also affected by reactive oxygen species (ROS) and secreted hyaluronidases (HYALs), which fragment HA to various sizes. Significant levels of ROS can be generated during times of oxidative stress and these are considered critical in cancer initiation, promotion and progression (Karihtala *et al.*, 2007). ROS are produced in response to extracellular stimuli such as bacterial infections and environmental toxins, but can also be produced by cellular metabolism (Yu *et al.*, 2011). Five HYALs fragment HA: HYAL-1-3, PH-20 and HYAL-5. The HYALs differ in their cellular location and enzymatic properties. HYAL-1 and 2 are the major HYALs produced by somatic tissues whereas HYAL-3 is expressed mostly in bone marrow and testes. Both PH-20 and HYAL-5 expression are normally restricted to testes but PH20 is aberrantly expressed in BCA (Stern, 2008). HYAL-1 and 2 cooperate to degrade HMW HA in a coordinated fashion. HYAL-2, which is GPI anchored to the cell surface, degrades extracellular HA to fragments of 20 kDa, which are then taken up into endocytic vesicles. HYAL-1 present in the lysosome further degrades intracellular HA into tetrasaccharides (Tammi *et al.*, 2001, Stern, 2008, Simpson and Lokeshwar, 2008). Coordinated breakdown of HA by HYALs increases the rate of HA metabolism and this appears to be an important factor in tumourigenesis (Veiseh and Turley, 2011). For example, co-expression of HAS3 and HYAL-1 increases the aggressiveness and spread of prostate cancer cells compared to expression of either alone (Bharadwaj *et al.*, 2009). In BCA, HYAL-1 and HYAL-2 are often coordinately overexpressed compared to non-malignant breast tissue. Knockdown of HYAL-1, which is overexpressed in MDA-MB-231 and MCF-7 BCA lines, reduces tumour xenograft size (Tan *et al.*, 2010).

3. HA receptors detect oligosaccharides and fragments: Control of key signalling pathways by HA fragments

3.1 CD44

CD44 is a class I transmembrane receptor, which binds to HA via a link domain and is expressed by a variety of cells, including fibroblasts, endothelial and epithelial cells, smooth muscle, and haematopoietic cells. A vital role of CD44 is recruiting cells, including immune cells and fibroblasts, to sites of inflammation through HA-mediated signalling. Under homeostatic conditions, CD44 is in a low HA binding state, but during injury and tumourigenesis its binding affinity is increased and it mediates the inflammatory and tissue repair responses (Thorne *et al.*, 2004, Naor *et al.*, 2008). CD44 is expressed as many different isoforms due to extensive splicing in a region proximal to the transmembrane domain (Thorne *et al.*, 2004). The smallest CD44 isoform, CD44s (standard form), skips this variable region. The role of CD44s and variants in BCA progression is still controversial. For example, CD44s expression in CD44[low] MCF-7 human BCA cells results in xenograft metastasis to the liver (Ouhtit *et al.*, 2007) while CD44-/- mice develop more lung metastases than wildtype animals in response to polyomavirus middle T (Lopez *et al.*, 2005). Importantly, a recent study by Brown *et al.* (2011) demonstrated that CD44s expression is elevated and required for epithelial-mesenchymal transition of immortalized human mammary epithelial cells and for recurrence of HER2/*neu* induced murine mammary tumours (Lopez *et al.*, 2005). HA synthesis is elevated in CD44+ BCAs compared to CD44- and both CD44+ and HER2+ BCAs are amongst the most aggressive and invasive subtypes of BCA with poor prognosis.   Expression of variant exons, in particular exon v6, is associated with increased *in vitro* cell migration and invasion of human BCA cells (Herrera-Gayol and Jothy, 1999). Although CD44v6 expression has been correlated with multiple clinicopathological features (primary tumour size, axillary nodal status, histological grade and pTNM stage) it is not an independent prognostic factor (Ma *et al.*, 2005). A study by Rys *et al.* (2003) found a correlation between the expression of CD44 v3 and the presence of BCA metastasis. Additionally, high CD44s expression correlates with increased disease free survival in node negative invasive BCA (Diaz *et al.*, 2005). The controversies surrounding CD44 and its role in BCA progression may be caused by a limited number of patient samples in some of these studies, heterogeneity of BCA, and CD44 expression by cancer stem cells. The latter, in particular, has raised much recent interest in CD44 since several groups have identified CD44 as a potential marker for BCA stem cells. This is a highly tumourigenic population of cancer cells that, although only representing a small percentage of cells in the tumour, are thought to be responsible for tumour recurrence, metastasis and treatment failure. Aggressive BCA and BCA tumour progenitor cells have enhanced CD44 expression, associated with an increase in HA synthesis and CD44-HA binding affinity (Heldin *et al.*, 2008).

In BCA cells, HA triggers CD44 interactions with a variety of signalling mediators involved in cell proliferation, migration and chemo-resistance. Ankyrin is a membrane-associated component of the cytoskeleton that is involved in regulation of cytoskeleton turnover and IP3 receptor-mediated regulation of intracellular Ca^{2+}. CD44-HA interactions induce CD44-ankyrin coupling and modify receptor-dependent Ca^{2+} mobilization (Bourguignon *et al.*, 2008). CD44 also localizes ankyrin and IP3 receptor to lipid rafts, which are cholesterol and caveolin rich signalling microdomains in the plasma membrane (Fig. 3). The Rho GTPases, RhoA, Rac and CDC42, are key regulators of cell migration and HA stimulates RhoA in BCA cells. RhoA activity is regulated by RhoGEF, a guanine nucleotide exchange factor that forms a complex with CD44 in BCA cells. One of the downstream RhoA targets, ROK, phosphorylates the cytoplasmic domain of CD44 thereby increasing CD44-ankyrin interactions. Other targets of ROK are myosin phosphatase and myosin light chain, two important mediators of actin-myosin dependent membrane ruffling required for cell migration. HA also activates the PI3 kinase/AKT pathway: Gab-1 phosphorylation by ROK stimulates PI3 kinase and AKT activation, leading to increased cell proliferation, invasion and cytokine production (Bourguignon *et al.*, 2008). Additionally, ROK phosphorylates and activates NHE1, a Na^+-H^+ exchanger, causing intracellular and extracellular acidification leading to HYAL-2 driven HA degradation, ECM breakdown and tumour progression. CD44-HA interactions stimulate signalling through Rac1, another RhoGTPase, via the GEF Tiam1. In MDA-MB-231 cells, CD44-HA interactions also activate c-Src kinase resulting in activation and nuclear translocation of the transcription factor Twist, miR-10b expression and down-regulation of the tumour suppressor gene HOXD10 (Bourguignon *et al.*, 2010 Toole, 2004). CD44 undergoes sequential proteolytic cleavages resulting in the release of its ectodomain from the cell surface and formation of a CD44 intracellular domain fragment, which is translocated to the nucleus, acting as a transcription co-regulator (Nagano and Saya, 2004). CD44 ectodomain cleavage is mediated by MT1-MMP and is stimulated by multiple factors, including HA fragments and TGF-β (Kuo *et al.*, 2009, Sugahara *et al.*, 2006) which, contribute to tumour cell migration and invasion (Fig. 3).

3.2 RHAMM/HMMR

Receptor for HA Mediated Motility (RHAMM/HMMR) belongs to a group of proteins that are found intracellularly as well as extracellularly. RHAMM does not contain a transmembrane domain or classical export signal and is likely exported through an unconventional mechanism that does not involve the Golgi/ER. RHAMM is expressed as multiple isoforms and one of these, an N-terminal truncation that lacks the first 163 aa residues, is transforming in mesenchymal cells (Hall *et al.*, 1995). On the cell surface, RHAMM interacts with HA and forms complexes with transmembrane receptors such as CD44, PDGFR, and RON (Maxwell *et al.*, 2008). Interestingly, CD44 surface display is reduced in mesenchymal cells isolated from RHAMM-/- mice, demonstrating functional interplay between these two HA receptors (Tolg *et al.*, 2006). RHAMM is elevated in most types of cancer in particular breast, ovarian, and prostate cancer, as well as in MM, AML and CML. In BCA, RHAMM is a tumour marker, novel susceptibility factor and prognostic factor for poor outcome (Maxwell *et al.*, 2008). Consistent with these clinical correlations, RHAMM has tumourigenic properties in experimental systems that have been linked to its ability to bind HA. In BCA cells, RHAMM/CD44/HA complexes sustain phosphorylation and activation of the Ras/MAPK (ERK1,2) signalling pathway, leading to BCA progression and constitutively high rates of motility and invasion (Hamilton *et al.*, 2007). The relationship between RHAMM and ERK1,2 activation has recently been confirmed in BCA samples where concomitant upregulation of phosphorylated ERK1,2 and RHAMM in tumour samples correlates with a high tumour grade (Ward C., in preparation). Intracellularly, RHAMM binds directly to tubulin and is involved in regulation of microtubule stability and turnover as a result of its association with ERK1,2. In mesenchymal cells, the absence of RHAMM increases microtubule stability resulting in reduced cell migration and aberrant mitotic spindle formation (Tolg *et al.*, 2010, Groen *et al.*, 2004). RHAMM interacts directly with ERK1, inferring that RHAMM may act as a scaffolding protein that directs ERK1 to its substrates including microtubule associated proteins that regulate microtubule stability (Tolg *et al.*, 2010). Interestingly, RHAMM expression is downregulated by p53, an important tumour suppressor gene, suggesting that RHAMM may be involved in p53 loss-induced tumour progression (Buganim and Rotter, 2008, Godar and Weinberg, 2008, Sohr and Engeland, 2008). RHAMM also acts on the BRCA1, pathway and may play an important role in BCA tumours arising from loss or inactivation of BRCA1 (Joukov *et al.*, 2006)

3.3 TLR2 and TLR4

Toll like receptors (TLR) are part of a cellular defence mechanism that is based on pattern recognition. TLRs recognize and bind bacterial lipopolysaccharides, DNA, and, in the case of TLR2,4, small HA fragments. In general, HA-TLR2,4 interactions control innate immunity through several mechanisms. For example, TLR 2,4 activation results in cytokine and chemokine release and leads to expression of metalloproteinases (MMPs) in immune cells (Voelcker *et al.*, 2008). Versican, which is associated with poor prognosis and relapse in BCA, interacts with HA polymers to form cord-like structures that link TLR2 on endothelial cells and fibroblasts. This, in turn, causes the secretion of pro-inflammatory cytokines (Theocharis *et al.*, 2010). HA-TLR2,4 interactions also stimulate NFκB signalling and activate TNFα. In BCA cells, TLR 2,4 interact with CD44 and act as co-receptors to stimulate signalling through HA and CD44 regulated pathways which may play a role in breast tumour cell migration/infiltration. The human BCA cell line MDA-MB-231 expresses mainly TLR4, and siRNA mediated knock-down of TLR4 significantly reduces cell survival and expression of the cytokines Il-6 and Il-8, suggesting that TLR4 is a promising target for BCA therapy (Yang *et al.*, 2010).

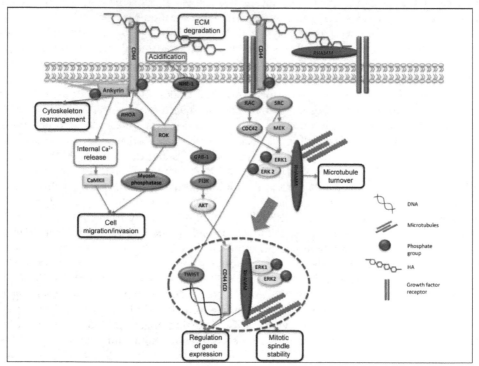

Fig. 3. HA initiates the signalling of RHAMM and CD44 regulated pathways, resulting in a variety of pro-tumourigenic outcomes.

3.4 LYVE-1

HA links the two main functions of the lymphatic system: draining of interstitial fluids and immune surveillance. These functions are achieved through its interaction with the receptor LYVE-1, present in lymphatic endothelia (Jackson, 2009). LYVE-1 is a type I integral membrane polypeptide that exhibits high homology with CD44 (Banerji *et al.*, 1999) and is a homeostatic HA receptor required for liver and lymphatic vessel formation. Its expression does not change as frequently in malignancy as HA receptors involved in response to injury, for example CD44 and RHAMM/HMMR. This does not rule out a role in injury and tumour progression however, as lymphangiogenesis is an important processes in both events, and elevated accumulation of HA in stroma results in lymphangiogenesis *via* signalling through LYVE-1 (Gale *et al.*, 2007).

To further demonstrate the association of LYVE-1 with tumour dissemination through the lymphatic system, (Du *et al.*, 2010) expressed LYVE-1 in COS-7 kidney cells and performed cell adhesion assays with the BCA cell line HS-578T which produces HA. These two cell lines had enhanced adhesion over the control cells, COS-7 not expressing LYVE-1. This suggests that LYVE-1 plays a role in tumour cell adhesion which is dependent on HA-LYVE-1 interaction. Apart from its effect on tumour cell adhesion, LYVE-1 has also been proven to be a prognostic factor in tongue squamous cell carcinoma and decreased levels of LYVE-1 in the invasive front of tumours predicts cervical lymph node metastasis (Matsumoto et al., 2010).

4. HA expression and signalling in different cell types and its relationship to BCA

4.1 HA, inflammation, and the role of inflammatory cells in tumourigenesis
4.1.1 Macrophages

HA has a major role in macrophage biology during inflammation, wound repair, and tumourigenesis and at least part of the detrimental effects of HA accumulation during tumourigenesis is due to the activation of tumour associated macrophages (TAMs). For instance, TAMs preferentially traffic to stromal compartments formed within HA producing tumours (Kobayashi et al., 2010). Macrophages are classed into type 1 and 2 according to the adaptive immune polarization with which they associate. Type 1 macrophages are antigen-presenting cells which promote the cytotoxic response, resulting in tumour cell killing. Type 2 macrophages, however, are classically associated with tissue remodelling, angiogenesis, and scavenging/phagocytosis. TAMs are similar to type 2 polarized macrophages which have decreased or inhibited cytotoxic activity (Mytar et al., 2003). Kuang et al. (2007) found that overexpression of HAS2 was able to polarize macrophages towards a malignant TAM phenotype. Additionally, exposure to solid tumour cell culture supernatant elicits a pro-inflammatory response in monocytes and their subsequent TAM-like polarization, showing that the tumour cells themselves are responsible for the immunosuppressive macrophage phenotype observed in solid tumours (Kuang et al., 2007). The importance of TAM recruitment in BCA dissemination was additionally illustrated by CSF-1 null mice crossed with the MMTV transgenic mouse model of BCA. In these mice, a failure to recruit macrophages into the primary tumour results in delayed primary tumour invasion and metastasis to the lungs compared to wildtype MMTV mice. The addition of exogenous CSF-1 rescues macrophage recruitment and restores tumour and metastasis development to baseline levels (Lin et al., 2001). After injury, or during tissue inflammation, small fragments of HA associate with TLR4 and control macrophage cytokines and chemokines (Termeer et al., 2000). For example, BCA cell associated HA promotes the production of pro-inflammatory cytokines and chemokines, such as TNF-α and IL-12, as well as ROS, by TAMs, an effect which can be alleviated by either blocking CD44 receptors on monocytes, or by the addition of non-BCA cell associated HA (Mytar et al., 2001). HA regulation of pro-inflammatory cytokine production also occurs in monocytes pre-exposed to a variety of solid tumour cell types and culture supernatants, including the BCA line MCF-7 (Mytar et al., 2003, del Fresno et al., 2005), modulating the IRAK family of NFκB regulatory molecules, this further downregulating TNF-α and IL-12 production. HA-mediated CD44 cross-linking induces this activity and is prevented by the addition of exogenous HYAL (Mytar et al., 2003). TAMs are recruited and regulated in response to NFκB, whose activation is often HA-mediated through TLR4 (del Fresno et al., 2005) and NFκB overexpression results in tumour metastasis (Mantovani et al., 2007). Nitric oxide, which is the product of nitric oxide synthase 2 (NOS), is stimulated by hypoxia and CSF-1, among others, and is a signalling molecule integrated within the NFκB inflammatory pathway. NOS2 signals the upregulation of CD44, c-Myc, MMP, and VEGF, which are all involved in promoting tumourigenesis. In BCA, NOS2 expression within tumour cells themselves is correlated with increased tumour grade and angiogenesis (Ambs and Glynn, 2011).

4.1.2 T Cells

T cells orient their cytoskeleton and migrate towards sites of inflammation, such as those present in a tumour microenvironment (TME), in a PKC-dependent manner as a direct result of CD44 crosslinking by HA (Fanning *et al.*, 2005). In BCA, CD8+ T cells are most predominant in advanced cancer stages where their presence in proliferating tumours is a good prognostic indicator. T cells are able to participate in either a Th1 or Th2 polarized immune response and, when polarized to a Th1 response, they express and secrete IFNγ, TGFβ, TNFα, IL-2, resulting in cytotoxic cooperation (T cells and M1). Th2 polarized CD4+ T cells secrete IL-4,5,6,10,13 which leads to an increase in B cell mediated immunity (DeNardo and Coussens, 2007). Because of the anti-tumour effects of T cells, the activation of cytotoxic T cells against HA receptors as immunotherapy in leukemias is currently undergoing clinical trials and will be discussed later in this chapter. On the other hand, the presence of CD4+ T cells correlates with disease progression and metastasis; however, it has been shown by different groups that CD4+ T cells are crucial for mounting an immune response against cancer. For example, tumour growth of EL4 lymphoma cells inoculated into mice is inhibited by the presence of dendritic cells primed against RHAMM protein. This interaction, however, is dependent on CD4+ T cells, as the effect of DC killing of the tumour is significantly reduced with a reduced CD4+ T cell population (Fukui *et al.*, 2006). Furthermore, Rakhra *et al.* (2010) showed that in ALL and B-cell leukemia, CD4+ cells were necessary for sustained tumour regression. In mouse models, inhibition of MYC or BCR-ABL rescues tumours from oncogene addiction; however, tumours regress in the presence of TSP-1 induced CD4+ T cells, and knockdown of TSP-1 impairs this ability (Rakhra *et al.*, 2010).

Regulatory T cells (Treg; CD4+/CD25+/FOXP3+) play controversial roles in tumour progression and can have both anti- and pro-tumourigenic effects, depending on the chemokines or cytokines produced and the type of solid tumour. Treg cells may be activated in an immunosuppressive manner, preventing cytotoxic immune responses, and allowing the tumours to evade immune attack. For example, in CLL, a large Treg population dampens specific CD8+ T cell responses against tumour associated antigens (Giannopoulos *et al.*, 2010). The same may be true for solid tumours. When coordinated, however, with a high T cell density, they may indicate good prognosis and inhibition of metastasis (Camus *et al.*, 2009, Carreras *et al.*, 2006).

4.1.3 B Cells

Immunoglobulin deposition by B cells in BCA stroma can be detrimental to disease progression and the accumulation of autoantibodies produced by B cells and deposited in the stroma correlates with poor prognosis (Fernandez Madrid *et al.*, 2005). An increase in serum IgG correlates with an increase in TAM numbers which, in turn, promotes angiogenesis in mouse mammary carcinoma, a process associated with poor clinical outcome. A proposed mechanism for the involvement of TAMs in B cell processes is the phagocytosis of IgG by macrophages. IgG engages Fcγ receptors, which stimulates VEGF secretion, increases angiogenesis and promotes tumour growth rate (Barbera-Guillem *et al.*,

2002). The majority of stromal B cells localize to perivascular regions within tumours and chronic B cell activation promotes tumours by recruiting macrophages and activating an innate immune response. However, the role of B cells in BCA progression is complicated since, for example, B cells may also recruit antigen presenting cells, such as CD8+ T cells and dendritic cells which help to eradicate neoplasms.

4.1.4 Dendritic cells and mast cells

Dendritic cells (DC) can also exhibit HA dependent characteristics that either promote or inhibit tumourigenesis. HA or chondroitin sulphate, in conjunction with CSF-1, activate DC from an immature to differentiated state via an NFκB regulated process, illustrating the importance of HA in eliciting an immune response (Yang *et al.*, 2002). Pedroza-Gonzalez *et al* (2011) recently showed that human BCA produces thymic stromal lymphopoietin (TSLP) which induces expression of OX40L on DCs, polarizing them towards a Th2 inflammatory response. *In vitro* this drives the production of IL-13 and TNF by Th2 polarized T cells (Pedroza-Gonzalez *et al.*, 2011). DC also become tumour insensitive and, as a result, do not mature and differentiate into cytotoxic cells. Furthermore, HA fragment build ups are at least partly responsible for preventing DC maturation in tumour bearing animals (Kuang *et al.*, 2008).

In BCA, c-kit expression by mast cells, a protein which is usually only present in specific tissue types, such as germ cells, predicts primary tumour recurrence (Khazaie *et al.*, 2011). However, an abundance of stromal mast cells in invasive BCA is associated with good prognosis (Rajput *et al.*, 2008). The mast cell line HMC-1 expresses high levels of CD44s and, through an interaction with HA, adheres to stromal tissue (Fukui *et al.*, 2000). Therefore, in both mast cells and DC, a CD44-HA interaction may result in anti-tumour responses.

4.2 HA regulation of a pro-inflammatory environment by non-immune cells
4.2.1 Breast cancer cells and their contribution to a pro-inflammatory environment

BCA cells secrete a variety of cytokines and chemokines which promote tumour progression. Studies by Tafani *et al.* (2010), showed that MCF-7 cells upregulate pro-inflammatory gene transcription and translation *in vitro*, and a pro-inflammatory gene expression profile can be seen in human BCA tumours even in the absence of an immune infiltrate. This illustrates that BCA cells themselves contribute to the pro-inflammatory/pro-tumourigenic TME. One or both of HER2 and ERα, which are often expressed on BCA cells, promote the expression and secretion of CXCL8 (IL-8) through the PI3K and ERK pathways. CXCL8 is a pro-angiogenic chemokine and secretion of CXCL8 by the MCF7 BCA line (which express both HER2 and ERα) is additive upon stimulation of both of these receptors (Haim *et al.*, 2008). The pro-inflammatory chemokines CCL2 and CCL5 are also secreted by BCA cells (Ben-Baruch, 2003) and expression and secretion of all three chemokines requires HA fragment/CD44 interactions on TAMs, tumour associated fibroblasts (TAFs) and BCA tumour cells. Both CCL2 and CCL5 are monocyte-recruiting chemokines and their expression in BCA tumours is correlated with poor prognosis, and in the case of CCL2, pro-angiogenesis factors and vascular invasion (Soria and Ben-Baruch, 2008). TNF-α secretion by TAMs activates a positive feedback loop in BCA tumour cells, stimulating further secretion of growth promoting chemokines (Ben-Baruch *et al.*, 2003). Eck *et al* (2009) also showed that conditioned media from BCA cells stimulates the expression of pro-inflammatory genes in normal mammary fibroblasts, polarizing them towards a TAF phenotype. Furthermore, TAF migration is increased, along with the secretion of MMP-1 and CXCR4 (IL-1/SDF-1 receptor), both of which are important factors in BCA progression (Eck *et al.*, 2009).

4.2.2 HA/stromal fibroblast/epithelial cell interaction and tumour progression

To begin to define the role played by TAFs in tumour progression, Micke *et al.* (2007) conducted cDNA microarray analyses comparing the transcriptome of TAFs from basal cell carcinoma with normal dermal fibroblasts (Micke *et al.*, 2007). This study showed that TAFs overexpress multiple growth factors such as PDGF, EGF, and VEGF, chemokines such as SDF1 and CXCL12 and matrix proteins such as MMP11, LAMA2 and COL5A2. In fact, these TAFs are known to secrete IGF-2, FGF-7, TGF-β, leptin, and NGF, which bind to their cognate receptors on BCA cells to stimulate HA production (Szabo *et al.*, 2011). This then promotes expression of cytokines such as TGF-β that attract and stimulate TAFs to proliferate. This paracrine effect is a positive feedback mechanism, because proliferating TAFs secrete additional growth factors, cytokines, chemokines, and MMPs that sustain BCA transformation and promote BCA progression. Additionally, VEGF, produced by TAFs, and HA oligosaccharides induce angiogenesis. HA itself also impairs immune surveillance, and/or activates TAMs and neutrophils that have tumour enhancing potential. Overexpression of HAS in a non-transformed rat fibroblast, 3Y1, increases high MW HA production and the resultant pericellular HA coat provides cells with a proliferation advantage that is accompanied by loss of contact inhibition of growth. This is achieved through HA-mediated activation of PI3 kinase. Lower MW HA also increases proliferation in these cells but has no effect on the HA matrix (Itano *et al.*, 2002). TAFs affect not only BCA cells but also normal cells in which the tumour is embedded. For example, TAFs induce stem cell-like behaviour and aberrant differentiation in normal fibroblasts, which can affect BCA progression. TAFs promote the expression of stem-cell markers such as Oct4 and Sox2 in 3T3 cells (Szabo *et al.*, 2011) and stimulate trans-differentiation of normal fibroblasts into myofibroblasts when they are confronted with primary BCA cells.

4.2.3 HA, adipocytes and adipose tissue

Adipose tissue in mammary glands is important for its secretory and endocrinal functions as well as metabolism, energy homeostasis and stem cell compartment. Adipocytes contribute to the mammary tissue ECM and this effect is at least partly regulated by HA. There are not many studies that focus on HA and its relationship to adipocytes, however, the importance of this polysaccharide on adipose-stromal interactions in the breast tissue is becoming apparent. For example, HA increases the crosslinking of collagen-HA matrices, supports proliferation and differentiation of pre-adipocytes and induces a higher proportion of cycling cells (Davidenko *et al.*, 2010).

Chen *et al.* (2007) also showed that HA extends the lifespan, reduces cellular senescence and enhances differentiation potential of murine adipose-derived stromal cells (mADSCs) *in culture*. Collectively, these results provide preliminary evidence for a key role of HA in controlling the adipose component of the breast tissue and allude to a potential role of this regulation in BCA (Chen *et al.*, 2007).

5. HA regulates mammary cell functions that promote BCA progression

5.1 Cell migration

Considerable evidence indicates that HA fragmentation is required for immune cell trafficking, fibroblast migration, stem cell migration from niches to the wound site and endothelial cell migration during angiogenesis. For example, acellular hydrogel matrix composed of fibronectin and HA, which simulates a wound microenvironment, supports proliferation, migration and spreading of human dermal fibroblasts *in vitro*. HA seems to regulate motility via a variety of mechanisms that include indirect and direct effects on the migrating cell population. An example of an indirect effect was provided by a study of the role of HA on fibroblast migration using a porcine skin wound model. The wound matrix, which contained HA, promoted cell migration and recruitment of fibroblasts. This was shown to be in part due to wounding produced HA, which promotes collagen fibril formation, thus indirectly affecting cell motility (Docherty *et al.*, 1989). Direct effects of HA on cell motility can result from its structural properties and from its ability to activate motogenic signalling cascades such as ERK1,2 and PI3 kinase. Both of these effects have been related to an association of HA with cell surface receptors such as CD44 and RHAMM. For example, extracellular HA accumulation induces penetration of stromal cells by increasing turgidity and hydration or disrupting cell-to-cell junctions. These effects may be a result of interactions with CD44 and RHAMM (Itano *et al.*, 2008). HA fragments bind to CD44 and/or RHAMM to induce activation of MAPK (ERK1,2) that results in enhanced BCA cell migration and invasion (Hamilton *et al.*, 2007). Moreover, upon HA-mediated activation of PI3 kinase, increased HAS2 production induces faster migration in scratch wound assays (Itano *et al.*, 2002).

5.2 Angiogenesis

Hypoxic conditions within tumours require neovascularisation of the microenvironment for the tumour to continue to grow and metastasize. Hypoxia, a condition often found within the TME, induces the activation, as seen by nuclear translocation, of either or both of NFκB and HIF-1α. This effect has been shown both *in vitro* in MCF-7 BCA cells, and *in vivo* (Tafani *et al.*, 2010). Invasion, migration, and proliferation of endothelial cells, as well as tissue remodelling, are essential processes during angiogenesis, which directly and indirectly help to promote tumour growth and metastasis. Necrotic cells, which have died as a result of hypoxia, also release chemokines that recruit macrophages and a pro-inflammatory response conducive to tissue remodelling. Hypoxia may produce ROS which in turn cause HA fragmentation and Noble *et al.* (1996) showed that NFκB transcription in macrophages is activated by HA fragments (Noble *et al.*, 1996). Later, Rockey *et al.* (1998) were the first to show in hepatocytes that HA activation of NFκB induces NOS2 production, which can be synergistically increased in the presence of cytokines such as IFN-γ (Rockey *et al.*, 1998). It has since been shown that HA fragments activate the NFκB pathway through TLR4 in both DC and macrophages (Termeer *et al.*, 2002). Hypoxia induced activation of HIF-1α and NFκB induces pro-inflammatory gene expression and both mRNA and protein levels of inflammatory mediators such as RAGE, PTX3, NOS2, COX2, and CXCR4 are increased. Increased expression of CXCR4, which is the receptor for SDF-1, is seen on MCF-7 cells subjected to hypoxic conditions (Tafani *et al.*, 2010). This increases the migratory and invasive capacity of these cells, which are usually non-invasive. In these same studies it was found that nuclear translocation of NFκB is at least partly dependent on HIF-1α, indicating that it may be under hypoxic regulation, as inhibition of HIF-1α decreases nuclear localisation of NFκB, and in turn RAGE and P2X7R expression, inhibiting cell invasion (Tafani *et al.*, 2010).

In general, high MW HA inhibits angiogenesis while fragments promote angiogenesis. Overexpression of HA and HYALs has been linked to an increase in angiogenesis in several types of cancers including breast (Tan *et al.*, 2010), bladder (Lokeshwar *et al.*, 2000, Golshani *et al.*, 2008), prostate (Ekici *et al*, 2004, Bharadwaj *et al.*, 2007), and endometrial (Paiva *et al.*, 2005). Koyama *et al.* (2007) demonstrated that an increase in HAS2 expression by genetic modifications in a mouse model of BCA causes a higher incidence of adenocarcinoma accompanied by an increase in angiogenesis (Koyama *et al.*, 2007). An increase in HA by overexpression of HAS2 in transgenic mice induces a more aggressive BCA phenotype and an increase in blood and lymphatic vessels (Kobayashi *et al.*, 2010). In these tumours, the stromal cells also secrete a variety of pro-angiogenic factors. Furthermore, HA concentration in stroma and blood vessels is increased, as well as the amount of small HA fragments.

The pro-angiogenic effects of HA fragments result from the display of CD44 and RHAMM (Wang *et al.*, 2011, Slevin *et al.*, 2007) on the surfaces of endothelial, BCA or leukocyte cells. and Interaction of HA fragments with these cells produces the factors required for stimulating endothelial cells to form new blood vessels. HA fragments stimulate endothelial cell proliferation, migration and tube formation. Increased expression of HYALs in conjunction with MMPs and Cathepsin-D induce a more invasive phenotype in the endothelial cell line ECV-304 as detected by matrigel invasion assay (Wang *et al.*, 2009). Additionally, pro-inflammatory cytokines, secreted by leukocytes activated by CD44-HA mediated interactions, stimulate endothelial cells to produce HA. When HUVEC cells are stimulated with IL-1B, TNF-α and β1, they secrete HA. CD44-HA interaction stimulates early morphogenic events, such as tube formation and proliferation in HUVECs (Wang *et al.*, 2011). Furthermore, HA works synergistically with macrophage recruitment to promote vascular formation and HA in the stroma promotes lymphangiogenesis at the invasive tumour front in BCA through the activation of endothelial LYVE-1 (Itano *et al.*, 2002).

6. HA and multi-drug resistance in BCA

Most tumours initially respond to chemotherapy treatment but later acquire resistance, resulting in treatment failure and tumour recurrence. Some mechanisms by which tumour cells acquire resistance include inhibition of apoptosis, stimulation of cell proliferation and enhanced expression and activity of drug export pumps, particularly ATP driven pumps (ABC transporters), which reduce the intracellular, and therefore active, concentration of several chemotherapeutic agents. HA fragments augment expression and activity of MDR1, a member of the ABC drug transporter family, in primary BCA cells (Toole and Slomiany, 2008). This HA induced upregulation involves the Akt/PI3 kinase signalling pathway and is CD44 dependent. CD44-HA interactions stimulate MDR1 expression via multiple signalling mechanisms including epigenetic gene expression regulation. CD44-HA binding results in activation of PKCε as well as increased phosphorylation and nuclear translocation of Nanog, a stem cell specific transcription factor. Moreover, interaction of Nanog with Stat-3 in the nucleus increases Stat-3 regulated gene expression, resulting in increased expression of MDR1. Activation of Nanog also results in production of the micro RNA miR-21 and down-regulation of PDCD4, a tumour suppressor protein (Bourguignon *et al.*, 2008, 2009). CD44-HA interaction increases an association between MDR1 and the cytoskeletal protein ankyrin, resulting in enhanced drug export (Bourguignon *et al.*, 2008). Additionally, CD44-HA interactions upregulate the expression of the histone acetyl-transferase, p300, inducing the acetylation of β-catenin and NFκB. This stimulates expression of MDR1 and the anti-apoptotic protein, Bcl-x$_L$ (Bourguignon *et al.*, 2009). It is very likely that BCA tumours with high HA metabolisms are also highly resistant to treatment with drugs that can be exported by MDR1.

7. HA and receptor antagonists in clinical trials

Since it is evident that HA and its receptors play an important role in BCA and other tumours, it is unsurprising that reagents blocking HA metabolism are being assessed as therapeutic agents in certain types of cancer. In pre-clinical models, Kultti et al. (2009) demonstrated that the HAS inhibitor 4-MU (4-Methylumbelliferone) specifically depletes intracellular levels of UDP-Glc-UA (Kakizaki et al., 2004) by serving as a glucoronidation substrate in A2058 melanoma cells, MCF-7, MDA-MB-361 BCA cells, SKOV-3 ovarian, and UT-SCC118 squamous carcinoma cells. Additionally, Lokeswar et al. (2010) used 4-MU to block growth of human prostate cancer cell line xenografts in immunocompromised mice. 4-MU induces apoptosis in these tumours and also strongly inhibits cell proliferation, motility and invasion. These effects can be reversed by addition of HA, which demonstrates that, although 4-MU does not specifically block HAS and has other off target effects, its effects on tumour cell growth result from inhibition of HAS (Ekici et al., 2004).

HA has also proven to be a good adjunct therapeutic option in vivo in human cancers since it promotes targeting of active anti-cancer compounds. For example, when patients with Calmette-Guérin refractory bladder cancer were included in a Phase I clinical trial using Paclitaxel-HA (ONCOFID-P-B™) for treatment of their cancers, 60% of the patients treated exhibited a clinical response with minimal toxicity reported (Bassi et al., 2010). HA has been successfully used to carry/target other chemotherapeutics, thus reducing cytotoxic side effects of the active drug. Hyung et al. (2008) demonstrated the efficacy of HA-coated drug carriers by delivering doxorubicin to MDA-MB-231 and ZR-75-1 human BCA cell lines (Hyung et al., 2008). Similarly, after coating nanoparticles containing paclitaxel with HA, cytotoxicity is reduced while cellular uptake of the drug by S-180 sarcoma cell line is enhanced 9.5 fold in vitro and in a mouse model (He et al., 2009).

In light of fairly recent evidence for the display of CD44 on BCA tumour initiator cells, interest in developing CD44 targeted therapies has increased. Riechelmann et al. (2008) exploited the potential of CD44 in a Phase I clinical trial using an antimicrotubule agent (mertansine) and a monoclonal antibody to CD44v6 (bivatuzumab), (BIWI 1), to treat patients with recurrent or metastatic head and neck squamous cell carcinoma (Riechelmann et al., 2008). The response to the treatment was unexpectedly variable and the trials using these agents were stopped after one patient died of toxic epidermal necrolysis (Tijink et al., 2006). Targeting the HA binding ability of activated CD44 may result in decreased toxicity.

RHAMM peptide vaccination (e.g. R3, which is HLA-A2-restricted) has recently been assessed in PhaseI/II clinical trials for treatment of MM, AML, and CLL (Giannopoulos et al., 2010, Greiner et al., 2008, 2010, Schmitt et al., 2008). Additionally, vaccination with DC pre-stimulated against the same peptide has also undergone Phase I and II clinical trials for treatment of CLL (Hus et al., 2008). Vaccination with RHAMM peptide has the attractive advantage of very low toxicity because it is not expressed in healthy bone marrow tissue. RHAMM vaccination resulted in leukemic blast lysis, blast reduction in the bone marrow and avoided the need for blood transfusions for one patient. Furthermore, an immunological response, marked by an increase in T cell frequency, was observed in 70% of AML, MM, and MDS patients in an initial study (Schmitt et al., 2008). Subsequently, RHAMM peptide was shown to be non-toxic at high dosage (1000 µg/vaccination), however, there was no dose-dependent effect, indicating that RHAMM is an effective therapeutic target even at low levels (Greiner et al., 2010). A similar response was seen in CLL patients vaccinated with RHAMM peptide, as well as RHAMM peptide-stimulated DC.

Clinical response was correlated with an increase in CD8+ T cell proliferation and in some cases a decrease in Treg population. Interestingly, in B-CLL patients with clinical response to vaccination with stimulated DC cells, the CD8+ cytotoxic T cell and IL-12 anti-tumour response was increased, whereas the Treg cell population was decreased (Hus *et al.*, 2008). In a Phase I study of CLL patients vaccinated with RHAMM peptide, there was no correlation between clinical response and Treg population dynamics (Giannopoulos *et al.*, 2010). This strategy has not yet been used for BCA, although, as RHAMM is a prognostic marker for BCA. and overexpressed in many cases which currently do not have a specific targeted therapeutic option (e.g. basal subtype) and also given the magnitude of the response, along with such low toxicity, it is an approach which merits further consideration.

8. Conclusion

In summary, HA is a glycosaminoglycan that exerts a critical role in BCA progression by interacting with other ECM components and the tumour cells themselves. HA fragmentation induces inflammation and signalling that results in cancer and immune cell proliferation and migration, which can lead to poor outcome. The links between HA and cancer progression, as well as HA and inflammation have in some aspects been well established. Given the similarities in their signalling cascades and cellular processes, the relationship between HA stimulated innate immunity and the BCA microenvironment should be further considered.

9. Acknowledgments

We would like to thank Kenneth Esguerra and the Translational Breast Cancer Research Unit for their support and assistance.

10. References

Ambs S, Glynn SA. (2011). Candidate pathways linking inducible nitric oxide synthase to a basal-like transcription pattern and tumor progression in human breast cancer. *Cell cycle (Georgetown, Tex*, Vol.10, No.4, (Feb 15, 2011), pp. 619-24, ISSN 1551-4005

Banerji S, Ni J, Wang SX, et al. (1999). LYVE-1, a new homologue of the CD44 glycoprotein, is a lymph-specific receptor for hyaluronan. *The Journal of cell biology*, Vol.144, No.4, (Feb 22, 1999), pp. 789-801, ISSN 0021-9525

Barbera-Guillem E, Nyhus JK, Wolford CC, et al. (2002). Vascular endothelial growth factor secretion by tumor-infiltrating macrophages essentially supports tumor angiogenesis, and IgG immune complexes potentiate the process. *Cancer research*, Vol.62, No.23, (Dec 1, 2002), pp. 7042-9, ISSN 0008-5472

Bassi PF, Volpe A, D'Agostino D, et al. (2010). Paclitaxel-hyaluronic acid for intravesical therapy of bacillus Calmette-Guerin refractory carcinoma in situ of the bladder: results of a phase I study. *The Journal of urology*, Vol.185, No.2, (Feb, 2010), pp. 445-9, ISSN 1527-3792 (Electronic)

Ben-Baruch A. (2003). Host microenvironment in breast cancer development: inflammatory cells, cytokines and chemokines in breast cancer progression: reciprocal tumor-microenvironment interactions. *Breast Cancer Res*, Vol.5, No.1, 2003), pp. 31-6, ISSN 1465-542X (Electronic)

Bharadwaj, A.G., Rector K., Simpson M.A. (2007). Inducible hyaluronan production reveals differential effects on prostate tumor cell growth and tumor angiogenesis. *The Journal of biological chemistry*, Vol. 282, No. 28, (Jul 13, 2007), pp.20561-72, ISSN 0021-9258 (Print)

Bharadwaj AG, Kovar JL, Loughman E, et al. (2009). Spontaneous metastasis of prostate cancer is promoted by excess hyaluronan synthesis and processing. *The American journal of pathology*, Vol.174, No.3, (Mar, 2009), pp. 1027-36, ISSN 1525-2191

Bourguignon LY, Gilad E, Peyrollier K. (2007). Heregulin-mediated ErbB2-ERK signaling activates hyaluronan synthases leading to CD44-dependent ovarian tumor cell growth and migration. *The Journal of biological chemistry*, Vol.282, No.27, (Jul 6, 2007), pp. 19426-41, ISSN 0021-9258 (Print)

Bourguignon LY. (2008). Hyaluronan-mediated CD44 activation of RhoGTPase signaling and cytoskeleton function promotes tumor progression. *Seminars in cancer biology*, Vol.18, No.4, (Aug, 2008), pp. 251-9, ISSN 1096-3650 (Electronic)

Bourguignon LY, Spevak CC, Wong G, et al. (2009). Hyaluronan-CD44 interaction with protein kinase C(epsilon) promotes oncogenic signaling by the stem cell marker Nanog and the Production of microRNA-21, leading to down-regulation of the tumor suppressor protein PDCD4, anti-apoptosis, and chemotherapy resistance in breast tumor cells. *The Journal of biological chemistry*, Vol.284, No.39, (Sep 25, 2009), pp. 26533-46, ISSN 1083-351X (Electronic)

Bourguignon LY, Wong G, Earle C, et al. (2010). Hyaluronan-CD44 interaction promotes c-Src-mediated twist signaling, microRNA-10b expression, and RhoA/RhoC up-regulation, leading to Rho-kinase-associated cytoskeleton activation and breast tumor cell invasion. *The Journal of biological chemistry*, Vol.285, No.47, (Nov 19, 2010), pp. 36721-35, ISSN 1083-351X (Electronic)

Brown RL, Reinke LM, Damerow MS, et al. (2011). CD44 splice isoform switching in human and mouse epithelium is essential for epithelial-mesenchymal transition and breast cancer progression. *The Journal of clinical investigation*, Vol.121, No.3, (Mar 1, 2011), pp. 1064-74, ISSN 1558-8238 (Electronic)

Buganim Y, Rotter V. (2008). RHAMM in the complex p53 cell cycle network. *Cell cycle (Georgetown, Tex*, Vol.7, No.21, (Nov 1, 2008), pp. ISSN 1551-4005 (Electronic)

Camus M, Tosolini M, Mlecnik B, et al. (2009). Coordination of intratumoral immune reaction and human colorectal cancer recurrence. *Cancer research*, Vol.69, No.6, (Mar 15, 2009), pp. 2685-93, ISSN 1538-7445 (Electronic)

Carreras J, Lopez-Guillermo A, Fox BC, et al. (2006). High numbers of tumor-infiltrating FOXP3-positive regulatory T cells are associated with improved overall survival in follicular lymphoma. *Blood*, Vol.108, No.9, (Nov 1, 2006), pp. 2957-64, ISSN 0006-4971 (Print)

Chen PY, Huang LL, Hsieh HJ. (2007). Hyaluronan preserves the proliferation and differentiation potentials of long-term cultured murine adipose-derived stromal cells. *Biochemical and biophysical research communications*, Vol.360, No.1, (Aug 17, 2007), pp. 1-6, ISSN 0006-291X (Print)

Davidenko N, Campbell JJ, Thian ES, et al. (2010). Collagen-hyaluronic acid scaffolds for adipose tissue engineering. *Acta biomaterialia*, Vol.6, No.10, (Oct, 2010), pp. 3957-68, ISSN 1878-7568 (Electronic)

del Fresno C, Otero K, Gomez-Garcia L, et al. (2005). Tumor cells deactivate human monocytes by up-regulating IL-1 receptor associated kinase-M expression via CD44 and TLR4. *J Immunol*, Vol.174, No.5, (Mar 1, 2005), pp. 3032-40, ISSN 0022-1767

DeNardo DG, Coussens LM. (2007). Inflammation and breast cancer. Balancing immune response: crosstalk between adaptive and innate immune cells during breast cancer progression. *Breast Cancer Res*, Vol.9, No.4, 2007), pp. 212, ISSN 1465-542X

Diaz LK, Zhou X, Wright ET, et al. (2005). CD44 expression is associated with increased survival in node-negative invasive breast carcinoma. *Clin Cancer Res*, Vol.11, No.9, (May 1, 2005), pp. 3309-14, ISSN 1078-0432 (Print)

Docherty R, Forrester JV, Lackie JM, et al. (1989). Glycosaminoglycans facilitate the movement of fibroblasts through three-dimensional collagen matrices. *Journal of cell science*, Vol.92 (Pt 2), (Feb, 1989), pp. 263-70, ISSN 0021-9533 (Print)

Du Y, Liu Y, Wang Y, et al. (2010). LYVE-1 enhances the adhesion of HS-578T cells to COS-7 cells via hyaluronan. *Clinical and investigative medicine*, Vol.34, No.1, 2010), pp. E45-54, ISSN 1488-2353 (Electronic)

Eck SM, Cote AL, Winkelman WD, et al. (2009). CXCR4 and matrix metalloproteinase-1 are elevated in breast carcinoma-associated fibroblasts and in normal mammary fibroblasts exposed to factors secreted by breast cancer cells. *Mol Cancer Res*, Vol.7, No.7, (Jul, 2009), pp. 1033-44, ISSN 1557-3125 (Electronic)

Ekici S, Cerwinka WH, Duncan R, et al. (2004). Comparison of the prognostic potential of hyaluronic acid, hyaluronidase (HYAL-1), CD44v6 and microvessel density for prostate cancer. *International journal of cancer*, Vol.112, No.1, (Oct 20, 2004), pp. 121-9, ISSN 0020-7136 (Print)

Fanning A, Volkov Y, Freeley M, et al. (2005). CD44 cross-linking induces protein kinase C-regulated migration of human T lymphocytes. *International immunology*, Vol.17, No.4, (Apr, 2005), pp. 449-58, ISSN 0953-8178 (Print)

Fernandez Madrid F. (2005). Autoantibodies in breast cancer sera: candidate biomarkers and reporters of tumorigenesis. *Cancer letters*, Vol.230, No.2, (Dec 18, 2005), pp. 187-98, ISSN 0304-3835 (Print)

Fukui M, Whittlesey K, Metcalfe DD, et al. (2000). Human mast cells express the hyaluronic-acid-binding isoform of CD44 and adhere to hyaluronic acid. *Clinical immunology (Orlando, Fla*, Vol.94, No.3, (Mar, 2000), pp. 173-8, ISSN 1521-6616 (Print)

Fukui M, Ueno K, Suehiro Y, et al. (2006). Anti-tumor activity of dendritic cells transfected with mRNA for receptor for hyaluronan-mediated motility is mediated by CD4+ T cells. *Cancer Immunol Immunother*, Vol.55, No.5, (May, 2006), pp. 538-46, ISSN 0340-7004 (Print)

Gale NW, Prevo R, Espinosa J, et al. (2007). Normal lymphatic development and function in mice deficient for the lymphatic hyaluronan receptor LYVE-1. *Molecular and cellular biology*, Vol.27, No.2, (Jan, 2007), pp. 595-604, ISSN 0270-7306 (Print)

Giannopoulos K, Dmoszynska A, Kowal M, et al. (2010). Peptide vaccination elicits leukemia-associated antigen-specific cytotoxic CD8+ T-cell responses in patients with chronic lymphocytic leukemia. *Leukemia*, Vol.24, No.4, (Apr, 2010), pp. 798-805, ISSN 1476-5551 (Electronic)

Godar S, Weinberg RA. (2008). Filling the mosaic of p53 actions: p53 represses RHAMM expression. *Cell cycle (Georgetown, Tex*, Vol.7, No.22, (Nov 15, 2008), pp. 3479, ISSN 1551-4005 (Electronic)

Goentzel BJ, Weigel PH, Steinberg RA. (2006). Recombinant human hyaluronan synthase 3 is phosphorylated in mammalian cells. *The Biochemical journal*, Vol.396, No.2, (Jun 1, 2006), pp. 347-54, ISSN 1470-8728 (Electronic)

Golshani, R., Lopez L., Estrella V., Kramer M., Iida N., Lokeshwar V.B. (2008). Hyaluronic acid synthase-1 expression regulates bladder cancer growth, invasion, and angiogenesis through CD44. *Cancer research*, Vol. 68, No. 2, (Jan 15, 2008), pp.483-91, ISSN 1538-7445 (Electronic)

Greiner J, Bullinger L, Guinn BA, et al. (2008). Leukemia-associated antigens are critical for the proliferation of acute myeloid leukemia cells. *Clin Cancer Res*, Vol.14, No.22, (Nov 15, 2008), pp. 7161-6, ISSN 1078-0432 (Print)

Greiner J, Schmitt A, Giannopoulos K, et al. (2010). High-dose RHAMM-R3 peptide vaccination for patients with acute myeloid leukemia, myelodysplastic syndrome and multiple myeloma. *Haematologica*, Vol.95, No.7, (Jul, 2010), pp. 1191-7, ISSN 1592-8721 (Electronic)

Groen, A.C., Cameron L.A., Coughlin M., Miyamoto D.T., Mitchison T.J., Ohi R. (2004). XRHAMM functions in ran-dependent microtubule nucleation and pole formation during anastral spindle assembly. *Curr Biol*, Vol. 14, No. 20, (Oct 26, 2004), pp.1801-11, ISSN 0960-9822 (Print)

Haim K, Weitzenfeld P, Meshel T, et al. (2008). Epidermal Growth Factor and Estrogen Act by Independent Pathways to Additively Promote the Release of the Angiogenic Chemokine CXCL8 by Breast Tumor Cells. *Neoplasia (New York, NY*, Vol.13, No.3, (Mar, 2008), pp. 230-43, ISSN 1476-5586 (Electronic)

Hall CL, Yang B, Yang X, et al. (1995). Overexpression of the hyaluronan receptor RHAMM is transforming and is also required for H-ras transformation. *Cell*, Vol.82, No.1, (Jul 14, 1995), pp. 19-26, ISSN 0092-8674 (Print)

Hamilton SR, Fard SF, Paiwand FF, et al. (2007). The hyaluronan receptors CD44 and Rhamm (CD168) form complexes with ERK1,2 that sustain high basal motility in breast cancer cells. *The Journal of biological chemistry*, Vol.282, No.22, (Jun 1, 2007), pp. 16667-80, ISSN 0021-9258 (Print)

He M, Zhao Z, Yin L, et al. (2009). Hyaluronic acid coated poly(butyl cyanoacrylate) nanoparticles as anticancer drug carriers. *International journal of pharmaceutics*, Vol.373, No.1-2, (May 21, 2009), pp. 165-73, ISSN 1873-3476 (Electronic)

Heldin P, Karousou E, Bernert B, et al. (2008). Importance of hyaluronan-CD44 interactions in inflammation and tumorigenesis. *Connective tissue research*, Vol.49, No.3, 2008), pp. 215-8, ISSN 1607-8438 (Electronic)

Herrera-Gayol A, Jothy S. (1999). CD44 modulates Hs578T human breast cancer cell adhesion, migration, and invasiveness. *Experimental and molecular pathology*, Vol.66, No.1, (Apr, 1999), pp. 99-108, ISSN 0014-4800 (Print)

Hus I, Schmitt M, Tabarkiewicz J, et al. (2008). Vaccination of B-CLL patients with autologous dendritic cells can change the frequency of leukemia antigen-specific CD8+ T cells as well as CD4+CD25+FoxP3+ regulatory T cells toward an antileukemia response. *Leukemia*, Vol.22, No.5, (May, 2008), pp. 1007-17, ISSN 1476-5551 (Electronic)

Hyung W, Ko H, Park J, et al. (2008). Novel hyaluronic acid (HA) coated drug carriers (HCDCs) for human breast cancer treatment. *Biotechnology and bioengineering*, Vol.99, No.2, (Feb 1, 2008), pp. 442-54, ISSN 1097-0290 (Electronic)

Itano N, Sawai T, Yoshida M, et al. (1999). Three isoforms of mammalian hyaluronan synthases have distinct enzymatic properties. *The Journal of biological chemistry*, Vol.274, No.35, (Aug 27, 1999), pp. 25085-92, ISSN 0021-9258 (Print)

Itano N, Atsumi F, Sawai T, et al. (2002). Abnormal accumulation of hyaluronan matrix diminishes contact inhibition of cell growth and promotes cell migration. *Proceedings of the National Academy of Sciences of the United States of America*, Vol.99, No.6, (Mar 19, 2002), pp. 3609-14, ISSN 0027-8424 (Print)

Itano N, Sawai T, Atsumi F, et al. (2004). Selective expression and functional characteristics of three mammalian hyaluronan synthases in oncogenic malignant transformation. *The Journal of biological chemistry*, Vol.279, No.18, (Apr 30, 2004), pp. 18679-87, ISSN 0021-9258 (Print)

Itano N, Kimata K. (2008). Altered hyaluronan biosynthesis in cancer progression. *Seminars in cancer biology*, Vol.18, No.4, (Aug, 2008), pp. 268-74, ISSN 1096-3650 (Electronic)

Itano, N., Zhuo L., Kimata K. (2008). Impact of the hyaluronan-rich tumor microenvironment on cancer initiation and progression. *Cancer science*, Vol. 99, No. 9, (Sep, 2008), pp.1720-5, ISSN 1349-7006 (Electronic)

Jackson DG. (2009). Immunological functions of hyaluronan and its receptors in the lymphatics. *Immunological reviews*, Vol.230, No.1, (Jul, 2009), pp. 216-31, ISSN 1600-065X (Electronic)

Jiang, D., Liang J., Noble P.W. (2007). Hyaluronan in tissue injury and repair. *Annual review of cell and developmental biology*, Vol. 23, No. 2007), pp.435-61, ISSN 1081-0706 (Print)

Insert 'Joukov V, Groen AC, et al. (2006). The BRCA1/BARD1 heterodimer modulates ran-dependent mitotic spindle assembly. *Cell*, Vol.127, No.3, (Nov, 2006), pp. 539-52, ISSN 0092-8674 (Electronic)'

Kakizaki I, Kojima K, Takagaki K, et al. (2004). A novel mechanism for the inhibition of hyaluronan biosynthesis by 4-methylumbelliferone. *The Journal of biological chemistry*, Vol.279, No.32, (Aug 6, 2004), pp. 33281-9, ISSN 0021-9258 (Print)

Karihtala P, Soini Y, Auvinen P, et al. (2007). Hyaluronan in breast cancer: correlations with nitric oxide synthases and tyrosine nitrosylation. *J Histochem Cytochem*, Vol.55, No.12, (Dec, 2007), pp. 1191-8, ISSN 0022-1554 (Print)

Karousou E, Kamiryo M, Skandalis SS, et al. (2010). The activity of hyaluronan synthase 2 is regulated by dimerization and ubiquitination. *The Journal of biological chemistry*, Vol.285, No.31, (Jul 30, 2010), pp. 23647-54, ISSN 1083-351X (Electronic)

Khazaie K, Blatner NR, Khan MW, et al. (2011). The significant role of mast cells in cancer. *Cancer metastasis reviews*, Vol.30, No.1, (Mar, 2011), pp. 45-60, ISSN 1573-7233

Kobayashi N, Miyoshi S, Mikami T, et al. (2010). Hyaluronan deficiency in tumor stroma impairs macrophage trafficking and tumor neovascularization. *Cancer research*, Vol.70, No.18, (Sep 15, 2010), pp. 7073-83, ISSN 1538-7445 (Electronic)

Koyama H, Hibi T, Isogai Z, et al. (2007). Hyperproduction of hyaluronan in neu-induced mammary tumor accelerates angiogenesis through stromal cell recruitment: possible involvement of versican/PG-M. *The American journal of pathology*, Vol.170, No.3, (Mar, 2007), pp. 1086-99, ISSN 0002-9440 (Print)

Kuang DM, Wu Y, Chen N, et al. (2007). Tumor-derived hyaluronan induces formation of immunosuppressive macrophages through transient early activation of monocytes. *Blood*, Vol.110, No.2, (Jul 15, 2007), pp. 587-95, ISSN 0006-4971 (Print)

Kuang DM, Zhao Q, Xu J, et al. (2008). Tumor-educated tolerogenic dendritic cells induce CD3epsilon down-regulation and apoptosis of T cells through oxygen-dependent pathways. *J Immunol*, Vol.181, No.5, (Sep 1, 2008), pp. 3089-98, ISSN 1550-6606

Kultti A, Pasonen-Seppanen S, Jauhiainen M, et al. (2009). 4-Methylumbelliferone inhibits hyaluronan synthesis by depletion of cellular UDP-glucuronic acid and downregulation of hyaluronan synthase 2 and 3. *Experimental cell research*, Vol.315, No.11, (Jul 1, 2009), pp. 1914-23, ISSN 1090-2422 (Electronic)

Kuo YC, Su CH, Liu CY, et al. (2009). Transforming growth factor-beta induces CD44 cleavage that promotes migration of MDA-MB-435s cells through the up-regulation of membrane type 1-matrix metalloproteinase. *International journal of cancer*, Vol.124, No.11, (Jun 1, 2009), pp. 2568-76, ISSN 1097-0215 (Electronic)

Lin EY, Nguyen AV, Russell RG, et al. (2001). Colony-stimulating factor 1 promotes progression of mammary tumors to malignancy. *The Journal of experimental medicine*, Vol.193, No.6, (Mar 19, 2001), pp. 727-40, ISSN 0022-1007 (Print)

Lokeshwar, V.B., Obek C., Pham H.T., Wei D., Young M.J., Duncan R.C., Soloway M.S., Block N.L. (2000). Urinary hyaluronic acid and hyaluronidase: markers for bladder cancer detection and evaluation of grade. *The Journal of urology*, Vol. 163, No. 1, (Jan, 2000), pp.348-56, ISSN 0022-5347 (Print)

Lokeshwar, V.B., Selzer M.G. (2008). Hyalurondiase: both a tumor promoter and suppressor. *Seminars in cancer biology*, Vol. 18, No. 4, (Aug, 2008), pp.281-7, ISSN 1096-3650

Lokeshwar, V.B., Lopez L.E., Munoz D., Chi A., Shirodkar S.P., Lokeshwar S.D., Escudero D.O., Dhir N., Altman N. (2010). Antitumor activity of hyaluronic acid synthesis inhibitor 4-methylumbelliferone in prostate cancer cells. *Cancer research*, Vol. 70, No. 7, (Apr 1, 2010), pp.2613-23, ISSN 1538-7445 (Electronic)

Lopez JI, Camenisch TD, Stevens MV, et al. (2005). CD44 attenuates metastatic invasion during breast cancer progression. *Cancer research*, Vol.65, No.15, (Aug 1, 2005), pp. 6755-63, ISSN 0008-5472 (Print)

Ma, W., Deng Y., Zhou L. (2005). The prognostic value of adhesion molecule CD44v6 in women with primary breast carcinoma: a clinicopathologic study. *Clinical oncology (Royal College of Radiologists (Great Britain))*, Vol. 17, No. 4, (Jun, 2005), pp.258-63, ISSN 0936-6555 (Print)

Mantovani A, Marchesi F, Porta C, et al. (2007). Inflammation and cancer: breast cancer as a prototype. *Breast (Edinburgh, Scotland)*, Vol.16 Suppl 2, (Dec, 2007), pp. S27-33, ISSN 0960-9776 (Print)

Matsumoto N, Mukae S, Tsuda H, et al. (2010). Prognostic value of LYVE-1-positive lymphatic vessel in tongue squamous cell carcinomas. *Anticancer research*, Vol.30, No.6, (Jun, 2010), pp. 1897-903, ISSN 1791-7530 Maxwell, C.A., Mccarthy J., Turley E. (2008). Cell-surface and mitotic-spindle RHAMM: moonlighting or dual oncogenic functions? *Journal of cell science*, Vol. 121, No. Pt 7, (Apr 1, 2008), pp.925-32, ISSN 0021-9533 (Print)

Maxwell, C.A., McCarthy J., Turley E. (2008). Cell-surface and mitotic-spindle RHAMM: moonlighting or dual oncogenic functions? *Journal of cell sciences*, Vol. 121, No. Pt 7, (Apr 1, 2008), pp.925-32, ISSN 0021-9533 (print)

Micke P, Kappert K, Ohshima M, et al. (2007). In situ identification of genes regulated specifically in fibroblasts of human basal cell carcinoma. *The Journal of investigative dermatology*, Vol.127, No.6, (Jun, 2007), pp. 1516-23, ISSN 1523-1747 (Electronic)

Mintz B, Illmensee K. (1975). Normal genetically mosaic mice produced from malignant teratocarcinoma cells. *Proceedings of the National Academy of Sciences of the United States of America*, Vol.72, No.9, (Sep, 1975), pp. 3585-9, ISSN 0027-8424 (Print)

Mytar B, Siedlar M, Woloszyn M, et al. (2001). Cross-talk between human monocytes and cancer cells during reactive oxygen intermediates generation: the essential role of hyaluronan. *International journal of cancer*, Vol.94, No.5, (Dec 1, 2001), pp. 727-32, ISSN 0020-7136 (Print)

Mytar B, Woloszyn M, Szatanek R, et al. (2003). Tumor cell-induced deactivation of human monocytes. *Journal of leukocyte biology*, Vol.74, No.6, (Dec, 2003), pp. 1094-101, ISSN 0741-5400 (Print)

Nagano O, Saya H. (2004). Mechanism and biological significance of CD44 cleavage. *Cancer science*, Vol.95, No.12, (Dec, 2004), pp. 930-5, ISSN 1347-9032 (Print)

Naor, D., Wallach-Dayan S.B., Zahalka M.A., Sionov R.V. (2008). Involvement of CD44, a molecule with a thousand faces, in cancer dissemination. *Seminars in cancer biology*, Vol. 18, No. 4, (Aug, 2008), pp.260-7, ISSN 1096-3650 Noble PW, McKee CM, Cowman M, et al. (1996). Hyaluronan fragments activate an NF-kappa B/I-kappa B alpha autoregulatory loop in murine macrophages. *The Journal of experimental medicine*, Vol.183, No.5, (May 1, 1996), pp. 2373-8, ISSN 0022-1007 Ouhtit A, Abd Elmageed ZY, Abdraboh ME, et al. (2007). In vivo evidence for the role of CD44s in promoting breast cancer metastasis to the liver. *The American journal of pathology*, Vol.171, No.6, (Dec, 2007), pp. 2033-9, ISSN 0002-9440 (Print)

Noble, P.W., McKee C.M., et al. (1996). Hyaluronan fragments activate an NF-kappa B/I-kappa B alpha autoregulatory loop in murine macrophages. *Journal of Experimental Medicine*, Vol.183, No.5, (May 1996), pp.2373-8, ISSN 0022-1007 (Print)

Ouhtit, A., Abd Elmageed Z.Y., Abdraboh M.E., Lioe T.F., Raj M.H. (2007). In vivo evidence for the role of CD44s in promoting breast cancer metastasis to the liver. *The American journal of pathology*, Vol. 171, No. 6, (Dec, 2007), pp.2033-9, ISSN 0002-9440

Paiva, P., Van Damme M.P., Tellbach M., Jones R.L., Jobling T., Salamonsen L.A. (2005). Expression patterns of hyaluronan, hyaluronan synthases and hyaluronidases indicate a role for hyaluronan in the progression of endometrial cancer. *Gynecologic oncology*, Vol. 98, No. 2, (Aug, 2005), pp.193-202, ISSN 0090-8258 (Print)

Pedroza-Gonzalez A, Xu K, Wu TC, et al. (2011). Thymic stromal lymphopoietin fosters human breast tumor growth by promoting type 2 inflammation. *The Journal of experimental medicine*, Vol.208, No.3, (Mar 14, 2011), pp. 479-90, ISSN 1540-9538

Rajput AB, Turbin DA, Cheang MC, et al. (2008). Stromal mast cells in invasive breast cancer are a marker of favourable prognosis: a study of 4,444 cases. *Breast cancer research and treatment*, Vol.107, No.2, (Jan, 2008), pp. 249-57, ISSN 1573-7217 (Electronic)

Rakhra K, Bachireddy P, Zabuawala T, et al. (2010). CD4(+) T cells contribute to the remodeling of the microenvironment required for sustained tumor regression upon oncogene inactivation. *Cancer cell*, Vol.18, No.5, (Nov 16, 2010), pp. 485-98, ISSN 1878-3686 (Electronic)

Riechelmann H, Sauter A, Golze W, et al. (2008). Phase I trial with the CD44v6-targeting immunoconjugate bivatuzumab mertansine in head and neck squamous cell carcinoma. *Oral oncology*, Vol.44, No.9, (Sep, 2008), pp. 823-9, ISSN 1368-8375 (Print)

Rockey DC, Chung JJ, McKee CM, et al. (1998). Stimulation of inducible nitric oxide synthase in rat liver by hyaluronan fragments. *Hepatology (Baltimore, Md*, Vol.27, No.1, (Jan, 1998), pp. 86-92, ISSN 0270-9139 (Print)

Rys J, Kruczak A, Lackowska B, et al. (2003). The role of CD44v3 expression in female breast carcinomas. *Pol J Pathol*, Vol.54, No.4, 2003), pp. 243-7, ISSN 1233-9687 (Print)

Schmitt M, Schmitt A, Rojewski MT, et al. (2008). RHAMM-R3 peptide vaccination in patients with acute myeloid leukemia, myelodysplastic syndrome, and multiple myeloma elicits immunologic and clinical responses. *Blood*, Vol.111, No.3, (Feb 1, 2008), pp. 1357-65, ISSN 0006-4971 (Print)

Simpson, M.A., Lokeshwar V.B. (2008). Hyaluronan and hyaluronidase in genitourinary tumors. *Front Biosci*, Vol. 13, No. 2008), pp.5664-80, ISSN 1093-4715 (Electronic)

Slevin M., Krupinski J., Gaffney J., Matou S., West D., Delisser H., Savani R.C., Kumar S. (2007). Hyaluronan-mediated angiogenesis in vascular disease: uncovering RHAMM and CD44 receptor signaling pathways. *Matrix Biol*, Vol. 26, No. 1, (Jan, 2007), pp.58-68, ISSN 0945-053X (Print)

Sohr S, Engeland K. (2008). RHAMM is differentially expressed in the cell cycle and downregulated by the tumor suppressor p53. *Cell cycle (Georgetown, Tex*, Vol.7, No.21, (Nov 1, 2008), pp. 3448-60, ISSN 1551-4005 Soria G, Ben-Baruch A. (2008). The inflammatory chemokines CCL2 and CCL5 in breast cancer. *Cancer letters*, Vol.267, No.2, (Aug 28, 2008), pp. 271-85, ISSN 1872-7980 Spicer AP, Tien JL, Joo A, et al. (2002). Investigation of hyaluronan function in the mouse through targeted mutagenesis. *Glycoconjugate journal*, Vol.19, No.4-5, (May-Jun, 2002), pp. 341-5, ISSN 0282-0080 (Print)

Soria G, Ben-Baruch A. (2008). The inflammatory chemokines CCL2 and CCL5 in breast cancer. *Cancer letters*, Vol.267, No.2, (Aug 28 2008), pp.271-85, ISSN 1872-7980

Stern R. (2008). Hyaluronidases in cancer biology. *Seminars in cancer biology*, Vol.18, No.4, (Aug, 2008), pp. 275-80, ISSN 1096-3650 (Electronic)

Sugahara KN, Hirata T, Hayasaka H, et al. (2006). Tumor cells enhance their own CD44 cleavage and motility by generating hyaluronan fragments. *The Journal of biological chemistry*, Vol.281, No.9, (Mar 3, 2006), pp. 5861-8, ISSN 0021-9258 (Print)

Szabo P, Kolar M, Dvorankova B, et al. (2011). Mouse 3T3 fibroblasts under the influence of fibroblasts isolated from stroma of human basal cell carcinoma acquire properties of multipotent stem cells. *Biology of the cell / under the auspices of the European Cell Biology Organization*, (Feb 28, 2011), pp. ISSN 1768-322X (Electronic)

Tafani M, Russo A, Di Vito M, et al. (2010). Up-regulation of pro-inflammatory genes as adaptation to hypoxia in MCF-7 cells and in human mammary invasive carcinoma microenvironment. *Cancer science*, Vol.101, No.4, (Apr, 2010), pp. 1014-23, ISSN 1349-7006 (Electronic)

Tammi R, Rilla K, Pienimaki JP, et al. (2001). Hyaluronan enters keratinocytes by a novel endocytic route for catabolism. *The Journal of biological chemistry*, Vol.276, No.37, (Sep 14, 2001), pp. 35111-22, ISSN 0021-9258

Tammi RH, Kultti A, Kosma VM, et al. (2008). Hyaluronan in human tumors: pathobiological and prognostic messages from cell-associated and stromal hyaluronan. *Seminars in cancer biology*, Vol.18, No.4, (Aug, 2008), pp. 288-95, ISSN 1096-3650 (Electronic)

Tan JX, Wang XY, Li HY, et al. (2010). HYAL1 overexpression is correlated with the malignant behavior of human breast cancer. *International journal of cancer*, Vol.128, No.6, (Mar 15, 2010), pp. 1303-15, ISSN 1097-0215 Termeer CC, Hennies J, Voith U, et al. (2000). Oligosaccharides of hyaluronan are potent activators of dendritic cells. *J Immunol*, Vol.165, No.4, (Aug 15, 2000), pp. 1863-70, ISSN 0021-1767 (Print)

Termeer CC, Hennies J, Voith U, et al. (2000). Oligosaccharides of hyaluronan are potent activators of dendritic cells. *Journal of Immunology*, Vol.165, No.4, (Aug 15 2000), pp.1863-70, ISSN 0021-1767 (Print)

Termeer C, Benedix F, Sleeman J, et al. (2002). Oligosaccharides of Hyaluronan activate dendritic cells via toll-like receptor 4. *The Journal of experimental medicine*, Vol.195, No.1, (Jan 7, 2002), pp. 99-111, ISSN 0022-1007 (Print)

Theocharis, A.D., Skandalis S.S., Tzanakakis G.N., Karamanos N.K. (2010). Proteoglycans in health and disease: novel roles for proteoglycans in malignancy and their pharmacological targeting. *The FEBS journal*, Vol. 277, No. 19, (Oct, 2010), pp.3904-23, ISSN 1742-4658 (Electronic)

Thorne RF, Legg JW, Isacke CM. (2004). The role of the CD44 transmembrane and cytoplasmic domains in co-ordinating adhesive and signalling events. *Journal of cell science*, Vol.117, No.Pt 3, (Jan 26, 2004), pp. 373-80, ISSN 0021-9533 (Print)

Tijink BM, Buter J, de Bree R, et al. (2006). A phase I dose escalation study with anti-CD44v6 bivatuzumab mertansine in patients with incurable squamous cell carcinoma of the head and neck or esophagus. *Clin Cancer Res*, Vol.12, No.20 Pt 1, (Oct 15, 2006), pp. 6064-72, ISSN 1078-0432 (Print)

Tolg C, Hamilton SR, Nakrieko KA, et al. (2006). Rhamm-/- fibroblasts are defective in CD44-mediated ERK1,2 motogenic signaling, leading to defective skin wound repair. *The Journal of cell biology*, Vol.175, No.6, (Dec 18, 2006), pp. 1017-28, ISSN 0021-9525 (Print)

Tolg C, Hamilton SR, Morningstar L, et al. (2010). RHAMM promotes interphase microtubule instability and mitotic spindle integrity through MEK1/ERK1/2 activity. *The Journal of biological chemistry*, Vol.285, No.34, (Aug 20, 2010), pp. 26461-74, ISSN 1083-351X (Electronic)

Toole, B.P. (2004). Hyaluronan: from extracellular glue to pericellular cue. *Nature reviews*, Vol. 4, No. 7, (Jul, 2004), pp.528-39, ISSN 1474-175X (Print)

Toole BP, Slomiany MG. (2008). Hyaluronan, CD44 and Emmprin: partners in cancer cell chemoresistance. *Drug Resist Updat*, Vol.11, No.3, (Jun, 2008), pp. 110-21, ISSN 1532-2084 (Electronic)

Toole, B.P., Slomiany M.G. (2008). Hyaluronan: a constitutive regulator of chemoresistance and malignancy in cancer cells. *Seminars in cancer biology*, Vol. 18, No. 4, (Aug, 2008), pp.244-50, ISSN 1096-3650 (Electronic)

Turley, E.A., Veiseh M., Radisky D.C., Bissell M.J. (2008). Mechanisms of disease: epithelial-mesenchymal transition--does cellular plasticity fuel neoplastic progression? *Nature clinical practice*, Vol. 5, No. 5, (May, 2008), pp.280-90, ISSN 1743-4262 (Electronic)

Udabage L, Brownlee GR, Waltham M, et al. (2005). Antisense-mediated suppression of hyaluronan synthase 2 inhibits the tumorigenesis and progression of breast cancer. *Cancer research*, Vol.65, No.14, (Jul 15, 2005), pp. 6139-50, ISSN 0008-5472 (Print)

Unger K, Wienberg J, Riches A, et al. (2009). Novel gene rearrangements in transformed breast cells identified by high-resolution breakpoint analysis of chromosomal aberrations. *Endocrine-related cancer*, Vol.17, No.1, (Mar, 2009), pp. 87-98, ISSN 1479-6821 (Electronic)

Veiseh, M., Turley E.A. (2011). Hyaluronan metabolism in remodeling extracellular matrix: probes for imaging and therapy of breast cancer. *Integr Biol (Camb)*, Vol. 3, No. 4, (Apr 1, 2011), pp.304-15, ISSN 1757-9708 Vigetti D, Genasetti A, Karousou E, et al. (2010). Proinflammatory cytokines induce hyaluronan synthesis and monocyte adhesion in human endothelial cells through hyaluronan synthase 2 (HAS2) and the nuclear factor-kappaB (NF-kappaB) pathway. *The Journal of biological chemistry*, Vol.285, No.32, (Aug 6, 2010), pp. 24639-45, ISSN 1083-351X (Electronic)

Vigetti, D., Genasetti A., Karousou E, et al. (2010). Proinflammatory cytokines induce hyaluronan synthesis and monocyte adhesion in human endothelial cells through hyaluronan synthase 2 (HAS2) and the nuclear factor-kappaB (NF-kappaB) pathway. *The Journal of biological chemistry*, Vol.285, No.32, (Aug 6 2010), pp.24639-45, ISSN 1083-351X (electronic)

Voelcker, V., Gebhardt C., Averbeck M., Saalbach A., Wolf V., Weih F., Sleeman J., Anderegg U., Simon J. (2008). Hyaluronan fragments induce cytokine and metalloprotease upregulation in human melanoma cells in part by signalling via TLR4. *Experimental dermatology*, Vol. 17, No. 2, (Feb, 2008), pp.100-7, ISSN 1600-0625 0906

Wang XY, Tan JX, Vasse M, et al. (2009). Comparison of hyaluronidase expression, invasiveness and tubule formation promotion in ER (-) and ER (+) breast cancer cell lines in vitro. *Chinese medical journal*, Vol.122, No.11, (Jun 5, 2009), pp. 1300-4, ISSN 0366-6999 (Print)

Wang YZ, Cao ML, Liu YW, et al. (2011). CD44 mediates oligosaccharides of hyaluronan-induced proliferation, tube formation and signal transduction in endothelial cells.

Experimental biology and medicine (Maywood, NJ, Vol.236, No.1, (Jan, 2011), pp. 84-90, ISSN 1535-3699 (Electronic)

Weigel PH, DeAngelis PL., (2007) Hyaluronan syntheases: a decade-plus of novel glycosyltransferases. *The Journal of biological chemistry*, Vol.282, No.51, (Dec 21, 2007), pp. 36777-81, ISSN 0021-9258 (Print)

Weigelt, B., Bissell M.J. (2008). Unraveling the microenvironmental influences on the normal mammary gland and breast cancer. *Seminars in cancer biology*, Vol. 18, No. 5, (Oct, 2008), pp.311-21, ISSN 1096-3650 (Electronic)

Yang R, Yan Z, Chen F, et al. (2002). Hyaluronic acid and chondroitin sulphate A rapidly promote differentiation of immature DC with upregulation of costimulatory and antigen-presenting molecules, and enhancement of NF-kappaB and protein kinase activity. *Scandinavian journal of immunology*, Vol.55, No.1, (Jan, 2002), pp. 2-13, ISSN 0300-9475 (Print)

Yang, H., Zhou H., Feng P., Zhou X., Wen H., Xie X., Shen H., Zhu X. (2010). Reduced expression of Toll-like receptor 4 inhibits human breast cancer cells proliferation and inflammatory cytokines secretion. *J Exp Clin Cancer Res*, Vol. 29, No. 2010), pp.92, ISSN 1756-9966 (Electronic)

Yu H, Li Q, Zhou X, et al. (2011). Role of hyaluronan and CD44 in reactive oxygen species-induced mucus hypersecretion. *Molecular and cellular biochemistry*, (Feb 10, 2011), pp. ISSN 1573-4919 (Electronic)

Part 3

Breast Cancer Stem Cells

11

Breast Cancer Stem Cells

Fengyan Yu, Qiang Liu, Yujie Liu, Jieqiong Liu and Erwei Song
Department of Breast Tumor Center, Sun Yat-Sen Memorial Hospital
Sun Yat-Sen University, Guangzhou
People's Republic of China

1. Introduction

Over 150 years ago, Cohnheim and Durante formalized the concept that cancers might arise from a small subset of cells with stem cell properties [1-3], and in 1961, Till and McCulloch demonstrated for the first time that the existence of hematopoietic stem cells (HSC) in the bone marrow, which was postulated that stem-like cells might be the origin of cancer [4]. However, only recently did an increased interest in cancer stem cells (CSC) occur, thus spurring great advances in cancer stem cell biology. The CSC model was first developed in 1994 when malignant initiating cells were discerned in human acute myeloid leukemia (AML) [5]. Afterwards, similar CSC model was extended to some solid tumors that originated in the breast, brain, lung, prostate, colon, head and neck, and pancreas [6-12]. Most importantly, the development of CSC hypothesis has fundamental implications in terms of understanding the biology of muti-step tumorigenesis, the prevention of cancer, and the creation of novel effective strategies for cancer therapy.

1.1 The definition of cancer stem cells

It is well documented that tumors contain cancer cells with heterogeneous phenotypes reflecting aspects of their apparent state of differentiation. In a tumor, the mutable expression of normal differentiation markers by cancer cells implies that some of the heterogeneity arises as a result of this altered manifestation. Also, cancer is known to be the product of the accumulation of multiple genetic mutations and epigenetic alterations in a single target cell, the occurrences of which can sometimes take place over many decades. Furthermore, chemotherapy and radiation therapy for cancers have limited effectiveness in long-term scenarios, and the possible recurrence of tumors after years of disease-free survival exists in great majority of cancers. All these observations provide persuasive evidence that tumors are not mere monoclonal expansions of cells but might contain a subset of long-lived tumor-initiating cells with the ability to self-renew indefinitely and to regenerate the phenotypic diversity of original tumor [13]. This subpopulation is now widely termed as cancer stem cells (CSCs), also named tumor-initiating cells (T-IC). The exist of CSCs within a tumor was also supported by *in vitro* "clonogenic assays" that showed subpopulations of tumor cells (with increased proliferative capacity) using cells isolated from tumor specimens, as well as by *in vivo* self-renewal assays that indicated only a small specific subset of cancer cell population had tumorigenic potential when injected into immunodeficient mice [13, 14].

The definition of CSCs is defined by two main properties: 1) self-renewal that drives tumorigenesis: the ability to form new CSCs with potential for proliferation, expansion, and differentiation; 2) multipotent differentiation, which contributes to the cellular heterogeneity of a tumor: the ability to give rise to a heterogeneous progeny of tumor cells, which diversify in a hierarchical manner.

When distinguished from the majority of differentiated cancer cells, CSCs are resistant to many current cancer treatments, including chemo- and radiation therapy [15-20]. This suggests that lots of cancer treatments, while targeting the majority of tumor cells, may fail in the end due to not eliminating CSCs, which survive by developing new tumors. However, this would open avenues for developing novel effective drugs targeting CSCs. Although CSCs share several properties (i.e. the ability to self-renew and to differentiate, increased membrane transporter activity, the capacity for migration and metastasis, the same intrinsic signaling pathways (Notch, Wnt, Hedgehog etc) for regulation of self-renewal etc) with the normal stem cells [21], they are found to have some particular characteristics. For instance, the proliferation and self-renewal of CSCs are uncontrolled and unlimited (sometimes referred to as "immortality"), and the CSCs always differentiate into abnormal cancer cells, thus they cannot give rise to mature somatic cells [22]. This reveals that therapies targeted at extrinsic signals generated in the microenvironment (such as CXCR1, endothelial cell-initiated signaling, IL-6 and CXCL7) [23-25] or microRNAs (see Part 3 of this chapter) [26-29], which are found to specifically regulate self-renewal and/or differentiation of CSCs, might achieve clinical success with little adverse effects in cancer treatment.

1.2 Leukemia stem cells: The first cancer stem cells identified

In the early 1990s, Dick and his colleagues started a series of groundbreaking investigations to understand whether the functional hierarchy observed in normal hematopoiesis was conserved in leukemia [5, 30]. They used magnetic separation techniques and purified cells from AML patients into several groups according to different surface markers. These groups of cells were then implanted into immunocompromised mice and assessed for the ability to produce leukemic colony forming units. Interestingly, only the CD34+ CD38- subpopulation of leukemic cells had the ability to generate substantially more leukemic colonies *in vivo*. As well, they found that CD34+ CD38- leukemic stem cells retained differentiative capacity, giving rise to CD38+ and Lin+ populations. These observations provided the first compelling evidence that in a human cancer, there was a small population of self-renewing, tumorigenic stem cells.

1.3 Solid tumor stem cells

Subsequent experiments extended the leukemic stem cell model to human solid tumors. In the year 2003, Al-Hajj *et al* reported the identification of CSCs in human breast cancer, the first solid tumor that the existence of a functional hierarchy stem cell system had been demonstrated [7]. In their experiments, human breast cancer specimens obtained from primary or metastatic sites in nine different patients all engrafted in the NOD/SCID (non-obese diabetic/severe combined immune deficiency) mice. They observed that in most human breast cancers, only a minority subset of the tumor clones (defined as CD44+, CD24-/low and representing 11%–35% of total cancer cells) is endowed with the capacity to maintain tumor growth when xenografted in NOD/SCID mice. Importantly, tumors grown from the CD44+, CD24-/low cells were shown to contain mixed populations of epithelial tumor cells, recreating the phenotypic heterogeneity of the parent tumors. The small subpopulation of cells was further enriched by sorting for those that expressed epithelial surface antigen (ESA). More interestingly, 200 of the enriched ESA+CD44+CD24−/low cells were able to form a tumor following injection into a NOD/SCID mouse, while 20,000 of the CD44+CD24+ cells failed to do so [7]. In summery, these results opened a new chapter in the understanding of the biology of CSCs in human solid tumors.

Soon after, Michael F. Clarke's group published similar data about CSCs in brain tumors [8, 31]. They carried out studies to enrich tumorigenic cells in glioblastoma multiforme and medulloblastoma by sorting for those that express positive / high levels of CD133, a neural cell surface stem cell antigen. CD133high cells formed numerous colonies in suspension culture, and injection of as few as 1000 of these cells into an immunocompromised mouse successfully form a tumor. Conversely, CD133low cells showed very limited proliferative potential *in vitro*, and as many as 10,000 of these cells failed to seed tumors in host mice [8]. Furthermore, tumors developing from orthotopic, intracerebral injection of the minority of CD133+/high cells (about 5% - 30% of total tumor cells) reproduced the phenotypic diversity and differentiation pattern of the parent tumors [31].

As mentioned earlier, comparable results have been obtained in other solid tumors, like lung, prostate, colon, head and neck, as well as pancreatic [6, 9-12].

2. Isolation and identification of breast cancer stem cells

In most tumor tissues, including breast cancer, CSCs are rare. As we know, breast cancer is a histologically and molecularly heterogeneous disease, with six different subtypes, including luminal A, luminal B, normal breast-like, basal-like, claudinlow and HER2 overexpressing, which are characterized by distinct histology, gene expression patterns, and genetic alterations [32-35]. The molecular heterogeneity between breast cancers has been revealed to issue from different targets of transformation. Recent studies found that basal-like breast cancers with BRCA1 mutations were more likely to arise from luminal progenitors rather than the basal stem cells [36, 37]. However, further studies that focus on breast CSCs and mammary stem/progenitor cells as well as their potential relationship are needed for determining the exact origin of luminal versus basal-like cancers, with the aim of developing targeted therapies for different subtypes of breast cancers. Moreover, CSCs was found to be the main culprit for the failure of chemo- and radiation therapy, as well as the seeds for the distant metastasis and relapse in breast cancers [20, 32, 38-40]. Taken together, in order to better understand the properties and biology of breast CSCs and eventually cure breast carcinoma, it is absolutely necessary and important to identify and separate breast CSCs prospectively.

2.1 Isolation of breast CSCs with cell-surface marker profiles

Since Dick, *et al* isolated a specific subpopulation of leukemia cells (that expressed surface markers similar to normal hematopoietic stem cells) which was consistently enriched for clonogenic activity in NOD/SCID immunocompromised mice from acute myeloid leukemias in the 1990s [5, 30], scientists attempted to see if they could enrich CSCs in human solid tumors by sorting for different cellular markers. CD24, a ligand for P-selectin in both mouse and human cells, was identified as a significant marker for human breast carcinoma invasion and metastasis [41, 42], and another adhesion molecular CD44 was found to correlate with cellular differentiation and lymph node metastasis in human breast cancers [43, 44], whereas B3.8 was described as a breast / ovarian cancer-specific marker [45]. Based on these observations, in 2003, Al-Hajj *et al* tried to determine whether these surface markers could distinguish tumorigenic from nontumorigenic cells, and flow cytometry was used to isolate cells that were positive or negative for each marker. They demonstrated that a small population of tumorigenic cells, isolated from human breast tumors and characterized by the expression of the cell surface markers CD44+CD24−/lowLineage−, was capable of regenerating the phenotypic heterogeneity of the original tumor when injected subcutaneously into NOD/SCID mice [7]. They showed that as few as 100 cells with CD44+CD24−/low phenotype could form tumors in immunodeficient mice, while thousands of cells with fungible phenotypes failed to do so. Since then, CD44 and CD24 are widely accepted as surface markers for breast CSCs, and lots of studies have focused on roles of CD44+CD24− tumor cells in breast cancers. For example, Abraham *et al.* conducted immunohistochemical studies of CD44+CD24− tumor cells in human breast tumors and showed that breast tumors containing a high proportion of CD44+CD24− cells were associated with distant metastases [46].

Nevertheless, besides CD24 and CD44, there are other surface marker candidates for the enrichment of breast CSCs. Ginestier *et al.* reported that they separated breast cancer stem/progenitor cells by sorting for Aldehyde dehydrogenase 1 (ALDH1), a detoxifying enzyme responsible for the oxidation of intracellular aldehydes [47, 48], and they found that fewer ALDH1-positive than CD44+CD24− tumor cells are required to produce tumors in immunodeficient mice [49]. Additionally, recent studies revealed that ALDH1-positive seemed to be a more significantly predictive marker than CD44+CD24− for the identification of breast CSCs, in terms of resistance to chemotherapy and more metastatic [39, 50]. Moreover, it has been reported that the surface marker CD133 could isolate a group of breast CSCs that doesn't overlap with CD44+CD24− cells [51]; and another recent study demonstrated that in a basal breast cancer cell line MDA-MB-231 (known as triple-negative), PROCR and ESA, instead of CD44+CD24−/low and ALDH, could be used to highly enrich breast cancer stem/progenitor cell populations which exhibited the ability to self renew and divide asymmetrically [52].

2.2 Separation of breast CSCs by selecting for side-population (SP) cells

Advances in the separation of breast CSCs was accelerated by the identification of side population (SP) cells, due to lack of dye retention and chemotherapy efflux [53]. The method is based on cells incubated with Hoechst dye 33342 or rhodamine, after which the cells are analyzed by flow cytometry for dye exclusion and size, and SP cells would not retain dye. Isolation of SP cells facilitates purification of adult tissue stem cells comprising human and murine hematopoietic stem cells and a population of putative mammary epithelial stem cells [54-57]. Moreover, because some evidence revealed that breast CSCs and mammary epithelial stem cells represent biologically related entities [58], scientists thought to apply this technique to isolate breast CSCs. In 2005, Patrawala *et al* successfully isolated SP cells from an ER-positive human breast cancer cell line MCF-7, and they demonstrated that these small subset (0.2%) SP cells preferentially express stemness-associated genes (such as Notch1 and β-catenin) and verapamil-sensitive ATP-binding cassette (ABC) transporter ABCG2 mRNA [59]. More interestingly, MCF-7 SP cells were highly tumorigenic, whereas MCF-7 non-SP cells could not give rise to tumors in mice at al[59]. Researchers then took advantage of similar method to separate SP cells with stem cell properties from an ER-negative human breast cancer cell line Cal-51 and an triple-negative human breast cancer cell line MDA-MB-231, respectively, and they both found the SP cells expressed high levels of ABCG2 [60, 61]. Previous studies showed that SP cells takes advantage of their ability to pump out the fluorescent dye Hoechst 33342 (H33342) through the ABCG2 (also known as breast cancer resistance protein-1), which was regarded as a major mediator of dye efflux in various stem cells [54, 62]. As the ability to efflux substrates is particularly important for the protection of CSCs, and CSCs survive after chemotherapy partially by effluxing cytotoxic drugs, ABCG2 seems to protect stem cells from toxins. This is evident in *ABCG2* knockout mice that are more sensitive to compounds such as vinblastine, ivermectin, topotecan, and mitoxantrone [63-65]. Taken together, SP cells have the capacity to efflux toxic substances out of breast cancer stem like cells via an ABCG2-mediated cytoprotective mechanism and seem to contribute to chemotherapy-resistance. In addition, it is important to consider that identification of cancer stem like cells by selecting for SP cells is not limited to breast carcinomas. Similar observations have been made in other solid tumors (such as glioma, ovarian and pancreatic cancers) where the isolated SP cells proliferated infinitely and could regenerate heterologous NSP cells in culture [59, 66-68].

2.3 Propagation of breast CSCs by isolating "mammospheres" from suspension cultures

Colonial growth in nonadherent culture was used to test for self-renewal capacity in cultures of neural cell in 1996, and in the experiment, suspension culture led to formation of "neurospheres", which consisted of 4% - 20% normal neural stem cells [69]. Based on this approach, Galli *et al.* succeeded in the characterization and isolation from human glioblastoma multiform of "cancer neurospheres", which were highly enriched in long-term self-renewing, multi-lineage-differentiating, and tumor-initiating cells [70]. According to these successful procedures, researchers tried to extend this technology to the identification and propagation of mammary epithelial stem cells and breast CSCs. In 2003, Dontu *et al.* demonstrated that nonadherent mammospheres are enriched in human mammary epithelial progenitor/stem cells and able to differentiate along all three mammary epithelial lineages and to clonally generate complex functional structures in reconstituted 3D culture systems [55]. More encouragingly, two years later (2005), Ponti and colleagues reported the isolation and *in vitro* propagation of spherical clusters of self-replicating cells ("mammospheres") with stem/progenitor cell properties in suspension cultures from three breast cancer lesions and from an established breast carcinoma cell line MCF-7 [71]. They found that the isolated cells which overexpressed neoangiogenic and cytoprotec-tive factors showed CD44+CD24- and Cx43-, and expressed the stem cell marker OCT-4, and could form tumors *in vivo* when as few as 10^3 cells were implanted. This was the first time showing that breast tumorigenic cells with stem/progenitor cell properties can be propagated *in vitro* as nonadherent mammospheres, and accordingly, this experimental system was then frequently used by researchers for isolating and studying the breast tumor–initiating cells (BT-IC) [72-74].

2.4 Novel strategies for enrichment of breast CSCs

As we mentioned in the first part of this chapter, the cancer stem cell hypothesis suggests that many cancers are maintained in a hierarchical organization of rare, slowly dividing CSCs (or T-IC), rapidly dividing amplifying cells (early precursor cells, EPC) and post-mitotic differentiated tumor cells [22]. Thus, the complex scheme which operates in most tumor tissues seems to be that the slowly dividing CSCs give birth to EPC, which then undertake a program of exponential growth for a limited period of time before the descendant cells differentiate and become post-mitotic (Figure 1). Although the above three classical methods are widely used for the isolation and identification of breast CSCs, these methods purify both T-IC and some EPC [7] [59, 71]. To study the breast CSCs more accurately, our group was trying to search for new strategies to enrich more purified breast CSCs. We found that breast carcinomas from chemo-treated patients were highly enriched for cells with the properties of BT-IC. We then sequentially passaged tumor cells in epirubicin-treated NOD/SCID mice to get a highly malignant breast cancer cell line (SK-3rd) using the chemo-therapeutic resistance of BT-IC. Our SK-3rd cell line showed all the tentatively defined properties of BT-IC, including enhanced mammosphere formation, multipotent differentiation, chemo-therapy resistance, as well as BT- IC phenotype(OCT4+CD44+CD24−lin−)[76] (Figure 2). We assess that about 16% of SK-3rd cells were T-IC, while the rest cells (also CD44+CD24−) were mostly EPC, and mammospheric SK-3rd cells were ~100-fold more tumorigenic *in vivo* than the parent cell line, metastasize, and can be serial xenotransplanted[26]. Additionally, SK-3rd cells was capable of providing unlimited numbers of cells for BT-IC studies. This method of *in vivo* chemotherapy may provide researchers a novel approach of selecting CSCs from other breast cancer lines or possibly for other cancers.

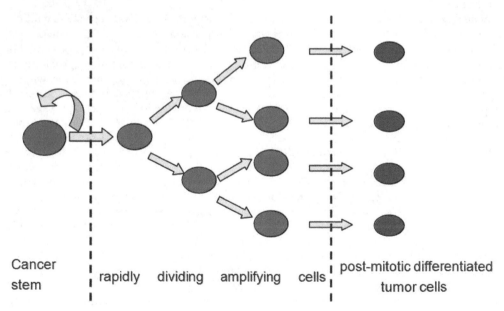

Cancer
stem

rapidly   dividing   amplifying   cells

post-mitotic differentiated
tumor cells

Fig. 1. A Model of the Cellular Hierarchies that May Exist in Human Cancers.

Besides our strategy, there might be other new approaches for generating breast CSCs. The epithelial-mesenchymal transition (EMT) is a key developmental program that is often activated during cancer progression, invasion and metastasis. Associations between the breast CSCs and EMT hypothesis of cancer were established recently as similarities in these two ideas were noted (will be discussed in Part 4 of this chapter). Several very recent studies have found that the EMT could generate mammary epithelial stem cells and breast CSCs [77-79]. This may provide potential novel methods to generate and enrich relatively unlimited numbers of breast CSCs, whose biology may then be studied with far greater facility.

The complex scheme which operates in most tumor tissues seems to be that the slowly dividing CSCs give birth to the rapidly dividing amplifying cells (early precursor cells, EPC), which then differentiate into post-mitotic tumor cells after a small number of cell divisions.

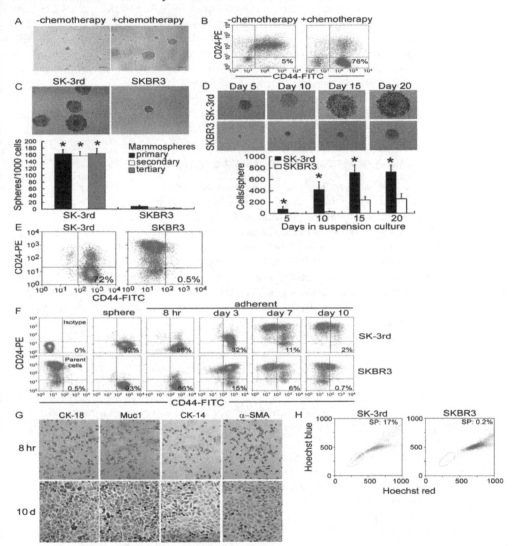

Fig. 2. Breast Cancer Cells under Pressure of Chemotherapy Are Enriched for BT-IC.

(A and B) 1°breast cancers from patients who received neoadjuvant chemotherapy are substantially enriched for self-renewing cells with the expected properties of BT-IC. Representative images show increased numbers of mammospheres after 15 days of culture (A) and a higher percentage of CD44+CD24- cells in freshly isolated tumors (B) from a patient who received chemotherapy. (C) Similarly, passaging the human breast cancer line SKBR3 in epirubicin-treated NOD/SCID mice enriches for cells with BT-IC properties.

Shown are numbers of 1°, 2°and 3°mammospheres on day 15 from 1000 cells. (D) Mammospheres generated from single-cell cultures of SK-3rd and SKBR3, imaged on indicated day of suspension culture. (E) The majority of freshly isolated SK-3rd cells are CD44+CD24-, while cells with this phenotype are rare in SKBR3. (F) SK-3rd and SKBR3 cells cultured as spheres are CD44+CD24-. When they differentiate in adherent cultures, they gradually assume the parental SBKR3 phenotype, but somewhat more rapidly for SKBR3 mammospheres. (G) When SK-3rd spheres are removed from growth factors, and plated on collagen for 8 hr (top), they do not express luminal (Muc1 and CK-18) or myoepithelial (CK-14 and a-SMA) differentiation markers, while after further differentiation (bottom), they develop into elongated cells with subpopulations staining for either differentiated subtype. (H) Freshly isolated SK-3rd cells are enriched for Hoechst[low] SP cells compared with SKBR3 cells[26]. Adapted from Yu F, et al.*Cell*, 2007: 131:1109-23.

3. The dysregulation of MicroRNAs in breast cancer stem cells

MicroRNAs (miRNAs) are endogenously synthesized small non-coding RNAs, 19-25 nucleotides in length that negatively regulate gene expression by repressing translation of target mRNAs or targeting them for degradation[80]. The active miRNA is produced by the RNase III enzyme Dicer in the cytosol from a precursor-miRNA (pre-miRNA) by removing the loop of the pre-miRNA stem-loop. The Dicer-processed miRNA is then taken up by the RNA-induced silencing complex (RISC), which becomes activated when one strand (the antisense or guide strand) is incorporated into the complex and the other strand separates and is discarded. The activated RISC complex can then seek out target mRNAs, which have partially complementary sequences to the guide strand (often in their 3'-UTR), and suppress their translation into protein[81].

MiRNA expression is altered in cancer cells and can be used to predict tumor type and prognosis. Cancer-associated miRNAs are frequently deleted, mutated or associated with satellite DNA expansions in cancers, suggesting that these molecules serve as important regulators of tumor development[82]. Emerging evidence has made it clear that miRNAs also function as important regulators of stemness, collaborating in the maintenance of the pluripotency, control of self-renewal, and differentiation of both normal stem cells and CSCs[83]. Except for certain miRNAs have high level transcripts, the global downregulation of miRNAs are present in CSCs when compared to their differentiated counterparts[82]. Dysregulation of miRNAs may result in excessive self-renewal and survival of CSCs which is a likely cause for the chemo-resistance and relapse in tumor patients.

MiRNAs can serve as either tumor suppressors or oncogenes depend on their expression levels in CSCs. Tumor suppressor miRNAs are supposed to inhibit tumor progression while their expression is downregulated. Oncogenic miRNAs are often called oncomiRs and are upregulated in the cancer cells[84].

3.1 Tumor suppressors

Let-7 is the first human miRNA to be discovered and its expression has been observed to be reduced in a number of tumor cell lines including lung and breast cancer[85]. Recent research indicated let-7 acted as tumor repressor playing an important role in the self-renewal potential of cancer stem cells. Yu and colleagues demonstrated that let-7 family was not expressed by breast CSCs generated from cell lines or 1°patient tumors and increased with differentiation. By expressing of let-7 in breast CSCs or antagonizing let-7 in more differentiated cells, it was found that let-7 regulated the key features of breast CSCs—self renewal in vitro, multipotent differentiation, and the ability to form tumors. Because the two targets of let-7 RAS and HMGA2 were responsible for the self renewal and multipotent differentiation, respectively, aberrant expression of let-7 in breast CSCs helps to maintain their stemness[26].

Recently, Yu et al. found that similar to let-7, the expression of miR-30 was reduced in breast cancer stem-like cells (BT-ICs), and its target genes, Ubc9, an E2-conjugating enzyme essential for sumoylation, and integrin ß3(ITGB3), were upregulated at protein levels. Overexpression of miR-30 in BT-ICs inhibited their self-renewal ability by repressing Ubc9 and promoted apoptosis by inhibiting Ubc9 and ITGB3. Furthermore, ectopic expression of mir-30 or blocking the expression of Ubc9 in BT-ICs xenografts reduced their tumor-forming capacity and metastasis in NOD/SCID mice, while miR-30 inhibitor enhanced tumorigenesis and metastasis of SKBR3 breast cancer cells with low metastasis potential[86]. These results suggested that miR-30 could be one of the important miRNAs in regulating the stem-like features of breast cancer

MiR-15/ miR-16 are also tumor suppressors. It was first identified in B cell chronic lymphocytic leukaemia (B-CLL) that miR-15/ miR-16 was lower in their expression level while their target protein the anti-apoptosis Bcl-2 was overexpressed[87]. The downregulation or deletion of miR-15/miR-16 was also found in other cancer types, such as prostate cancer[88], pituitary adenomas[89], non-small cell lung cancer (NSCLC)[90], and ovarian cancer[91]. Expression of these miRNAs inhibited cell proliferation, promoted apoptosis, and suppressed tumorigenicity both in vitro and in vivo by targeting multiple oncogenes, including Bcl-2, MCL1, CCND1, Wnt3A and Bmi-1. There has been growing evidence illustrated that the pivotal signaling pathways of the "stem cell genes": Notch, Hedgehog, Wnt, HMGA2, Bcl-2 and Bmi-1 were involved in the self-renewal of CSCs[92]. Since the oncogenic activation of Bmi-1, Bcl-2 and Wnt3A were frequently correlated with the downregulation of miR-15/miR-16, it was strongly suggested miR-15/miR-16 played a key role in the regulation of CSCs.

MiR-34 has been implicated in cell cycle control related to p53[93]. In p53 deficient human gastric cancer cells, restoration of functional miR-34 inhibited the formation of tumorsphere in vitro and tumor initiation in vivo[94]. In parallel, miR-34 was reported to be involved in pancreatic CSCs self-renewal[95]. The mechanism of miR-34 mediated suppression of self-renewal of CSCs was potentially related to the direct modulation of downstream targets Bcl-2 and Notch, suggesting that miR-34 might play an important role in gastric and pancreatic CSCs' self-renewal and/or cell fate determination. However, reduced expression of miR-34a in prostate cancer stem cells facilitated tumor development and metastasis by directly regulating CD44. Accordingly, CD44 knockdown inhibited prostate cancer growth and metastasis[96]. These results provided a solid experimental basis for developing miR-34a as a promising therapeutic agent against prostate CSCs.

MiR-128 is also a tumor suppressor involved in CSCs. Its expression was dramatically reduced in high grade gliomas, while application of miR-128 inhibited glioma proliferation and self-renewal by targeting Bmi-1 oncogene/stem cell renewal factor[97]. Same result was found in neural tumor medulloblastoma that miR-128a had growth suppressive activity in medulloblastoma and this activity was partially mediated by targeting Bmi-1 and thereby increasing the steady-state levels of superoxide and promoting cellular senescence. This data has implications for the modulation of redox states in CSCs, which are thought to be resistant to therapy due to their low ROS states[98].

miR-200 is an evolutionary conserved family which were found to be strongly suppressed in CD44+/CD24− lineage human breast cancer cells[27] and poorly differentiated pancreatic adenocarcinomas[99]. Recent research conducted in an inducible oncogenesis model showed that inhibition of miR-200b expression resulted in enrichment of the CSC population, and CSC or mammosphere growth was blocked by overexpression of miR-200b. Meanwhile one of its target Suz12 subunit of PRC2 was increased in CSC which in turn repress the transcription of E-cadherin. Thus, miR-200b acts as a tumor suppressor that blocks the formation and maintenance of mammospheres by targetting Suz12-E-cadherin pathway[100]. These results identified miR-200 microRNA family as a critical regulator for CSC growth and function.

3.2 Oncogenes

The miR-17-92 polycistron which is composed of 7 members is found to be overexpressed in multiple tumors, including lung[101], lymphoma[102], myeloid leukemias[103], hepatocellular carcinomas[104], medulloblastoma[105] and colorectal[106]. It's known to function as oncogenes to promotes cell proliferation and tumor progression. Introduction of miR-17-92 into hematopoietic stem cells was shown to significantly accelerated the formation of lymphoid malignancies partly by inhibiting apoptosis[101]. Also Wang et al found members of the miR-17 family were notably more abundant in a mouse model of MLL leukemia stem cells compared with their normal counterpart granulocyte-macrophage progenitors and myeloblast precursors. Forced expression of miR-17-19b in leukemia cells, was consistent with a higher frequency of leukemia stem cell, reduced differentiation and increased proliferation. The oncogenic effects of miR17-92 on leukemia stem cell self-renewal in MLL-associated leukemia in part due to modulating the expression of p21, a known regulator of normal stem cell function[103]. Taken together, these studies implicated the miR-17-92 cluster as a potential human oncogene that played a role in cancer stem cells.

The miR-181 has an oncogenic role within cancers as well. MiR-181 family members were up-regulated in EpCAM(+)AFP(+) hepatocellular carcinoma(HCCs) and in EpCAM(+) HCC cells isolated from AFP(+) tumors which have the cancer stem/progenitor cell features. Downregulation of miR-181 reduced EpCAM(+) HCC cell quantity and tumorigenesis, whereas enforced expression of miR-181 in HCC cells resulted in an enrichment of EpCAM(+) HCC cells. The mechamism underlying the regulation of miR-181 on the stemness of EpCAM(+) HCC cells was partially by negatively regulating two hepatic transcriptional regulators of differentiation and an inhibitor of Wnt/_-catenin signaling (nemo-like kinase [NLK])[107]. Other evidence also showed miR-181 was elevated in breast cancer stem cells. Overexpression of miR-181a/b, or depletion of its target ataxia telangiectasia mutated(ATM), was sufficient to induce sphere formation in breast cancer cells and promote tumorgenesis[108].

3.3 EMT

The epithelial-mesenchymal transition (EMT) is a vital developmental process that is often activated during cancer invasion and metastasis. During EMT, epithelial cells lose its epithelial characteristics including cell polarity and acquire mesenchymal phenotypes. On the molecular level, cells undergoing EMT down-regulated epithelial markers such as E-cadherin and up-regulated mesenchymal markers such as N-cadherin, vimentin, and fibronectin[109]. Mani and colleagues were the first group to demonstrated that the immortalized human mammary epithelial cells (HMLEs) undergoing EMT displayed not only mesenchymal traits, also cancer stem cell like properties as characterized by their CD44[high]/CD24[low] phenotype and increased ability to form mammospheres. On the other hand, HMLE mammospheres expressed markers similar to those of HMLEs that have undergone an EMT[77]. These findings illustrated EMT cells have cancer stem cell features and CSCs exhibit mesenchymal phenotype.

MiR-200 is the most discussed family that involved in the regulation of EMT process. Several studies have demonstrated suppression of endogenous miR-200 family members was sufficient to induce EMT, whereas their ectopic expression induces MET in normal and cancer cell lines through direct targeting of ZEB1/2[110]. While in CSCs with EMT phenotypes, miR-200 was also detected to be aberrant or absent in breast, pancreas and prostate. Wellner et al showed ZEB1 not only promoted tumor cell dissemination, but also was necessary for the maintaining a stem cell phenotype of pancreatic and colorectal cancer cells by inversely inhibiting the stemness-inhibiting miR-200 family members[111]. Hence, ZEB/miR-200 feedback loop is a driving force for cancer progression towards metastasis by controlling the state of CSCs. MiR-200 and let-7 both were differentiation associated miRNAs, sometimes they work together regulating the EMT status of CSCs. It has been shown in prostate cancer cells the expression of miR-200 and/or let-7 was decreased in EMT phenotypic tumor cells which also expressed stem-like cell features as defined by increased expression of Sox2, Nanog, Oct4, Lin28B and/or Notch1. Restoration of miR-200 in prostate cancer cells inhibited the EMT process, as well as the clonogenic and sphere (prostasphere)-forming ability and tumorigenecity in mice which was consistent with the inhibition of Notch1 and Lin28B expression. Along with the decreased expression of Lin28, let-7 was increased which further repressed self-renewal capability[112].

As discussed above miRNAs are critically involved in the regulation of CSCs and EMT which were considered the "root causes" of chemo-resistant and tumor relapse. Therefore, targeting specific miRNAs could be a very promising therapeutic approach for the treatment optimization aiming at restoring the sensitivity of drug-resistant cells to chemotherapy. If it was possible to introduce miRNA mimics and/or antagonists into CSCs, it could in principle result in reversal of the some of the cells' tumorigenic properties. However, from a clinical/translational research point of view, the critical hurdle to developing this type of approach for cancer therapy is to find an efficient way to selectively deliver miRNAs into CSCs or just cancer cells, but not normal tissues. So far the effective and safe therapeutics are still to be studied.

4. References

[1] J, C. Ueber entzundung und eiterung. Path Anat Physiol Klin Med 40, 1-79. (1867).
[2] J, C. Congenitales, quergestreiftes Muskelsarkon der Nireren. Virchows Arch, 64-65. (1875).
[3] F, D. Nesso fisio-pathologico tra la struttura dei nei materni e la genesi di alcuni tumori maligni. Arch Memor Observ Chir Pract 11, 217-226. (1874).
[4] Till, J. E. & Mc, C. E. A direct measurement of the radiation sensitivity of normal mouse bone marrow cells. Radiat Res 14, 213-22 (1961).
[5] Lapidot, T. et al. A cell initiating human acute myeloid leukaemia after transplantation into SCID mice. Nature 367, 645-8 (1994).
[6] Li, C. et al. Identification of pancreatic cancer stem cells. Cancer Res 67, 1030-7 (2007).

[7] Al-Hajj, M., Wicha, M. S., Benito-Hernandez, A., Morrison, S. J. & Clarke, M. F. Prospective identification of tumorigenic breast cancer cells. Proc Natl Acad Sci U S A 100, 3983-8 (2003).

[8] Singh, S. K. et al. Identification of a cancer stem cell in human brain tumors. Cancer Res 63, 5821-8 (2003).

[9] Kim, C. F. et al. Identification of bronchioalveolar stem cells in normal lung and lung cancer. Cell 121, 823-35 (2005).

[10] Xin, L., Lawson, D. A. & Witte, O. N. The Sca-1 cell surface marker enriches for a prostate-regenerating cell subpopulation that can initiate prostate tumorigenesis. Proc Natl Acad Sci U S A 102, 6942-7 (2005).

[11] O'Brien, C. A., Pollett, A., Gallinger, S. & Dick, J. E. A human colon cancer cell capable of initiating tumour growth in immunodeficient mice. Nature 445, 106-10 (2007).

[12] Prince, M. E. et al. Identification of a subpopulation of cells with cancer stem cell properties in head and neck squamous cell carcinoma. Proc Natl Acad Sci U S A 104, 973-8 (2007).

[13] Reya, T., Morrison, S. J., Clarke, M. F. & Weissman, I. L. Stem cells, cancer, and cancer stem cells. Nature 414, 105-11 (2001).

[14] Clarke, M. F. A self-renewal assay for cancer stem cells. Cancer Chemother Pharmacol 56 Suppl 1, 64-8 (2005).

[15] Gupta, P. B. et al. Identification of selective inhibitors of cancer stem cells by high-throughput screening. Cell 138, 645-59 (2009).

[16] Bao, S. et al. Glioma stem cells promote radioresistance by preferential activation of the DNA damage response. Nature 444, 756-60 (2006).

[17] Dean, M., Fojo, T. & Bates, S. Tumour stem cells and drug resistance. Nat Rev Cancer 5, 275-84 (2005).

[18] Diehn, M. et al. Association of reactive oxygen species levels and radioresistance in cancer stem cells. Nature 458, 780-3 (2009).

[19] Li, X. et al. Intrinsic resistance of tumorigenic breast cancer cells to chemotherapy. J Natl Cancer Inst 100, 672-9 (2008).

[20] Woodward, W. A. et al. WNT/beta-catenin mediates radiation resistance of mouse mammary progenitor cells. Proc Natl Acad Sci U S A 104, 618-23 (2007).

[21] Wicha, M. S., Liu, S. & Dontu, G. Cancer stem cells: an old idea--a paradigm shift. Cancer Res 66, 1883-90; discussion 1895-6 (2006).

[22] Dalerba, P., Cho, R. W. & Clarke, M. F. Cancer stem cells: models and concepts. Annu Rev Med 58, 267-84 (2007).

[23] Ginestier, C. et al. CXCR1 blockade selectively targets human breast cancer stem cells in vitro and in xenografts. J Clin Invest 120, 485-97 (2010).

[24] Krishnamurthy, S. et al. Endothelial cell-initiated signaling promotes the survival and self-renewal of cancer stem cells. Cancer Res 70, 9969-78 (2010).

[25] Liu, S. et al. Breast cancer stem cells are regulated by mesenchymal stem cells through cytokine networks. Cancer Res 71, 614-24 (2011).

[26] Yu, F. et al. let-7 regulates self renewal and tumorigenicity of breast cancer cells. Cell 131, 1109-23 (2007).

[27] Shimono, Y. et al. Downregulation of miRNA-200c links breast cancer stem cells with normal stem cells. Cell 138, 592-603 (2009).

[28] Liu, C. et al. The microRNA miR-34a inhibits prostate cancer stem cells and metastasis by directly repressing CD44. Nat Med 17, 211-5 (2011).

[29] Yu, F. et al. MiR-30 reduction maintains self-renewal and inhibits apoptosis in breast tumor-initiating cells. Oncogene 29, 4194-204 (2010).

[30] Bonnet, D. & Dick, J. E. Human acute myeloid leukemia is organized as a hierarchy that originates from a primitive hematopoietic cell. Nat Med 3, 730-7 (1997).

[31] Singh, S. K. et al. Identification of human brain tumour initiating cells. Nature 432, 396-401 (2004).

[32] McDermott, S. P. & Wicha, M. S. Targeting breast cancer stem cells. Mol Oncol 4, 404-19 (2010).

[33] Perou, C. M. et al. Molecular portraits of human breast tumours. Nature 406, 747-52 (2000).

[34] Sorlie, T. et al. Gene expression patterns of breast carcinomas distinguish tumor subclasses with clinical implications. Proc Natl Acad Sci U S A 98, 10869-74 (2001).

[35] Troester, M. A. et al. Gene expression patterns associated with p53 status in breast cancer. BMC Cancer 6, 276 (2006).

[36] Lim, E. et al. Aberrant luminal progenitors as the candidate target population for basal tumor development in BRCA1 mutation carriers. Nat Med 15, 907-13 (2009).

[37] Chaffer, C. L. & Weinberg, R. A. Cancer cell of origin: spotlight on luminal progenitors. Cell Stem Cell 7, 271-2 (2010).

[38] Nguyen, N. P. et al. Molecular biology of breast cancer stem cells: potential clinical applications. Cancer Treat Rev 36, 485-91 (2010).

[39] Tanei, T. et al. Association of breast cancer stem cells identified by aldehyde dehydrogenase 1 expression with resistance to sequential Paclitaxel and epirubicin-based chemotherapy for breast cancers. Clin Cancer Res 15, 4234-41 (2009).

[40] Charafe-Jauffret, E. et al. Aldehyde dehydrogenase 1-positive cancer stem cells mediate metastasis and poor clinical outcome in inflammatory breast cancer. Clin Cancer Res 16, 45-55 (2010).

[41] Fogel, M. et al. CD24 is a marker for human breast carcinoma. Cancer Lett 143, 87-94 (1999).

[42] Schindelmann, S. et al. Expression profiling of mammary carcinoma cell lines: correlation of in vitro invasiveness with expression of CD24. Tumour Biol 23, 139-45 (2002).

[43] Friedrichs, K. et al. CD44 isoforms correlate with cellular differentiation but not with prognosis in human breast cancer. Cancer Res 55, 5424-33 (1995).

[44] Berner, H. S. & Nesland, J. M. Expression of CD44 isoforms in infiltrating lobular carcinoma of the breast. Breast Cancer Res Treat 65, 23-9 (2001).

[45] Kufe, D. W. et al. Biological behavior of human breast carcinoma-associated antigens expressed during cellular proliferation. Cancer Res 43, 851-7 (1983).

[46] Abraham, B. K. et al. Prevalence of CD44+/CD24-/low cells in breast cancer may not be associated with clinical outcome but may favor distant metastasis. Clin Cancer Res 11, 1154-9 (2005).

[47] Duester, G. Families of retinoid dehydrogenases regulating vitamin A function: production of visual pigment and retinoic acid. Eur J Biochem 267, 4315-24 (2000).

[48] Sophos, N. A. & Vasiliou, V. Aldehyde dehydrogenase gene superfamily: the 2002 update. Chem Biol Interact 143-144, 5-22 (2003).

[49] Ginestier, C. et al. ALDH1 is a marker of normal and malignant human mammary stem cells and a predictor of poor clinical outcome. Cell Stem Cell 1, 555-67 (2007).

[50] Charafe-Jauffret, E. et al. Breast cancer cell lines contain functional cancer stem cells with metastatic capacity and a distinct molecular signature. Cancer Res 69, 1302-13 (2009).

[51] Wright, M. H. et al. Brca1 breast tumors contain distinct CD44+/CD24- and CD133+ cells with cancer stem cell characteristics. Breast Cancer Res 10, R10 (2008).

[52] Hwang-Verslues, W. W. et al. Multiple lineages of human breast cancer stem/progenitor cells identified by profiling with stem cell markers. PLoS One 4, e8377 (2009).

[53] Goodell, M. A. et al. Dye efflux studies suggest that hematopoietic stem cells expressing low or undetectable levels of CD34 antigen exist in multiple species. Nat Med 3, 1337-45 (1997).

[54] Scharenberg, C. W., Harkey, M. A. & Torok-Storb, B. The ABCG2 transporter is an efficient Hoechst 33342 efflux pump and is preferentially expressed by immature human hematopoietic progenitors. Blood 99, 507-12 (2002).

[55] Dontu, G. et al. In vitro propagation and transcriptional profiling of human mammary stem/progenitor cells. Genes Dev 17, 1253-70 (2003).

[56] Alvi, A. J. et al. Functional and molecular characterisation of mammary side population cells. Breast Cancer Res 5, R1-8 (2003).

[57] Clarke, R. B. et al. A putative human breast stem cell population is enriched for steroid receptor-positive cells. Dev Biol 277, 443-56 (2005).

[58] Liu, B. Y., McDermott, S. P., Khwaja, S. S. & Alexander, C. M. The transforming activity of Wnt effectors correlates with their ability to induce the accumulation of mammary progenitor cells. Proc Natl Acad Sci U S A 101, 4158-63 (2004).

[59] Patrawala, L. et al. Side population is enriched in tumorigenic, stem-like cancer cells, whereas ABCG2+ and ABCG2- cancer cells are similarly tumorigenic. Cancer Res 65, 6207-19 (2005).

[60] Christgen, M. et al. Identification of a distinct side population of cancer cells in the Cal-51 human breast carcinoma cell line. Mol Cell Biochem 306, 201-12 (2007).

[61] Hiraga, T., Ito, S. & Nakamura, H. Side population in MDA-MB-231 human breast cancer cells exhibits cancer stem cell-like properties without higher bone-metastatic potential. Oncol Rep 25, 289-96 (2011).

[62] Zhou, S. et al. The ABC transporter Bcrp1/ABCG2 is expressed in a wide variety of stem cells and is a molecular determinant of the side-population phenotype. Nat Med 7, 1028-34 (2001).

[63] Zhou, S. et al. Bcrp1 gene expression is required for normal numbers of side population stem cells in mice, and confers relative protection to mitoxantrone in hematopoietic cells in vivo. Proc Natl Acad Sci U S A 99, 12339-44 (2002).

[64] Petrides, M., Alivisatos, B. & Frey, S. Differential activation of the human orbital, mid-ventrolateral, and mid-dorsolateral prefrontal cortex during the processing of visual stimuli. Proc Natl Acad Sci U S A 99, 5649-54 (2002).

[65] Schinkel, A. H. et al. Disruption of the mouse mdr1a P-glycoprotein gene leads to a deficiency in the blood-brain barrier and to increased sensitivity to drugs. Cell 77, 491-502 (1994).

[66] Gao, Q., Geng, L., Kvalheim, G., Gaudernack, G. & Suo, Z. Identification of cancer stem-like side population cells in ovarian cancer cell line OVCAR-3. Ultrastruct Pathol 33, 175-81 (2009).

[67] Kabashima, A. et al. Side population of pancreatic cancer cells predominates in TGF-beta-mediated epithelial to mesenchymal transition and invasion. Int J Cancer 124, 2771-9 (2009).

[68] Szotek, P. P. et al. Ovarian cancer side population defines cells with stem cell-like characteristics and Mullerian Inhibiting Substance responsiveness. Proc Natl Acad Sci U S A 103, 11154-9 (2006).

[69] Reynolds, B. A. & Weiss, S. Clonal and population analyses demonstrate that an EGF-responsive mammalian embryonic CNS precursor is a stem cell. Dev Biol 175, 1-13 (1996).

[70] Galli, R. et al. Isolation and characterization of tumorigenic, stem-like neural precursors from human glioblastoma. Cancer Res 64, 7011-21 (2004).
[71] Ponti, D. et al. Isolation and in vitro propagation of tumorigenic breast cancer cells with stem/progenitor cell properties. Cancer Res 65, 5506-11 (2005).
[72] Zhang, M. et al. Identification of tumor-initiating cells in a p53-null mouse model of breast cancer. Cancer Res 68, 4674-82 (2008).
[73] Pece, S. et al. Biological and molecular heterogeneity of breast cancers correlates with their cancer stem cell content. Cell 140, 62-73 (2010).
[74] Karimi-Busheri, F., Rasouli-Nia, A., Mackey, J. R. & Weinfeld, M. Senescence evasion by MCF-7 human breast tumor-initiating cells. Breast Cancer Res 12, R31 (2010).
[75] Al-Hajj, M. Cancer stem cells and oncology therapeutics. Curr Opin Oncol 19, 61-4 (2007).
[76] Clarke, M. F. et al. Cancer stem cells--perspectives on current status and future directions: AACR Workshop on cancer stem cells. Cancer Res 66, 9339-44 (2006).
[77] Mani, S. A. et al. The epithelial-mesenchymal transition generates cells with properties of stem cells. Cell 133, 704-15 (2008).
[78] Santisteban, M. et al. Immune-induced epithelial to mesenchymal transition in vivo generates breast cancer stem cells. Cancer Res 69, 2887-95 (2009).
[79] Hennessy, B. T. et al. Characterization of a naturally occurring breast cancer subset enriched in epithelial-to-mesenchymal transition and stem cell characteristics. Cancer Res 69, 4116-24 (2009).
[80] Carthew, R. W. Gene regulation by microRNAs. Curr Opin Genet Dev 16, 203-8 (2006).
[81] Bushati, N. & Cohen, S. M. microRNA functions. Annu Rev Cell Dev Biol 23, 175-205 (2007).
[82] Lu, J. et al. MicroRNA expression profiles classify human cancers. Nature 435, 834-8 (2005).
[83] Navarro, A. & Monzo, M. MicroRNAs in human embryonic and cancer stem cells. Yonsei Med J 51, 622-32.
[84] Chen, C. Z. MicroRNAs as oncogenes and tumor suppressors. N Engl J Med 353, 1768-71 (2005).
[85] Takamizawa, J. et al. Reduced expression of the let-7 microRNAs in human lung cancers in association with shortened postoperative survival. Cancer Res 64, 3753-6 (2004).
[86] Yu, F. et al. MiR-30 reduction maintains self-renewal and inhibits apoptosis in breast tumor-initiating cells. Oncogene 29, 4194-204.
[87] Cimmino, A. et al. miR-15 and miR-16 induce apoptosis by targeting BCL2. Proc Natl Acad Sci U S A 102, 13944-9 (2005).
[88] Bonci, D. et al. The miR-15a-miR-16-1 cluster controls prostate cancer by targeting multiple oncogenic activities. Nat Med 14, 1271-7 (2008).
[89] Bottoni, A. et al. miR-15a and miR-16-1 down-regulation in pituitary adenomas. J Cell Physiol 204, 280-5 (2005).
[90] Bandi, N. et al. miR-15a and miR-16 are implicated in cell cycle regulation in a Rb-dependent manner and are frequently deleted or down-regulated in non-small cell lung cancer. Cancer Res 69, 5553-9 (2009).
[91] Bhattacharya, R. et al. MiR-15a and MiR-16 control Bmi-1 expression in ovarian cancer. Cancer Res 69, 9090-5 (2009).
[92] DeSano, J. T. & Xu, L. MicroRNA regulation of cancer stem cells and therapeutic implications. Aaps J 11, 682-92 (2009).
[93] He, L. et al. A microRNA component of the p53 tumour suppressor network. Nature 447, 1130-4 (2007).
[94] Ji, Q. et al. Restoration of tumor suppressor miR-34 inhibits human p53-mutant gastric cancer tumorspheres. BMC Cancer 8, 266 (2008).

[95] Ji, Q. et al. MicroRNA miR-34 inhibits human pancreatic cancer tumor-initiating cells. PLoS One 4, e6816 (2009).

[96] Liu, C. et al. The microRNA miR-34a inhibits prostate cancer stem cells and metastasis by directly repressing CD44. Nat Med 17, 211-5.

[97] Godlewski, J. et al. Targeting of the Bmi-1 oncogene/stem cell renewal factor by microRNA-128 inhibits glioma proliferation and self-renewal. Cancer Res 68, 9125-30 (2008).

[98] Venkataraman, S. et al. MicroRNA 128a increases intracellular ROS level by targeting Bmi-1 and inhibits medulloblastoma cancer cell growth by promoting senescence. PLoS One 5, e10748.

[99] Kent, O. A. et al. A resource for analysis of microRNA expression and function in pancreatic ductal adenocarcinoma cells. Cancer Biol Ther 8, 2013-24 (2009).

[100] Iliopoulos, D. et al. Loss of miR-200 inhibition of Suz12 leads to polycomb-mediated repression required for the formation and maintenance of cancer stem cells. Mol Cell 39, 761-72.

[101] Hayashita, Y. et al. A polycistronic microRNA cluster, miR-17-92, is overexpressed in human lung cancers and enhances cell proliferation. Cancer Res 65, 9628-32 (2005).

[102] He, L. et al. A microRNA polycistron as a potential human oncogene. Nature 435, 828-33 (2005).

[103] Wong, P. et al. The miR-17-92 microRNA polycistron regulates MLL leukemia stem cell potential by modulating p21 expression. Cancer Res 70, 3833-42.

[104] Connolly, E. et al. Elevated expression of the miR-17-92 polycistron and miR-21 in hepadnavirus-associated hepatocellular carcinoma contributes to the malignant phenotype. Am J Pathol 173, 856-64 (2008).

[105] Uziel, T. et al. The miR-17~92 cluster collaborates with the Sonic Hedgehog pathway in medulloblastoma. Proc Natl Acad Sci U S A 106, 2812-7 (2009).

[106] Monzo, M. et al. Overlapping expression of microRNAs in human embryonic colon and colorectal cancer. Cell Res 18, 823-33 (2008).

[107] Ji, J. et al. Identification of microRNA-181 by genome-wide screening as a critical player in EpCAM-positive hepatic cancer stem cells. Hepatology 50, 472-80 (2009).

[108] Wang, Y. et al. Transforming growth factor-beta regulates the sphere-initiating stem cell-like feature in breast cancer through miRNA-181 and ATM. Oncogene 30, 1470-80.

[109] Thiery, J. P. Epithelial-mesenchymal transitions in development and pathologies. Curr Opin Cell Biol 15, 740-6 (2003).

[110] Gregory, P. A. et al. An autocrine TGF-{beta}/ZEB/miR-200 signaling network regulates establishment and maintenance of epithelial-mesenchymal transition. Mol Biol Cell.

[111] Wellner, U. et al. The EMT-activator ZEB1 promotes tumorigenicity by repressing stemness-inhibiting microRNAs. Nat Cell Biol 11, 1487-95 (2009).

[112] Kong, D. et al. Epithelial to mesenchymal transition is mechanistically linked with stem cell signatures in prostate cancer cells. PLoS One 5, e12445.

12

The Microenvironment of Breast Cancer Stem Cells

Deepak Kanojia and Hexin Chen
University of South Carolina
USA

1. Introduction

Ernst Haeckel first described the term "stem" as a concept for the evolution or organisms. For representation purpose he described the ancestor organism as a "stem" from which all the other organisms evolved. Arthur Pappenheim later adopted this concept in the context of cells, and he elegantly placed the "stem cell" in the centre in cartoon from which all the blood cells arise describing hematopoiesis (Ramalho-Santos and Willenbring, 2007).

The concept was carried forward and the term "cancer stem cell" was first coined in 1980 (Carney *et al.*, 1982) where the authors described the stem cell origin of lung cancer cells. The difficulty in isolation and the absence of specific markers of cancer stem cell stalled the research in this area. However a decade later Bonnet and Dick successfully isolated CSC in AML which then incited the development in the field of cancer stem cells (Bonnet and Dick, 1997). Their discovery was later supported by many groups, which also resulted in isolation of CSC from a variety of malignancies including solid tumors.

Now a large body of evidence suggests that cancer comprises of different population of cells with various tumorogenic potentials. The tumor cells follow a hierarchy, where the subset capable of self-renewal, generate the tumor heterogeneity and are called cancer stem cells (CSC). Very low number of these cancer stem cells generates tumors in immunocompromised mice whereas large number of non-CSCs fails to generate tumors.

CSCs have been characterized based on their ability to form colonies in soft agar and their ability to form spheres in serum free media. The generation of tumors in immunocompromised mice however remains the gold standard. Another characteristic of CSC is their ability to resist the action of common chemotherapeutic drugs which is attributed to higher expression of ABC transporters and their slow cycling nature. Further it has also been documented that these CSCs have activated signaling pathways as in the case of normal stem cells. Hence CSCs are distinct from other non-CSC in many respects.

Cancer stem cells have been isolated based on membrane markers. One of the characteristics is their ability to efflux the Hoechst dye. However this ability to efflux the dye is also attributed to membrane ABC transporter ABCG2. ABCG5 has been used as a cancer stem cell marker as it pumps out the drug doxorubicin. ALDH1 has the ability to convert retinol to retinoic acid, which has diverse role in cell physiology, and this activity is used as a marker for CSC. CD 44, CD 133, EpCAM and CD 90 are also abundantly expressed in CSCs and are used to isolate or enrich CSC (Visvader and Lindeman, 2008). A number of groups have isolated CSC based on these markers however a robust marker for CSC still remains to be identified.

1.1 Origin of CSC

A number of theories have been proposed for the generation of these CSCs. (1)CSC can originate from genetic/ epigenetic alteration of normal stem cells or from the progenitor cells. (2) They can be derived from somatic tumor cells by de differentiation or reprogramming into a stem- like cell (Visvader and Lindeman, 2008). (3) And recently it has been suggested that CSC can be generated from non-CSC through production secretary molecules (Iliopoulos *et al.*, 2011).

2. Breast cancer stem cells

The existence of cancer stem cells was first demonstrated in solid tumors by Al Hajj et al., where CSCs were identified from human breast cancer tissue using CD44+ / CD24- Lin- as cellular markers (Al-Hajj *et al.*, 2003). They isolated the cells from primary breast cancer or metastatic pleural effusions and injected them directly in to mice or after cellular sorting with the above mentioned markers. They found that CD44+, CD24- were able to form tumors while CD44- , CD24- were unable to form tumors in immunocompromised mice. Further they performed repopulation assays where they found that the tumorigenic population (CD44+ / CD24- Lin-) was able to give rise to phenotypic heterogeneity of the initial tumor. This suggested that the breast cancer stem cells undergo self-renewal and differentiation as in the case of normal stem cells. After this report a large number of studies identified CSC from various other malignancies (Curley *et al.*, 2009; Fang *et al.*, 2005; Kondo *et al.*, 2004; Liu *et al.*, 2007; Prince *et al.*, 2007; Singh *et al.*, 2004).

The normal stem cells reside in a distinct environment called the "stem cell niche". This stem cell niche consists of complex composition of ECM, soluble factors, stromal cells, immune cells which are responsible for maintaining the self renewal ability of stem cells. Similarly the CSCs also depend on similar environment, which may be altered in many ways. Moreover in some of the tumors, the tumor niche has been shown to have a protective role from genotoxic insults (Garcia-Barros *et al.*, 2003). Although much research has been done on understanding the cancer stem cells, very few studies have been carried out on understanding the microenvironment of breast cancer stem cells and their targeting. We believe that understanding the breast cancer microenvironment will offer easily tractable solutions to cancer therapy.

2.1 Role of microenviroment in mammary gland development

The breast tissue is composed of multiple cell types for proper functioning of tissue and the primary function of which is production of milk. During lactation milk is produced by the luminal epithelial cells and secreted in the hollow cavity. The luminal epithelial cells are surrounded by myoepithelial cells, which synthesize the basement membrane. Together the luminal epithelia and the myoepithelia form the milk duct. Different cell types whose function is to maintain the homeostasis surround milk duct. These cells include fibroblasts, leucocytes and endothelial cells.

The environment of epithelial cells plays a critical role in shaping their function. For eg. When the epithelial cells from breast tissue were placed on plastic, they were unable to produce milk and exhibited different phenotype as compared to the cells when plated in 3 dimentional reconstituted basement membrane (Matrigel) which led to proper function of epithelial cells (Howlett and Bissell, 1993; Petersen *et al.*, 1992). Hence proper cellular interaction and spatial localization of cells with the right constituents are required for correct functioning of epithelial tissue. This was explained by the fact that invivo normal mammary gland are in contact with myoepithelial cells and not the basement membrane. Further luminal epithelial cells display apical–basal polarity as demonstrated by MUC 1, ESA and occludin expression on the apical membrane and ß4 integrin on the basolateral membrane. However such a polarity is observed when luminal cells are grown in matrigel but not in collagen(Gudjonsson *et al.*, 2002). The polarity is restored when the myoepithelial cells are co- cultured with luminal epithelial cells even in collagen, which is mediated by laminin 1 secreted by myoepithelial cells. These studies demonstrate the role of 3D environment and is important for optimal function of epithelial cells.

2.1.1 Microenvironment of breast cancer cells

A large number of reports demonstrate that breast tumor progression is facilitated by stromal cells and that their presence is critical for survival of cancer cells. However it is also important to note that the normal mammary gland microenvironment has inhibitory effect on breast cancer progression (DeCosse *et al.*, 1973). This indicates that cancer cells can maintain their properties only in an abnormal microenvironment. One of the recent reports underlies the role of mesenchymal stem cells in amplifying the metastatic potential of weakly metastatic cells. Karnoub A et al mixed a weakly metastatic cell line MDA MB 231 with bone marrow derived human MSC and found that the metastatic potential of the cell line is dramatically increased (Karnoub *et al.*, 2007). To further understand the mechanism of this increase in metastatic potential they used a cytokine array to identify soluble factors. They found CCL5 release, which was induced by physical interaction between breast cancer cells and the MSC, and that it renders the breast cancer cells more metastatic.

Another seminal report by Kaplan et al demonstrate that bone marrow- derived hematopoietic progenitors may localize to future sites of metastasis and "prepare" the sites for the arrival and growth of disseminated cancer cells (Kaplan *et al.*, 2005). This has been proposed a new concept in metastasis, which is called the "premetastatic niche". The precise mechanism and the factors responsible for such localization of bone marrow derived hematopoietic progenitors is unclear however it appears to be derived from the serum (Kaplan *et al.*, 2005).

One of the extensive study in understanding the breast cancer microenvironment, Allinen et al. performed genome wide gene expression analysis of stromal cells (Endothelial cells, infiltrating leukocytes, fibroblasts, and myofibroblasts) and breast epithelial cells (luminal epithelial and myoepithelial cells) from normal, insitu carcinoma and invasive carcinoma. The authors found that alterations in gene expression takes place in all cell types however clonally selected genetic alterations are confined to tumor epithelial cells. Further there were consistent and significant alterations in myoepithelial cells from DCIS as compared to normal myoepithelial cells and many of these changes were in secreted proteins and cell surface receptors (Allinen *et al.*, 2004). This further underlines the importance of soluble factors in breast cancer progression.

Although a large amount of literature is present on microenvironment of breast cancer cells, there are few studies on cancer stem cell microenviroenment. This is ascribed to the age of this new field however research in this direction will significantly impact the therapy of breast cancer.

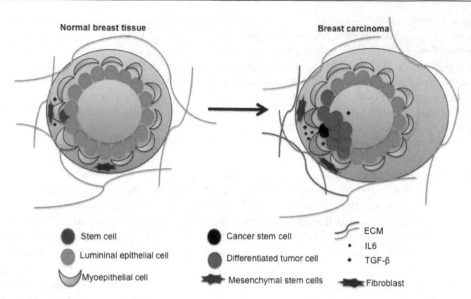

Fig. 1. Microenvironment of normal breast epithelium and breast cancer cells.

2.1.2 Influence of microenvironment on development of breast cancer stem cells

A limited number of factors have been studied to understand the interaction of microenvironment generated by tumors and its effect on development and maintenance of cancer stem cells. One of the widely studied environment which the solid tumors reside in, is hypoxia.

2.1.2.1 Hypoxia

It has been suggested that hypoxia contributes to the generation aggressive cancer by selecting tumor cells and results into growth of cells that can survive compromised levels of oxygen and nutrients (Graeber *et al.*, 1996). Further the growth of tumor results in hypoxic microenvironment, which is followed by periods of reoxygenation. Hence to mimic the invivo environment and to assess the fate of cells undergoing periods of hypoxia-reoxygenation Louie E etal., exposed breast cancer cells (MDA-MB-231 and BCM2) to cycles of hypoxia and nutrient deprivation. They discovered that after the first cycle of hypoxia a small fraction of cells survived and that repetitive exposure of the same cells to hypoxia and reoxygenation led to increased viability under hypoxia and to proliferate either as monolayer or tumor spheres. They also found increase in the number of cells expressing CD44+/CD24-/ESA+ cell surface markers, and hence the cancer stem cell content. Therefore repetitive cycling of hypoxia and re-oxygenation can increase the stem cell content of metastatic breast cancer cell lines indicating that microenvironment plays an important role in selectively increasing CSC (Louie *et al.*, 2010).

2.1.2.2 Stromal cells

Carcinoma associated fibroblasts (CAF)

For a long time scientist have primararily focused on epithelial component of breast cancer, however recently, the critical importance of tumor stroma has been realized. Literature documents important interaction between mammary epithelia and the adjacent tumor stroma. One of the reports demonstrates that CAF increases the number of CD44+CD24- cells in mammospheres, whereas normal fibroblasts (NFs) down-regulated it in mammospheres. They also demonstrate increase in the ability to form epithelial tumors in immunocompromised mice in presence of CAF. This indicates that CAFs can increase the cancer stem cell population in breast cancer (Huang et al., 2010). Furthermore since, CXCR4 expression on carcinoma cells is known to correlate with a poor prognosis for several types of carcinomas (Balkwill, 2004), the authors assessed CXCR4 gene expression in mamosphere co cultured with CAF. They found increase expression of CXCR4 and it was speculated that increase in cancer stem cell population could be because of CXCR4 signaling (Huang et al., 2010).

The normal fibroblasts on the contarary have a inhibitory effect on the tumor growth. For e.g Coculture studies using different mesenchymal cells and MCF10A and preneoplastic MCF10AT1-EIII8 mammary epithelial cells showed that fibroblasts derived from normal reduction mammoplasty inhibit or retard the morphological conversion and growth of MCF10A and EIII8 cells, whereas tumor derived fibroblasts evoke ductal-alveolar morphogenesis of both cell types (Shekhar et al., 2001). Further caveolin-1 deficient (Cav1-/-) mammary stromal fibroblasts were shown to mimic the effects of human breast cancer associated fibroblasts as they show similar profile of RB/ E2F-regulated genes that are up-regulated and confer a poor prognosis with enhanced epithelial-mesenchymal transition (EMT) (Sotgia et al., 2009).

Interestingly, genome-wide expression profiling of human breast cancer-associated fibroblasts and Cav-1 (-/-) mammary stromal fibroblasts indicates that they both show the upregulation of a number of ES-cell related genes and factors (Oct4, Nanog, Sox2 and Myc-target genes), indicating that they may behave like "cancer stem cells". Thus, the tumor stromal microenvironment may directly contribute to maintaining the "cancer stem cell" phenotype, leading to drug-resistance and treatment failure (Sotgia et al., 2009).

Fibroblast synthesize growth and survival factors which are critical for the tumor. In breast cancer, stromal fibroblasts evolve with the tumor epithelial cells and assist the growth of tumor cells. Inspite of much known about role of stromal cells the mechanistic basis of such a requirement of fibroblast remains elusive. PTEN is a tumor suppressor and is a critical regulator of PI3K signaling whose activation is associated with activation of tumor stroma (Cully et al., 2006). To understand the role of fibroblast in tumor formation Trimboli et al deleted PTEN from fibroblast in MMTV- ERBB2 mice model. They found that deletion of PTEN from fibroblast results in increase incidence and tumor load in the mice model. Extensive remodeling of ECM and increased recruitment of innate immune cells were some of the salient findings. Gene expression analysis revealed that PTEN deleted stromal fibroblasts consists of activation of Ets2 transcription factor. Further double transgenic mice having inactivation of Ets2 in mammary stroma reversed the increased malignancy caused by PTEN deficiency. These observations show the importance of the PTEN-Ets2 axis in stromal fibroblasts in the MMTV-ErbB2 model in suppressing breast cancer growth and indicate the stromal pathway contributes to the complexity of human breast cancer stroma (Trimboli et al., 2009).

Mesenchymal stem cells

Mesenchymal stem cells localize to the breast carcinoma and integrate into tumor associated stroma. A seminal report by Ling X et al., demonstrate that MSC overexpressing IFN-beta inhibit breast cancer growth and metastasis (Ling et al., 2010). They demonstrate that MSC are recruited to tumors and that IFN-beta inhibits tumor growth. (Ling X 2010). Such a reduction in tumor could also be attributable to decrease CSC content. Karnoub A et al., have shown increase in the metastatic potential of the breast cancer cells when they were mixed with bone marrow derived human MSC. Using a cytokine array they identified CCL5 is induced by physical interaction between breast cancer cells and the MSC, and that it renders the breast cancer cells more metastatic. These results indicate the importance of mesenchymal stem cells in rendering the cells more metastatic (Karnoub *et al.*, 2007).

2.1.2.3 Stromal factors

IL-6

IT has been documented that CSCs arise from mutant versions of normal stem cells. Alternatively, CSCs can also represent a stage in the path of transformation. CSCs are precursors of differentiated cancer cells (NSCCs), however CSCs can also be derived from NSCCs or can arise independently. The proportion of CSCs remains constant over multiple generations, but the basis of this phenomenon is unknown. Hence Iliopoulos D et al., assessed these issues using an inducible model of oncogenesis that MCF-10A cells which harbor a ligand-binding domain of estrogen receptor (ER-Src), a derivative of the Src kinase oncoprotein (v-Src) that is fused to the ligand-binding domain of the estrogen receptor. Treatment of these cells with tamoxifen (TAM) rapidly induces Src, results in transformation within 24-26 h. This property of the model helps in understanding the transition between normal and transformed cells. The authors then discovered that induction of CSC from non-CSC through activation of v-src. They also document that CSC formation depends on transformation however it is not required for transformation. Moreover because of the fact that breast CSCs have an enhanced inflammatory feedback loop compared with NSCCs, they treated the cells with IL6 which resulted in generation of CSC fron non-CSC (Iliopoulos *et al.*, 2011). This indicates the critical role of microenvironment as the CSC itself secrete IL6 which can maintain the stemness of a cancer cell population. Further the fact that macrophages and dendritic cells are potent IL-6 producers, which can be activated by molecular "danger" signals by cancer cells it is important to control the IL6 signaling to regenerate the CSC .

TGF beta

One of the elegant studies by Mani et al demonstrates the role of TGF beta in cancer stem cell through induction of EMT. The authors treated the immortalized HMEC cells with TGF beta which resulted in fibroblast like, mesenchymal like phenotype with concomitant downregulation of ephtielial markers like E-cadherin and upregulation of mesenchymal markers like vimentin, fibronectin and N-cadherin. Similar results were obtained through ectopic expression of TWIST or SNAI1. They further assessed the CD44 and CD24 population of these cells and found that CD44+ and CD24 low cells were increased which TGF beta treatment/ TWIST, SNAI1 expression. The rise in CD44+ and CD24 low population was accompanied by approximately 30-40 fold enrichment in mamosphere forming capability (Mani *et al.*, 2008). This was a clear demonstration of TGF beta induction of cancer stem cell population.

Yin X et al., showed that the activating transcription factor 3 (ATF3) is induced by TGF beta in breast cancer and is important for increasing the migration potential of the breast cancer cells. Further ATF3 can be induced by a number of stromal factors like TGF beta, IFN alpha, TNF alpha and hypoxia. And the fact that ectopic expression of ATF3 increases the cancer stem cell content of breast cancer cells (CD 24[low]/ CD 44[high]), it was hypothesized that tumor microenvironment has a significant effect in the development of cancer (Yin *et al.*, 2010).

2.1.2.4 Embryonic microenvironment

Four decades back it was documented that embryonic microenvironment can reprogram the cancer cells to a benign phenotype; however, the mechanisms underlying this phenomenon remains unclear (Hendrix *et al.*, 2007). The human embryonic stem cells (hESC) and cancer cells have various common features however hESC do not form tumors owing to the ability to differentiate in response to signals from the microenvironment. Normally the stem cell microenvironment or the stem cell niche controls the fate of the stem cells and that it provides the necessary constituents for maintaining homeostasis of tissue (Fuchs *et al.*, 2004). In cancer cells such control is lost and that restoring the niche may result in maintaining the homeostasis of growth and normal differentiation.

Hence to understand the mechanism Lynne-Marie Postovit et al (2006) developed an in vitro 3D model to investigate the capacity of hESC-derived factors to epigenetically influence metastatic cancer cells. They showed exposure of melanoma cells to a hESC microenvironment results in the reexpression of melanocyte-specific markers which are indicative of differentiation and a reduction in invasive potential.

Further (Lynne-Marie Postovit, 2006) they discovered that hESC microenvironments suppress the tumorigenic phenotype of human metastatic melanoma and breast carcinoma cells and that this effect is is brought about only by hESCs and not other stem cell types. Further they found that hESC microenvironment neutralize the aberrant expression of Nodal in metastatic melanoma and breast carcinoma cells and reprogram them to a less aggressive phenotype (Postovit *et al.*, 2006a; b). They also identified lefty which is sectreted by hESC (an inhibitor of Nodal signaling) as an important mediator of these phenomena. Hence the microenvironment of hESCs provides a previously unexplored therapeutic entity for the regulation of aberrantly expressed embryonic factor(s) in aggressive tumor cells (Postovit *et al.*, 2008).

3. Conclusion

CSC are rare cells and they are distinct from other bulk tumor cells. They generate the tumor and maintain the tumor hetrogenity. If the CSCs are elemiminated/differentiated to nonCSCs then cancer can be eradicated. The CSC niche maintains the CSC characteristics and increases the CSC potential, hence CSC niche offers a critical window treatment of cancer. Hence strategies that target the pathways critical for selfrenewal which are maintained through niche should be the focus of therapy. Notch, Wnt and Hedgehog pathways are known for maintaining self renewal of normal stem cells (Merchant and Matsui, 2010; Pannuti *et al.*, 2010; Takahashi-Yanaga and Kahn, 2010). These pathways offers targets in combination of other tumor specific markers for CSC targeting. For eg. Farnie, G et al., demonstrated that inhibiting notch signaling using gama secretase inhibitors in DCIS derived cells decreases their mamosphere forming efficiency (Farnie *et al.*, 2007). Further antibodies against the ECM Protein fibronectin receptor $\alpha4\beta1$ integrin prevented the interaction of cancer cells with premetastatic niches and reduce the minimal residual disease (Kaplan *et al.*, 2005). Moreover antibodies to fibronectin and $\beta1$ integrin promoted epithelial phenotype of invasive breast cancer cells in organotypic three dimentional cultures (Sandal *et al.*, 2007). Hence when formulating such therapeutic modalities a combination of inhibitors/biomolecules which can efficiently inhibit the cancer stem cells self renewal should be considered.

4. Acknowledgment

This work was in part supported by the Elsa U. Pardee Cancer Foundation grant (B94AFFAA), the American Cancer Society Research Award (RSG-10-067-01-TBE) and NIH grant (3P20RR017698-08) to HC.

5. References

Al-Hajj, M.; Wicha, M. S.; Benito-Hernandez, A.; Morrison, S. J., and Clarke, M. F. (2003). Prospective identification of tumorigenic breast cancer cells. *Proc Natl Acad Sci U S A* 100, 3983-3988.

Allinen, M.; Beroukhim, R.; Cai, L.; Brennan, C.; Lahti-Domenici, J.; Huang, H.; Porter, D.; Hu, M.; Chin, L.; Richardson, A.; Schnitt, S.; Sellers, W. R., and Polyak, K. (2004). Molecular characterization of the tumor microenvironment in breast cancer. *Cancer Cell* 6, 17-32.

Balkwill, F. (2004). Cancer and the chemokine network. *Nat Rev Cancer* 4, 540-550.

Bonnet, D., and Dick, J. E. (1997). Human acute myeloid leukemia is organized as a hierarchy that originates from a primitive hematopoietic cell. *Nat Med* 3, 730-737.

Carney, D. N.; Gazdar, A. F.; Bunn, P. A., Jr., and Guccion, J. G. (1982). Demonstration of the stem cell nature of clonogenic tumor cells from lung cancer patients. *Stem Cells* 1, 149-164.

Cully, M.; You, H.; Levine, A. J., and Mak, T. W. (2006). Beyond PTEN mutations: the PI3K pathway as an integrator of multiple inputs during tumorigenesis. *Nat Rev Cancer* 6, 184-192.

Curley, M. D.; Therrien, V. A.; Cummings, C. L.; Sergent, P. A.; Koulouris, C. R.; Friel, A. M.; Roberts, D. J.; Seiden, M. V.; Scadden, D. T.; Rueda, B. R., and Foster, R. (2009). CD133 expression defines a tumor initiating cell population in primary human ovarian cancer. *Stem Cells* 27, 2875-2883.

DeCosse, J. J.; Gossens, C. L.; Kuzma, J. F., and Unsworth, B. R. (1973). Breast cancer: induction of differentiation by embryonic tissue. *Science* 181, 1057-1058.

Fang, D.; Nguyen, T. K.; Leishear, K.; Finko, R.; Kulp, A. N.; Hotz, S.; Van Belle, P. A.; Xu, X.; Elder, D. E., and Herlyn, M. (2005). A tumorigenic subpopulation with stem cell properties in melanomas. *Cancer Res* 65, 9328-9337.

Farnie, G.; Clarke, R. B.; Spence, K.; Pinnock, N.; Brennan, K.; Anderson, N. G., and Bundred, N. J. (2007). Novel cell culture technique for primary ductal carcinoma in situ: role of Notch and epidermal growth factor receptor signaling pathways. *J Natl Cancer Inst* 99, 616-627.

Fuchs, E.; Tumbar, T., and Guasch, G. (2004). Socializing with the neighbors: stem cells and their niche. *Cell* 116, 769-778.

Garcia-Barros, M.; Paris, F.; Cordon-Cardo, C.; Lyden, D.; Rafii, S.; Haimovitz-Friedman, A.; Fuks, Z., and Kolesnick, R. (2003). Tumor response to radiotherapy regulated by endothelial cell apoptosis. *Science* 300, 1155-1159.

Graeber, T. G.; Osmanian, C.; Jacks, T.; Housman, D. E.; Koch, C. J.; Lowe, S. W., and Giaccia, A. J. (1996). Hypoxia-mediated selection of cells with diminished apoptotic potential in solid tumours. *Nature* 379, 88-91.

Gudjonsson, T.; Villadsen, R.; Nielsen, H. L.; Ronnov-Jessen, L.; Bissell, M. J., and Petersen, O. W. (2002). Isolation, immortalization, and characterization of a human breast epithelial cell line with stem cell properties. *Genes Dev* 16, 693-706.

Hendrix, M. J.; Seftor, E. A.; Seftor, R. E.; Kasemeier-Kulesa, J.; Kulesa, P. M., and Postovit, L. M. (2007). Reprogramming metastatic tumour cells with embryonic microenvironments. *Nat Rev Cancer* 7, 246-255.

Howlett, A. R., and Bissell, M. J. (1993). The influence of tissue microenvironment (stroma and extracellular matrix) on the development and function of mammary epithelium. *Epithelial Cell Biol* 2, 79-89.

Huang, M.; Li, Y.; Zhang, H., and Nan, F. (2010). Breast cancer stromal fibroblasts promote the generation of CD44+CD24- cells through SDF-1/CXCR4 interaction. *J Exp Clin Cancer Res* 29, 80.

Iliopoulos, D.; Hirsch, H. A.; Wang, G., and Struhl, K. (2011). Inducible formation of breast cancer stem cells and their dynamic equilibrium with non-stem cancer cells via IL6 secretion. *Proc Natl Acad Sci U S A* 108, 1397-1402.

Kaplan, R. N.; Riba, R. D.; Zacharoulis, S.; Bramley, A. H.; Vincent, L.; Costa, C.; MacDonald, D. D.; Jin, D. K.; Shido, K.; Kerns, S. A.; Zhu, Z.; Hicklin, D.; Wu, Y.; Port, J. L.; Altorki, N.; Port, E. R.; Ruggero, D.; Shmelkov, S. V.; Jensen, K. K.; Rafii, S., and Lyden, D. (2005). VEGFR1-positive haematopoietic bone marrow progenitors initiate the pre-metastatic niche. *Nature* 438, 820-827.

Karnoub, A. E.; Dash, A. B.; Vo, A. P.; Sullivan, A.; Brooks, M. W.; Bell, G. W.; Richardson, A. L.; Polyak, K.; Tubo, R., and Weinberg, R. A. (2007). Mesenchymal stem cells within tumour stroma promote breast cancer metastasis. *Nature* 449, 557-563.

Kondo, T.; Setoguchi, T., and Taga, T. (2004). Persistence of a small subpopulation of cancer stem-like cells in the C6 glioma cell line. *Proc Natl Acad Sci U S A* 101, 781-786.

Ling, X.; Marini, F.; Konopleva, M.; Schober, W.; Shi, Y.; Burks, J.; Clise-Dwyer, K.; Wang, R. Y.; Zhang, W.; Yuan, X.; Lu, H.; Caldwell, L., and Andreeff, M. (2010). Mesenchymal Stem Cells Overexpressing IFN-beta Inhibit Breast Cancer Growth and Metastases through Stat3 Signaling in a Syngeneic Tumor Model. *Cancer Microenviron* 3, 83-95.

Liu, R.; Wang, X.; Chen, G. Y.; Dalerba, P.; Gurney, A.; Hoey, T.; Sherlock, G.; Lewicki, J.; Shedden, K., and Clarke, M. F. (2007). The prognostic role of a gene signature from tumorigenic breast-cancer cells. *N Engl J Med* 356, 217-226.

Louie, E.; Nik, S.; Chen, J. S.; Schmidt, M.; Song, B.; Pacson, C.; Chen, X. F.; Park, S.; Ju, J., and Chen, E. I. (2010). Identification of a stem-like cell population by exposing metastatic breast cancer cell lines to repetitive cycles of hypoxia and reoxygenation. *Breast Cancer Res* 12, R94.

Mani, S. A.; Guo, W.; Liao, M. J.; Eaton, E. N.; Ayyanan, A.; Zhou, A. Y.; Brooks, M.; Reinhard, F.; Zhang, C. C.; Shipitsin, M.; Campbell, L. L.; Polyak, K.; Brisken, C.; Yang, J., and Weinberg, R. A. (2008). The epithelial-mesenchymal transition generates cells with properties of stem cells. *Cell* 133, 704-715.

Merchant, A. A., and Matsui, W. (2010). Targeting Hedgehog--a cancer stem cell pathway. *Clin Cancer Res* 16, 3130-3140.

Pannuti, A.; Foreman, K.; Rizzo, P.; Osipo, C.; Golde, T.; Osborne, B., and Miele, L. (2010). Targeting Notch to target cancer stem cells. *Clin Cancer Res* 16, 3141-3152.

Petersen, O. W.; Ronnov-Jessen, L.; Howlett, A. R., and Bissell, M. J. (1992). Interaction with basement membrane serves to rapidly distinguish growth and differentiation pattern of normal and malignant human breast epithelial cells. *Proc Natl Acad Sci U S A* 89, 9064-9068.

Postovit, L. M.; Margaryan, N. V.; Seftor, E. A.; Kirschmann, D. A.; Lipavsky, A.; Wheaton, W. W.; Abbott, D. E.; Seftor, R. E., and Hendrix, M. J. (2008). Human embryonic stem cell microenvironment suppresses the tumorigenic phenotype of aggressive cancer cells. *Proc Natl Acad Sci U S A* 105, 4329-4334.

Postovit, L. M.; Seftor, E. A.; Seftor, R. E., and Hendrix, M. J. (2006a). Influence of the microenvironment on melanoma cell fate determination and phenotype. *Cancer Res* 66, 7833-7836.

Postovit, L. M.; Seftor, E. A.; Seftor, R. E., and Hendrix, M. J. (2006b). A three-dimensional model to study the epigenetic effects induced by the microenvironment of human embryonic stem cells. *Stem Cells* 24, 501-505.

Prince, M. E.; Sivanandan, R.; Kaczorowski, A.; Wolf, G. T.; Kaplan, M. J.; Dalerba, P.; Weissman, I. L.; Clarke, M. F., and Ailles, L. E. (2007). Identification of a subpopulation of cells with cancer stem cell properties in head and neck squamous cell carcinoma. *Proc Natl Acad Sci U S A* 104, 973-978.

Ramalho-Santos, M., and Willenbring, H. (2007). On the origin of the term "stem cell". *Cell Stem Cell* 1, 35-38.

Sandal, T.; Valyi-Nagy, K.; Spencer, V. A.; Folberg, R.; Bissell, M. J., and Maniotis, A. J. (2007). Epigenetic reversion of breast carcinoma phenotype is accompanied by changes in DNA sequestration as measured by AluI restriction enzyme. *Am J Pathol* 170, 1739-1749.

Shekhar, M. P.; Werdell, J.; Santner, S. J.; Pauley, R. J., and Tait, L. (2001). Breast stroma plays a dominant regulatory role in breast epithelial growth and differentiation: implications for tumor development and progression. *Cancer Res* 61, 1320-1326.

Singh, S. K.; Hawkins, C.; Clarke, I. D.; Squire, J. A.; Bayani, J.; Hide, T.; Henkelman, R. M.; Cusimano, M. D., and Dirks, P. B. (2004). Identification of human brain tumour initiating cells. *Nature* 432, 396-401.

Sotgia, F.; Del Galdo, F.; Casimiro, M. C.; Bonuccelli, G.; Mercier, I.; Whitaker-Menezes, D.; Daumer, K. M.; Zhou, J.; Wang, C.; Katiyar, S.; Xu, H.; Bosco, E.; Quong, A. A.; Aronow, B.; Witkiewicz, A. K.; Minetti, C.; Frank, P. G.; Jimenez, S. A.; Knudsen, E. S.; Pestell, R. G., and Lisanti, M. P. (2009). Caveolin-1-/- null mammary stromal fibroblasts share characteristics with human breast cancer-associated fibroblasts. *Am J Pathol* 174, 746-761.

Takahashi-Yanaga, F., and Kahn, M. (2010). Targeting Wnt signaling: can we safely eradicate cancer stem cells? *Clin Cancer Res* 16, 3153-3162.

Trimboli, A. J.; Cantemir-Stone, C. Z.; Li, F.; Wallace, J. A.; Merchant, A.; Creasap, N.; Thompson, J. C.; Caserta, E.; Wang, H.; Chong, J. L.; Naidu, S.; Wei, G.; Sharma, S. M.; Stephens, J. A.; Fernandez, S. A.; Gurcan, M. N.; Weinstein, M. B.; Barsky, S. H.; Yee, L.; Rosol, T. J.; Stromberg, P. C.; Robinson, M. L.; Pepin, F.; Hallett, M.; Park, M.; Ostrowski, M. C., and Leone, G. (2009). Pten in stromal fibroblasts suppresses mammary epithelial tumours. *Nature* 461, 1084-1091.

Visvader, J. E., and Lindeman, G. J. (2008). Cancer stem cells in solid tumours: accumulating evidence and unresolved questions. *Nat Rev Cancer* 8, 755-768.

Yin, X.; Wolford, C. C.; Chang, Y. S.; McConoughey, S. J.; Ramsey, S. A.; Aderem, A., and Hai, T. (2010). ATF3, an adaptive-response gene, enhances TGF{beta} signaling and cancer-initiating cell features in breast cancer cells. *J Cell Sci* 123, 3558-3565.

13

Involvement of Mesenchymal Stem Cells in Breast Cancer Progression

Jürgen Dittmer, Ilka Oerlecke and Benjamin Leyh
Clinic for Gynecology, University of Halle
Germany

1. Introduction

For many reasons, mesenchymal stem cells (MSCs) have lately received much attention. Their plasticity, their tropism for wounds and cancer, their ability to assist in tissue regeneration, their immunomodulary activities, their effects on cancer development and finally their usefulness as drug-delivery vectors made MSCs a prime target for many researchers worldwide. Many aspects of MSC functions have been covered by recent reviews (Beyer Nardi & da Silva Meirelles, 2006; Kidd et al., 2008; Klopp et al., 2011; Krabbe et al., 2005; Patel et al., 2008; Uccelli et al., 2008; Wislet-Gendebien et al., 2005; Yen & Yen, 2008). In this review, we are summarizing the current knowledge on the communication of MSCs with breast cancer cells and its consequences for breast cancer progression.

2. General aspects of MSC biology

2.1 What are mesenchymal stem cells?

Mesenchymal stem cells, also called multipotent mesenchymal stromal cells, were first described as stromal cells residing in the bone marrow (Friedenstein et al., 1966). They have stem cell-like characteristics (Caplan, 1991; Friedenstein & Kuralesova, 1971), a fibroblast-like appearance and features different from cells of the haematopoietic lineages. Those features include the ability to differentiate to osteoblasts, chondrocytes and adipocytes (Friedenstein et al., 1974; Noth et al., 2002; Pittenger et al., 1999). MSCs may also play a role in haematopoiesis, as MSCs have been shown to be involved in forming niches for the haematopoietic stem cells and to regulate the activities of these cells (Ehninger & Trumpp, 2011; Mendez-Ferrer et al., 2010; Omatsu et al., 2010; Sacchetti et al., 2007). MSCs are rare in the bone marrow. Only 1 of 34,000 nucleated cells in this tissue were determined to be MSCs (Wexler et al., 2003). Though much is known about MSCs today, there are still no specific markers available that clearly define a cell as an MSC. In 2006, the International Society for Cellular Therapy published a list of minimal criteria instead (Dominici et al., 2006) that are now commonly used to identify MSCs. Among these criteria are two functional features, the potential to differentiate to osteoblasts, chondrocytes and adipocytes as mentioned above and the ability to adhere to plastic. The latter feature allows the separation of MSCs from the other bone marrow cell populations, as cells of the haematopoietic lineages are non-adherent cells (Beyer Nardi & da Silva Meirelles, 2006). Other critieria used to characterize

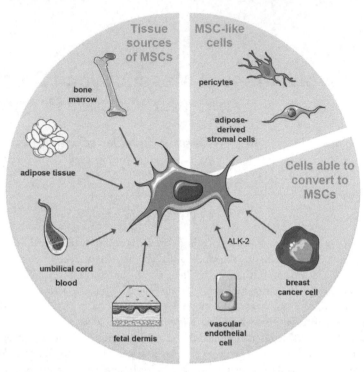

Fig. 1. Sources of MSCs. The cartoon depicts the different sources from which MSCs can be isolated (left), the cells that can convert to MSCs (right, bottom) and cells that display MSC-like features (right, top). Details are described in the text. ALK-2 = activin-like kinase-2.

MSCs are the expression profiles of certain proteins. MSCs express CD105 (endoglin), CD73 (ecto 5'-nucleotidase) and CD90 (Thy-1) and are deficient of CD45 (pan-leukocyte marker), CD34 (marker for primitive haematopoietic progenitors and endothelial cells), CD14 and CD11 (marker for monocytes and macrophages), CD79α and CD19 (marker for B-cells) and HLA-DR (MSCs not stimulated by IFN-γ). Bone marrow is not the only source of MSCs, other tissues are suitable to isolate MSCs as well (Fig. 1). Among these tissues are human adipose tissue (Zuk et al., 2002), umbilical cord blood (Sun et al., 2010), fetal dermis tissue (Qiao et al., 2008a), pancreatic tissue (Seeberger et al., 2006) and breast milk (Patki et al., 2010). More MSC sources are expected (Ding et al., 2011). Recently, menstrual blood and endometrium have been shown to contain MSCs. It is likely that most MSCs found in other tissues originated from the bone marrow. However, there is also evidence that some tissues, such as the adipose tissue, may produce their own MSCs (Bianco, 2011; Zhao et al., 2010). The MSC pool of a tissue may be expanded by dedifferentiation of differentiated cells (Fig. 1). This has been demonstrated for vascular endothelial cells that, under certain conditions, can undergo endothelial-to-mesenchymal transition to convert to MSCs (Medici et al., 2010). Some tissue-specific MSCs may be known for many years by other names (Fig. 1). Adipose-derived stromal cells or preadipocytes are likely to be MSCs residing in adipose tissue (Locke et al., 2011; Manabe et al., 2003; Zuk et al., 2002). Pericytes isolated from skeletal muscles or non-muscle tissues have recently be found to show the typical characteristics of

MSCs (Crisan et al., 2008). It is possible that MSCs from different sources may not be identical and may behave differently (Zhao et al., 2010). In fact, environmental conditions, such as the supply with growth factors or oxygen, have been shown to change the behavior of MSCs (Krinner et al., 2010; Sanchez et al., 2011). Even a population of MSCs derived from a single source may not be homogenous and may have different developmental potentials (Phinney, 2002). This hypothesis was confirmed by Wicha and his co-workers who demonstrated that MSCs from bone marrow contain at least two subpopulations, one that expresses and one that lacks the stem cell marker ALDH-1 (aldehyde dehydrogenase-1) (Liu et al., 2011). These two subpopulations behaved also functionally different (see 4.3).

2.2 Plasticity of MSCs

In addition to the ability to mature to osteoblasts, chondrocytes and adipocytes, MSCs are also capable of differentiating to fibroblasts (Mishra & Banerjee, 2011). This conversion may be of particular importance in cancer, where MSCs that colonize a cancerous lesion switch to a particular type of fibroblast-like cells, the carcinoma-associated fibroblast (CAF) (Mishra et al., 2008; Spaeth et al., 2009). This may have consequences for tumor progression (see 4.4). The differentiation potential of MSCs goes far beyond the ability to differentiate towards the mesodermal lineage (Uccelli et al., 2008). Differentiation of MSCs to cells of ectodermal and endodermal lineages have been demonstrated as well. E.g., MSCs derived from adipose tissue were shown to be able to differentiate to endothelial cells (Zuk et al., 2002), while pancreatic MSCs could become hepatocytes (Seeberger et al., 2006). In addition, MSCs from umbilical cord blood were shown to have the potential to switch to cells displaying features of neural cells (Li et al., 2005; Park et al., 2007; Tondreau et al., 2004), though, in some cases, the neural phenotype may have caused by fusions of MSCs with neurons (Krabbe et al., 2005; Wislet-Gendebien et al., 2005). Under certain conditions, MSCs can also become epithelial cells, such as lung or renal epithelium-like cells (Kale et al., 2003; Lin et al., 2003; Ortiz et al., 2003; Rojas et al., 2005).

3. Attracted to wounds and cancer

3.1 Tropism towards injured tissue: MSCs as "repair" cells

MSCs are believed to play an important role in wound healing. Chemokines and cytokines as secreted by inflammatory cells seem to chemoattract MSCs to injured tissues (Brooke et al., 2007). E.g., Kidd and his co-workers reported that, when inoculated into wounded mice, labeled MSCs were preferentially detected in wounds, whereas, in non-injured mice, MSCs settled in lung, liver and spleen (Kidd et al., 2009). MSCs are attracted to many types of organs after injury, such as heart after myocardial infarction (Barbash et al., 2003), kidney after glomeruli damage (Ito et al., 2001), injured muscles (Natsu et al., 2004), bleomycin-damaged lung (Ortiz et al., 2003) and brain after stroke (Chen et al., 2001; Mahmood et al., 2003). Interestingly, homing to the injured brain could be specifically blocked by an antibody directed to the chemokine MCP-1 (monocyte chemotactic protein-1)/CCL2 (Wang et al., 2002) suggesting that MCP-1/CCL2 is an important chemoattractant for MSCs. In the injured tissue, MSCs were found to help to regenerate this tissue. MSCs accomplish this goal partly by directly converting to those cells specifically needed to restore the function of the tissue. It is therefore tempting to consider the MSC as a general repair cell (Dittmer, 2010). Numerous reports support this hypothesis. E.g., bone marrow-derived MSCs were demonstrated to facilitate healing of injured muscles by differentiating to muscle progenitor cells (Natsu et al., 2004). In bleomycin-injured lung, MSCs switched to a phenotype typical for lung epithelial cells (Ortiz et al., 2003; Rojas et al., 2005). In the damaged myocardium, bone marrow-derived MSCs converted to cardiomyocytes (Toma et al., 2002; Wang et al., 2001). In ischemically injured renal tubules, MSCs are able to become tubular epithelial cells (Kale et al., 2003; Lin et al., 2003). In kidneys after anti-Thy1 antibody-induced glomerulonephritis, MSCs have been shown to mature to mesangial cells (Ito et al., 2001). And in diabetic mice, MSCs induced the number of pancreatic islets to increase and enhanced insulin production (Hess et al., 2003; Lee et al., 2006). The affinity of MSCs to injured tissue can be utilized for therapy (Brooke et al., 2007; Tocci & Forte, 2003). MSCs can be used as vectors to deliver drugs to injured tissues. Examples are BDNF (brain-derived neurotrophic factor)- or insulin-secreting MSCs to improve recovery from stroke (Kurozumi et al., 2004) or to treat diabetes (Xu et al., 2007), respectively. MSCs have also been used in clinical trials (Herberts et al., 2011). Most of the clinical trials with MSCs were carried out to treat patients with heart disease (Prockop & Olson, 2007). In many cases, patients' conditions improved suggesting that MSCs have positive effects on tissue repair also in humans.

3.2 Tropism towards cancer: MSCs are attracted to breast cancer lesions

Given the fact that MSCs are entering wounds to facilitate tissue repair, MSCs are of great value to maintain body functions. However, the affinity of MSCs to wounds may be of disadvantage to people who are suffering from cancer. In support of the view that a tumor is a wound that never heals (Dvorak, 1986), MSCs were also found to be attracted to cancerous lesions (Kidd et al., 2009) where they may promote tumor progression. Importantly, wounds and cancers secrete a similar cocktail of inflammatory cytokines and chemokines (Kidd et al., 2008). Among them are MSC-attracting factors, such as the growth factors PDGF (platelet-derived growth factor) and IGF-1 (insulin-like growth factor-1), the cytokines IL-6 (interleukin-6) and IL-8 as well as the chemokines MCP-1/CCL2, RANTES/CCL5, MDC (macrophage-derived chemokine)/CCL22 and SDF-1 (stromal-derived factor-1)/CXCL12 (Dwyer et al., 2007,Ponte, 2007 #228; Kim et al., 2011; Liu et al., 2011). It was confirmed that MSCs express the corresponding receptors for these ligands, i.e. PDGFR (PDGF receptor), IGFR (insulin growth factor receptor), IL-6R, gp130, CXCR1, CCR2, CCR3, CCR4 and CXCR4 (Dwyer et al., 2007,Ponte, 2007 #228; Kim et al., 2011; Liu et al., 2011). The susceptibility of MSCs to chemoattractants can be enhanced by certain factors. E.g., TNFα (tumor necrosis factor α) was shown to increase the response of MSCs to certain chemokines by upregulating the expression of the receptors CCR2, CCR3 and CCR4 (Ponte et al., 2007). Many studies demonstrated that MSCs are attracted by tumors. In one study, the bone marrow of a mouse was replaced by the bone marrow from a transgenic mouse that expressed beta-galactosidase and MSC migration monitored from the bone marrow towards a prostate tumor xenograft (Ishii et al., 2003). It was found that X-gal positive MSCs colonized the tumor and differentiated to fibroblasts and endothelial cells. In a similar experimental setting, Direkze and co-workers could show that MSCs enter pancreatic insulinoma and convert to myofibroblasts (Direkze et al., 2004). Also breast cancer cells have been shown to chemoattract MSCs *in vitro* as well as *in vivo* (Dittmer et al., 2009; Dwyer et al., 2007; Goldstein et al., 2010; Klopp et al., 2007; Lin et al., 2008; Ling et al., 2010; Liu et al., 2011; Mishra et al., 2008; Pulukuri et al., 2010; Rattigan et al., 2010; Ritter et al., 2008; Zielske et al., 2009). Most breast cancer studies with MSCs were performed with luminal A-type

MCF-7 cells and mesenchymal (basal-B)-type MDA-MB-231 cells. In some investigations, also luminal A-type T47D, basal A-type MDA-MB-468, murine 4T1 breast cancer cells and primary human breast cancer were used. In all cases, breast cancer cells stimulated MSC migration. However, the chemoattractive potency differed among the different breast cancer cell subtypes. E.g., the highly invasive MDA-MB-231 cells were more potent than the weakly invasive MCF-7 cells in stimulating migration of MSCs *in vitro* and *in vivo* (Dittmer et al., 2009; Goldstein et al., 2010; Ritter et al., 2008). Hence, it seems that MSCs have a higher affinity to more aggressive tumors. It is well established that factors secreted by breast cancer cells are responsible for MSC attraction (Fig. 2). IL-6 is one factor that is secreted by breast cancer cells and acts as a chemoattractant for MSCs (Liu et al., 2011; Rattigan et al., 2010). In response to IL-6, MSCs not only enhance their migratory activity, but also secrete chemokines, such as CXCL7 (see 4.3) (Liu et al., 2011). Interestingly, hypoxic conditions as often found in tumors trigger breast cancer cells to produce more IL-6 which further enhances migration of MSCs (Rattigan et al., 2010). Hypoxia also affects MSCs directly in

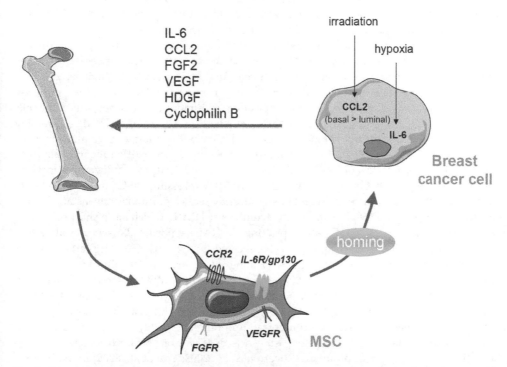

Fig. 2. Chemoattraction of MSCs to breast cancer cells. Breast cancer-derived cytokines and growth factors stimulate MSCs to migrate towards the tumor. Irradiation or hypoxia increase the CCL2 or IL-6 secretion, respectively, by breast cancer cells. Basal-type breast cancer cells seem to produce more CCL-2 than luminal A-type breast cancer cells. IL-6(R) = interleukin-6 (receptor), FGF(R) = fibroblast growth factor (receptor), VEGF(R) = vascular endothelial growth factor (receptor), HDGF = hepatoma-derived growth factor.

that it increases their proliferative activity and their expression of stem cell and differentiation markers (Grayson et al., 2006). Besides IL-6, breast cancer cell-derived FGF-2, VEGF (vascular endothelial growth factor), cyclophilin B and HDGF (hepatoma-derived growth factor) were demonstrated to induce migration of MSCs (Lin et al., 2003; Ritter et al., 2008). Another important tumor-derived chemoattractant was shown to be the chemokine MCP-1/CCL2 (Dwyer et al., 2007) which is recognized by MSCs via the receptor CCR2 (Lu et al., 2006; Wang et al., 2002). Interestingly, mesenchymal (basal B-type) MDA-MB-231 cells produce more MCP-1/CCL2 than luminal A-type T47D cells, which may explain why more aggressive breast cancer cells have a higher potential to stimulate MSC migration. In primary breast cancer, which contains both an epithelial and a stromal compartment, the stromal compartment seems to be the major source of MCP-1/CCL2 (Dwyer et al., 2007). Irradiation of tumors was found to increase the expression of MCP-1/CCL2 and, along with it, the potential to recruit MSCs to tumors (Zielske et al., 2009). This further supports the notion that MCP-1/CCL2 plays an important role in attracting MSCs to tumors. The efficiency of recruitment of MSCs to tumors may also depend on inherent features of MSCs. MSCs overexpressing uPA (urokinase plasminogen activator) have a higher ability to migrate towards breast and prostate cancer cells than their vector-treated counterparts (Pulukuri et al., 2010). Given their similar tropism to injuries and cancer (Kidd et al., 2009), MSCs are a promising tool for therapeutic intervention of cancer (Motaln et al., 2010) as much as they are for treating injuries. MSCs engineered to express anti-cancer drugs can be used as vectors to deliver toxic loads to tumor cells. In many studies with engineered MSCs, MSCs were forced to express TRAIL (tumor necrosis factor-related apoptosis-inducing ligand), a membrane protein that induces apoptosis of tumor cells, but not of normal cells (Walczak et al., 1999). Using mouse xenografts, it could be shown that TRAIL-expressing MSCs are able to eradicate many kinds of tumor cells, including glioma, cervival, pancreatic, colon and breast cancer cells (Grisendi et al., 2010; Loebinger et al., 2009; Menon et al., 2009; Sonabend et al., 2008; Yang et al., 2009). MSC-delivered TRAIL can induce apoptosis by upregulating caspase 8 (Grisendi et al., 2010). TRAIL-expressing MSCs were also able to attack metastatic breast cancer cells and to significantly reduce pulmonary metastatic load in mice (Loebinger et al., 2009). In contrast to recombinant TRAIL, which has a short half life in plasma, TRAIL-expressing MSCs allow prolonged TRAIL exposure (Grisendi et al., 2010). Other approaches use MSCs that were engineered to express IFN-β (interferon-β) or transduced with CRAds (conditionally replicating adenoviruses) (Dembinski et al., 2009; Ling et al., 2010; Stoff-Khalili et al., 2007). In another setting, MSCs were transfected with enzymes to locally convert a relatively non-toxic substance into a toxin. Examples are MSCs expressing HSV-TK (herpes simplex virus-thymidine kinase) which catalyses the conversion of the prodrug ganciclovir to a toxic compound (Conrad et al., 2011) and MSCs loaded with cytosine deaminase which induces the deamination of 5-fluorocytosine to the chemotherapeutic drug 5-fluorouracil (Kucerova et al., 2008; You et al., 2009). In both cases, the non-toxic prodrug was systemically administered to tumor-bearing mice. MSCs can also be engineered such that they boost immune responses to cancer cells. MSCs engineered to express Her2 (human epidermal receptor2), a receptor tyrosine kinase often overexpressed in breast cancer (Theillet, 2010), can act as antigen-presenting cells to induce an immune reaction against Her2-exposing breast cancer cells (Romieu-Mourez et al., 2010). However, it should be noted that caution should be exercised when using MSCs as therapeutic tools as

MSCs may be able to transform to sarcoma cells (Burns et al., 2008; Gjerstorff et al., 2009; Li et al., 2009; Mohseny & Hogendoorn, 2011; Riggi et al., 2008; Rosland et al., 2009). Currently, there is a debate about whether the MSC and not a primitive neuroectodermal cell is the cell of origin of Ewing's sarcoma (Lin et al., 2011).

3.3 Immunosuppression by MSCs: Consequences for wound healing and cancer progression

It is well established that MSCs act anti-inflammatory by modulating the activities of cells of the innate and the adaptive immune system (Rasmusson, 2006; Uccelli et al., 2008; Yagi et al., 2010). Among the affected cells are antigen-presenting dendritic cells, tumor cell-targeting natural killer cells, neutrophils and B- as well as T-lymphocytes. MSCs block antigen presentations by dendritic cells (Jiang et al., 2005; Ramasamy et al., 2007), inhibit the proliferation of activated T-lymphocytes (Bartholomew et al., 2002; Di Nicola et al., 2002; Krampera et al., 2003; Rasmusson et al., 2005), activate regulatory T cells (T_{regs}) that suppress T-effector cells (Aggarwal & Pittenger, 2005; Patel et al., 2010; Selmani et al., 2008), inhibit the activity of cytotoxic T-lymphocytes (Rasmusson et al., 2003) and block the proliferation of natural killer cells (Aggarwal & Pittenger, 2005; Sotiropoulou et al., 2006; Spaggiari et al., 2008). Direct and indirect interactions of MSCs with immune cells are made responsible for the anti-inflammatory activity of the MSCs (Uccelli et al., 2008). The indirect effects are mediated by a number of cyto- and chemokines as secreted by MSCs. Among them are TGFβ1 (transforming growth factor β1) which stimulates the proliferation of inhibitory T_{regs} (Patel et al., 2010), IL-6 shown to inhibit neutrophil proliferation (Raffaghello et al., 2008) and prostaglandin E2 that inhibits antigen presentation by dendritic cells as well as proliferation of T-effector cells (Aggarwal & Pittenger, 2005; Bartholomew et al., 2002; Di Nicola et al., 2002; Glennie et al., 2005; Jiang et al., 2005; Krampera et al., 2003; Ramasamy et al., 2007; Rasmusson et al., 2005; Selmani et al., 2008). In the mouse model, the anti-inflammatory effects of MSCs were also linked to increased phagocytosis and enhanced elimination of bacteria (Mei et al., 2010). However, due to differences in the anti-sepsis defense in mice and men, it is unclear whether these data allow the prediction of an MSC-induced anti-sepsis effect also in humans (Monneret, 2009). It is likely that, by down-modulating the immune response, MSCs prevent excessive inflammation in injuries. This is thought to be the second way by which MSCs facilitate regeneration of the injured tissue. While for that reason the anti-inflammatory effect of MSCs may be beneficial for a patient with an injury, it may be however detrimental to a cancer patient. By inducing local immunosuppression cancer-residing MSCs may help cancer cells to escape immune surveillance.

4. Communication between MSCs and breast cancer cells

4.1 The cytokine cocktail secreted by MSCs

MSCs secrete a plethora of cytokines and chemokines. In addition to the immuno-regulatory proteins, such as TGFβ1, IL-6 and prostaglandin E2, MSCs produce many other interleukins, including IL-7, IL-8 and IL-9, CC-type chemokines (CCL1, 2, 5, 8, 11, 15, 16, 20, 22, 26, and 27), CXC-type chemokines (CXCL1, 5, 6, 10, 11, 12, 13, and 16) and other factors, such as TIMP (tissue inhibitor of metalloproteases) -1 and -2, TNFα and β, PDGF A and B, G-CSF (granulocyte colony-stimulating factor), HGF (hepatocyte growth factor), VEGF and angiopoietin (Parekkadan et al., 2007). The syntheses of these factors can be further stimulated. E.g., IL-6 induces the expression of CXCL7, which further enhances the expression levels of IL-6, IL-8, CXCL5 and CXCL6 (Liu et al., 2011). TGFα (transforming growth factor α) was found to stimulate MSCs to secrete more IL-6, IL-8, angiopoietin-2, G-CSF, HGF, VEGF and PDGF-BB (De Luca et al., 2010). TNFα forced MSCs to increase their expression of CXCL9, CXCL10 and CXCL11 (Shin et al., 2010). Exposure of MSCs to conditioned medium from tumor cells also stimulate expression of chemokines, such as CXCL2 and CXCL12 (Menon et al., 2007). Direct interactions of cancer cells with MSCs may as well contribute to the rise of chemokine secretion by MSCs. Direct contacts of MSCs with MDA-MB-231 breast cancer cells were found to strongly upregulate the production of RANTES/CCL5 (Karnoub et al., 2007).

4.2 Modulatory effects of MSCs on breast cancer cell function

MCF-7 cells are ERα-positive luminal A-type breast cancer cells that show many features of normal breast epithelial cells, including the formation of E-cadherin-based cell-cell interactions and the ability to generate multicellular 3D-aggregates that can mature to lumen-containing spheroids (dit Faute et al., 2002; do Amaral et al., 2010). Decreased expression or complete loss of E-cadherin has been linked to epithelial-mesenchymal transition (EMT) and increased cellular migration of breast epithelial cells as well as to metastasis (Cano et al., 2000; Chua et al., 2007; Mani et al., 2008; Onder et al., 2008). We and others have shown that MSCs negatively interfere with the E-cadherin status of MCF-7 cells either by downregulation of the full length protein (Fierro et al., 2004; Hombauer & Minguell, 2000; Klopp et al., 2010) or by increasing E-cadherin shedding as triggered by the transmembrane protease ADAM10 (a disintegrin and metalloprotease 10) (Dittmer et al., 2009). It is noteworthy that as few as one MSC per 500 MCF-7 cells was sufficient to induce E-cadherin shedding. E-cadherin shedding leads to extracellular E-cadherin fragments that may block E-cadherin-based cell-cell contacts by competing with membrane-bound E-cadherin proteins (Ryniers et al., 2002). Hence, both downregulation of E-cadherin expression and increased E-cadherin shedding may decrease the strength of E-cadherin-based cell-cell interactions. With intercellular adhesions weakened cellular migration may increase. In fact, MSCs have been shown to significantly enhance the migratory activity of MCF-7 cells (Dittmer et al., 2009; Rhodes et al., 2010). Also along with the destabilization of cell-cell contacts, disruption of the architecture of MCF-7 spheroids was observed. It is interesting that, despite these changes in the E-cadherin status, MSCs did not induce EMT of MCF-7 cells, as indicated by the failure of MSCs to stimulate the expression of mesenchymal markers, such as vimentin or snail (Dittmer et al., 2009; Klopp et al., 2010). However, in the luminal A-type T47D breast cancer cell line, MSCs not only downregulated E-cadherin levels, but also increased expression of vimentin, snail, twist and N-cadherin (Martin et al., 2010) suggesting that, under certain conditions, MSCs can induce EMT of breast cancer cells. MSCs were also shown to increase the proliferation of MCF-7 cells in a dose-dependent manner (Fierro et al., 2004; Klopp et al., 2010; Rhodes et al., 2010; Sasser et al., 2007a). These effects may be mediated by IL-6, VEGF and/or SDF-1/CXCL12 as secreted by MSCs (Fig. 3) (Fierro et al., 2004; Sasser et al., 2007b). MSCs or similarly IL-6 induced the phosphorylation of STAT3 (signal transducer and activator of transcription 3) on tyrosine-705 in MCF-7 cells (Sasser et al., 2007b). Incubation of MSCs with TGFα, a ligand of the EGFR (epidermal growth factor receptor), further stimulated the secretion of IL-6 and other factors (De Luca et al., 2010). This suggests that TGFα-primed MSCs would even be more effective in promoting proliferation of MCF-7 cells. MSCs also enhanced the tumorigenic activity of

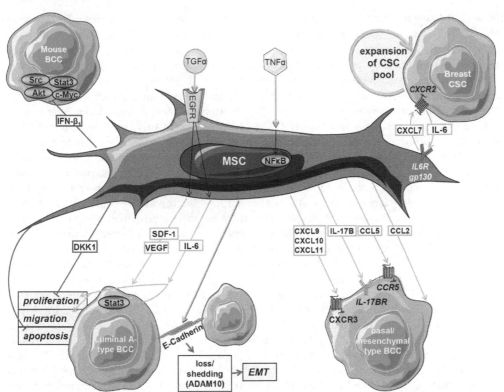

Fig. 3. Paracrine actions of MSCs on breast cancer cells (BCCs). The effects of MSCs on luminal A and basal/mesenchymal subtype BCCs, on murine BCCs and on cancer stem cells (CSCs) are separately displayed. IL-6/-17B(R) = interleukin-6/-17B (receptor), VEGF = vascular endothelial growth factor, SDF-1 = stromal-derived factor-1, DKK = dickkopf, INF-β₁ = interferon β₁, TGFα = transforming growth factor α, TNFα = tumor necrosis factor α, EGFR = epidermal growth factor receptor, NF-κB = nuclear factor kappa-light-chain-enhancer of activated B-cells, Stat3 = signal transducer and activator of transcription 3, ADAM10 = a disintegrin and metalloprotease 10, EMT = epithelial-to-mesenchymal transition.

MCF-7 cells. In mouse xenografts, MCF-7 tumor formation and growth were fostered by MSCs (Klopp et al., 2010). Though ERα-positive MCF-7 cells are dependent on estrogen for growth, MSCs may even trigger estrogen-independent proliferation of MCF-7 cells (Rhodes et al., 2009). The estrogen-independent growth may nevertheless be dependent on ER, as the proliferation-promoting effect of MSCs on MCF-7 cells was found to be blocked by ER-specific inhibitor ICI 182780 (Rhodes et al., 2010). It is thought that, by a yet unknown mechanism, MSCs activate ER which, in turn, stimulates the expression of SDF-1/CXCL12, a chemokine shown to trigger the proliferation of MCF-7 cells. Growth-stimulating effects of MSCs were also found on other ERα-positive breast cancer cell lines, including T47D, BT474 and ZR-75-1 (Sasser et al., 2007a) and may be dependent on similar mechanisms as those on MCF-7 cells. There are also two reports that show that MSCs are able to inhibit the proliferation of MCF-7 cells (Goldstein et al., 2010; Qiao et al., 2008a). Dickkopf-1 (DKK-1) secreted by MSCs and known to block differentiation and to promote proliferation of MSCs by an autocrine mechanism (Pinzone et al., 2009) may be responsible for this effect (Qiao et al., 2008a). As an inhibitor of the Wnt/β-catenin pathway, DKK-1 was shown to downregulate β-catenin activity and, concomitantly, to reduce the expression of proliferation-promoting proteins c-Myc and NF-κB (nuclear factor kappa-light-chain-enhancer of activated B-cells) in MCF-7 cells (Qiao et al., 2008a; Qiao et al., 2008b). Why some studies showed stimulatory while others demonstrated inhibitory effects of MSCs on MCF-7 cell proliferation is not clear yet. Qiao et al. used human fetal dermal tissue as a source to isolate MSCs for their study (Qiao et al., 2008a). In this case, the different MSC sources may have accounted for the contradictory results. Since MSCs are a heterogeneous population (Uccelli et al., 2008), a different environment may drive the selection of a certain subtype of MSCs with features distinct to the bone-marrow MSC population. In particular, types and amounts of chemokines/cytokines these MSC populations secrete might be different. The importance of environmental conditions for the ability of MSCs to interfere with breast cancer functions is nicely demonstrated in a study that compared serum-exposed MSCs with serum-deprived MSCs (Sanchez et al., 2011). Serum-deprived MSCs were found to be more effective than serum-exposed MSCs in protecting MCF-7 cells from apoptotic death by secreting pro-survival factors. MSCs also modulate the functions of highly aggressive ERα-negative MDA-MB-231 cells (Fig. 3). Two studies demonstrated that MSCs increase the invasive and metastatic behavior of these breast cancer cells (Goldstein et al., 2010; Karnoub et al., 2007). In one study, this effect was found to be mediated by IL-17B (Goldstein et al., 2010). In the other study, the chemokine RANTES/CCL5 was shown to be responsible (Karnoub et al., 2007). Paracrine feedback loops between breast cancer cells and MSCs seem to be important for these effects. It could be shown that MDA-MB-231 cells stimulate the expression of RANTES/CCL5 in MSCs by secreting osteopontin which binds to MSC surface integrins which then leads to the activation of AP-1, a transcription factor able to induce the transcription of the RANTES/CCL5 gene (Mi et al., 2011). MCP-1/CCL2 is another chemokine whose secretion can be stimulated when MSCs are co-cultured with MDA-MB-231 cells (Molloy et al., 2009). MCP-1/CCL2 belongs to those chemokines that enhance the motility of MDA-MB-231 cells. Other migration-promoting chemokines are CXCR3 ligands CXCL9, CXCL10 and CXCL11 (Shin et al., 2010). These CXCL chemokines also increase the activity of Rho GTPases and the expression of MMP-9 (matrix metalloprotease-9). These chemokines may be of particular importance when MSCs are exposed to TNFα which was found to induce CXCL gene transcription through a mechanism involving NF-κB (Fig. 3). One group also demonstrated inhibitory effects of MSCs on MDA-MB-231 cells (Sun et al., 2009; Sun et al., 2010). According to their data, MSCs suppress the proliferative, migratory, tumor-initiating and metastatic activities of MDA-MB-231 cells and induce apoptosis of these cells by interfering with the AKT/mTOR (mammalian target of rapamycin) pathway. Different to the other investigations, these studies were performed with MSCs isolated from human umbilical cord blood or adipose tissue. Hence, as discussed above, source-dependent features of MSC isolates may be responsible for these contradictory results. Also murine metastatic 4T1 breast cancer cells were shown to be affected by MSCs (Ling et al., 2010). Using a syngeneic, immunocompetent murine model, Ling and colleagues demonstrated that murine MSCs enter 4T1 tumors to deliver IFN-β to the tumor. This factor then inhibited cancer growth by inducing the inactivation of STAT3, Src and AKT and by triggering the downregulation of c-Myc and MMP-2 (matrix metalloprotease-2). Interestingly, human MSCs engineered to secrete IFN-β have also a suppressing effect on growth of MDA-MB-231 cells in mouse xenografts (Studeny et al., 2004). It may well be that the ratio of tumor-suppressing vs. tumor-promoting factors as secreted by MSCs determine whether MSCs promote or inhibit tumor growth. This ratio could be different among different MSC isolates.

4.3 MSCs, EMT and breast cancer stem cells
There is growing evidence that, in accordance with the hierarchical model of cancer development (Visvader & Lindeman, 2008), breast cancer is driven by cancer stem cells (CSCs) (Liu & Wicha, 2010). Breast CSCs are characterized by high expression of surface marker CD44 and low expression of CD24 (Fillmore & Kuperwasser, 2007). Another useful breast CSC marker is ALDH-1 (Ginestier et al., 2007). A recent study showed that MSCs increase the pool of CSCs in breast cancer lines, including MCF-7, SUM149 and SUM159 cells (Liu et al., 2011). Interestingly, bone marrow-derived MSCs themselves show also a hierarchical organization with only a minority of cells expressing the stem cell marker ALDH-1. And only those ALDH-1 positive MSCs were able to interfere with the CSC pool. Wicha and his co-workers showed that the MSC/breast cancer interaction generated a cytokine network which is initiated by IL-6 as secreted by breast cancer cells (Liu et al., 2011). IL-6 induces the production of CXCL7 in MSCs which, in turn, triggers the expression of a number of other cytokines and chemokines, namely IL-6, IL-8, CXCL6 and CXCL5, in both MSCs and breast cancer cells. This mixture of secreted factors then stimulates the expansion of the CSC pool. In line with the observation that MSCs induce the CSC pool to expand is the finding that MSCs stimulated mammosphere formation of normal mammary epithelial cells (Klopp et al., 2010). Evidence has been accumulated suggesting that the generation of mammospheres depends on the presence of mammary stem cells (Dontu et al., 2003). Hence, the number of mammospheres formed is supposed to be a measure of the number of mammary stem cells present (Charafe-Jauffret et al., 2008). A recent study on breast cancer patients support the notion of a link between MSCs and breast cancer stem cells (De Giorgi et al., 2011). It showed that the relative number of disseminated CD44+/CD24low/-/ALDH-1+ breast cancer stem cells correlated with the relative number of MSCs in the bone marrow. Recently, it has been found that epithelial cells after having undergone full EMT display stem cell-like characteristics, including expression of CD44 and ALDH-1 (Mani et al., 2008; May et al., 2011). EMT is linked to E-cadherin loss and the expression of mesenchymal markers. As mentioned above, MSCs have been shown to reduce E-cadherin expression or to induce E-cadherin shedding in luminal A-type, epitheloid breast cancer cells, such as MCF-7 and T47D. In T47D, this downregulation of E-cadherin was accompanied with increased expression of mesenchymal markers suggesting that MSCs may induce at least partial EMT of breast cancer cells. Hence, MSCs may not only be able to trigger the CSC pool to expand, but also to force new CSCs to be generated from the pool of non-CSC breast cancer cells by EMT. These MSC-induced new CSCs may have other features than the CSCs of the existing pool and may further contribute to tumor heterogeneity and progression (Visvader & Lindeman, 2008). Another interesting observation is that the gene expression profile of mesenchymal (basal-type) breast cancer cells show similarities to the expression profile of MSCs (Marchini et al., 2010) suggesting that this type of breast cancer cell and MSCs have also common functions. In support of this notion, a recent study showed that mesenchymal breast cancer cells generated by

transformation of human mammary epithelial cells by SV40 T-antigen and forced expression of EMT-inducing proteins had the potential to undergo adipogenic and chondrogenic differentiation. Also, these mesenchymal breast cancer cells were attracted to wounds and tumors, a feature typical for MSCs. The latter observation may shed a new light on a phenomenon called tumor-self seeding (Leung & Brugge, 2009). Tumor-self seeding describes the ability of metastasized cells to circulate back to the primary tumor. Chemoattraction to the primary tumor was shown to be driven by IL-6 and IL-8. As mentioned above, IL-6 is highly active on MSCs and triggers the production of a number of chemokines (Leung & Brugge, 2009). Based on these data, it is tempting to assume that MSCs are also generated from breast cancer cells (Fig. 1) and that these MSCs containing the mutations (and epigenetic changes) of the breast cancer cells they derived from play a role in breast cancer metastasis and tumor-self seeding. Nestin[+] - MSCs have been reported to share with haematopoietic stem cells the same niche in the bone marrow (Mendez-Ferrer et al., 2010). This niche might also be available for breast cancer-derived MSCs and allow these cells to survive in this tissue. An exciting hypothesis would be to assume that, at least in some cases of breast cancer, dormancy (Pantel et al., 2009; Willis et al., 2010) is caused by breast cancer-derived MSCs that are caught in these niches. The niches could fulfill two functions in order to maintain dormancy, preventing the cells from proliferating while, at the same time, protecting them from death-inducing signals. The bone marrow seems to be an attractive tissue for circulating tumor cells to home and form micrometastasis which is an early event in breast cancer development (Pantel et al., 2009). The number of such disseminated breast cancer cells in bone has been linked to prognosis of breast cancer patients. MSCs may also play a role in this early entry of breast cancer cells into bone marrow (Corcoran et al., 2008). MSCs were shown to facilitate the migration of MCF-7 and T47D breast cancer cells across bone marrow endothelial cells *in vitro* and to be in close contact with bone-metastasized breast cancer cells *in vivo*. Evidence was presented that these MSC/breast cancer cell interactions may require the chemokine receptor CXCR4 as well as its ligand SDF-1/CXCL12. Hence, it might be possible that breast cancer-derived MSCs not only would be able to home to the bone marrow and induce tumor dormancy, but also to help other breast cancer cells to enter this tissue and form micrometastasis. The breast cancer cell may not be the only non-stem cell which may be able to convert to an MSC. Vascular endothelial cells have been shown to become MSC-like cells as well as displaying typical MSC features, such as the ability to differentiate to osteoblasts, chondrocytes and adipocytes, upon treatment with ALK2 (activin-like kinase-2), TGFβ2 or BMP4 (bone morphognetic protein-4) (Medici et al., 2010). This suggests that certain non-stem cells under certain conditions can be an additonal source for generating MSCs. These cells may have different features compared to those MSCs that derived from the bone marrow.

4.4 MSCs and carcinoma-associated fibroblasts

Besides differentiating to osteoblast, chondrocytes and adipocytes, MSCs are able to convert to neural cells or to undergo transdifferentiation to different kinds of epithelial cells (Uccelli et al., 2008; Wislet-Gendebien et al., 2005). In tumors, MSCs can also differentiate to the carcinoma-associated fibroblasts (CAFs) (Mishra et al., 2008; Spaeth et al., 2009). These cells are different to normal fibroblasts/myofibroblasts in that they are able to stimulate tumor progression (Olumi et al., 1999) and show higher proliferative and migratory activity (Schor et al., 1988). Defined as myofibroblasts, CAFs share features with both smooth muscle cells and fibroblasts (Mueller & Fusenig, 2004). CAFs are found in many cancers, including breast cancer (Chauhan et al., 2003), and are linked to tumor invasion and proliferation (De Wever & Mareel, 2003; Tlsty & Coussens, 2006). They are responsible for a phenomenon called desmoplasia and promote angiogenesis and inflammation (Orimo et al., 2005; Tlsty & Coussens, 2006). Interestingly, CAFs secrete factors that are also produced by MSCs. In particular, CAFs and MSCs both secrete IL-6 and SDF-1/CXCL12, cytokines able to induce the proliferation of luminal A-type MCF-7 breast cancer cells (Bhowmick et al., 2004; Fierro et al., 2004; Mishra et al., 2008; Orimo et al., 2005; Sasser et al., 2007b). In addition, both cell types were found to interfere similarly with the response of MCF-7 and MDA-MB-231 breast cancer cells to inhibitors of mTOR and B-RAF (Dittmer et al., 2011). Differentiation of MSCs to CAFs requires the exposure of MSCs to conditioned medium from tumor cells over several weeks (Mishra et al., 2008; Spaeth et al., 2009). Conditioned medium from MDA-MB-231 breast cancer cells and from Skov-3 ovarian cancer cells were similar effective in inducing a MSC/CAF conversion which was accompanied by increased expression of CAF markers, such as tenascin-C, α-smooth muscle actin and IL-6. What are the consequences of this finding? As soon as MSCs enter a tumor, they will be bombarded with a cocktail of cytokines as produced by the tumor cells and may receive additional signals by direct cell-cell contacts. This may then force MSCs to lose their stemness and to undergo differentiation towards CAFs. By converting to CAFs, MSCs may not further be able to act also suppressive on tumor cells and may only keep their potency to promote tumor progression. Hence, the differentiation of MSCs to CAFs may be as much of a benefit for a progressing tumor as is the differentiation of MSCs to particular cells for an injured tissue to be repaired (Dittmer, 2010).

5. Conclusions

MSCs display an astounding plasticity and have shown to differentiate to cells as different as neurons and epithelial cells. The main function of MSCs is likely to promote tissue regeneration after injuries and, since tumors are probably wounds that never heal, also to support repair of tumoral lesions. However, tumors may misguide MSCs and "misuse" them for their "own benefit". Primary tumors may particularly profit from MSCs when they differentiate to tumor-promoting CAFs. MSCs may further facilitate breast cancer to metastasize by helping breast cancer cells to enter the bone marrow as well as by increasing the pool of metastasizing breast cancer stem cells. Most of the interactions between MSCs and tumor cells are mediated by cytokines as secreted by both cell types. Paracrine feedback mechanisms may further increase cytokine concentrations at places where these cells communicate with each other and may attract other cell types, such as macrophages, that are known to support tumor progression. To interfere with the interaction between MSCs and breast cancer cells treatments may be considered involving the inhibition of the activities of key cytokines, such as IL-6 (Liu & Wicha, 2010), which are important for both attraction of MSCs to breast cancer and expansion of the breast cancer stem cell pool by MSCs. On the other hand, there is also evidence that MSCs may have suppressive effects on breast cancer. Different sources from which MSCs were isolated may partially account for these contradictory results. Further studies are necessary to clarify this controversy, before conclusions can be drawn in terms of treatment of breast cancer patients. Certainly, when engineered to produce anti-tumor factors, MSCs possess anti-tumoral effects and may be used as trojan horses that enter and eradicate tumor cells. Drug-carrying MSCs may have a great advantage over "naked" drugs since they may deliver drugs more selectively and more efficiently at places where they are meant to act.

6. Acknowledgment

This work was supported by the Deutsche Krebshilfe (grant # 109271)

7. References

Aggarwal S. & Pittenger M. F. (2005). Human mesenchymal stem cells modulate allogeneic immune cell responses. *Blood,* Vol.105, No.4, pp. 1815-1822.

Barbash I. M.; Chouraqui P.; Baron J.; Feinberg M. S.; Etzion S.; Tessone A.; Miller L.; Guetta E.; Zipori D.; Kedes L. H.; Kloner R. A. & Leor J. (2003). Systemic delivery of bone marrow-derived mesenchymal stem cells to the infarcted myocardium: feasibility, cell migration, and body distribution. *Circulation,* Vol.108, No.7, pp. 863-868.

Bartholomew A.; Sturgeon C.; Siatskas M.; Ferrer K.; McIntosh K.; Patil S.; Hardy W.; Devine S.; Ucker D.; Deans R.; Moseley A. & Hoffman R. (2002). Mesenchymal stem cells suppress lymphocyte proliferation in vitro and prolong skin graft survival in vivo. *Exp Hematol,* Vol.30, No.1, pp. 42-48.

Beyer Nardi N. & da Silva Meirelles L. (2006). Mesenchymal stem cells: isolation, in vitro expansion and characterization. *Handb Exp Pharmacol,* No.174, pp. 249-282.

Bhowmick N. A.; Neilson E. G. & Moses H. L. (2004). Stromal fibroblasts in cancer initiation and progression. *Nature,* Vol.432, No.7015, pp. 332-337.

Bianco P. (2011). Back to the future: moving beyond "mesenchymal stem cells". *J Cell Biochem,* Vol.112, No.7, pp. 1713-1721.

Brooke G.; Cook M.; Blair C.; Han R.; Heazlewood C.; Jones B.; Kambouris M.; Kollar K.; McTaggart S.; Pelekanos R.; Rice A.; Rossetti T. & Atkinson K. (2007). Therapeutic applications of mesenchymal stromal cells. *Semin Cell Dev Biol,* Vol.18, No.6, pp. 846-858.

Burns J. S.; Abdallah B. M.; Schroder H. D. & Kassem M. (2008). The histopathology of a human mesenchymal stem cell experimental tumor model: support for an hMSC origin for Ewing's sarcoma? *Histol Histopathol,* Vol.23, No.10, pp. 1229-1240.

Cano A.; Perez-Moreno M. A.; Rodrigo I.; Locascio A.; Blanco M. J.; del Barrio M. G.; Portillo F. & Nieto M. A. (2000). The transcription factor snail controls epithelial-mesenchymal transitions by repressing E-cadherin expression. *Nat Cell Biol,* Vol.2, No.2, pp. 76-83.

Caplan A. I. (1991). Mesenchymal stem cells. *J Orthop Res,* Vol.9, No.5, pp. 641-650.

Charafe-Jauffret E.; Monville F.; Ginestier C.; Dontu G.; Birnbaum D. & Wicha M. S. (2008). Cancer stem cells in breast: current opinion and future challenges. *Pathobiology,* Vol.75, No.2, pp. 75-84.

Chauhan H.; Abraham A.; Phillips J. R.; Pringle J. H.; Walker R. A. & Jones J. L. (2003). There is more than one kind of myofibroblast: analysis of CD34 expression in benign, in situ, and invasive breast lesions. *J Clin Pathol,* Vol.56, No.4, pp. 271-276.

Chen J.; Li Y.; Wang L.; Zhang Z.; Lu D.; Lu M. & Chopp M. (2001). Therapeutic benefit of intravenous administration of bone marrow stromal cells after cerebral ischemia in rats. *Stroke*, Vol.32, No.4, pp. 1005-1011.

Chua H. L.; Bhat-Nakshatri P.; Clare S. E.; Morimiya A.; Badve S. & Nakshatri H. (2007). NF-kappaB represses E-cadherin expression and enhances epithelial to mesenchymal transition of mammary epithelial cells: potential involvement of ZEB-1 and ZEB-2. *Oncogene*, Vol.26, No.5, pp. 711-724.

Conrad C.; Husemann Y.; Niess H.; von Luettichau I.; Huss R.; Bauer C.; Jauch K. W.; Klein C. A.; Bruns C. & Nelson P. J. (2011). Linking transgene expression of engineered mesenchymal stem cells and angiopoietin-1-induced differentiation to target cancer angiogenesis. *Ann Surg*, Vol.253, No.3, pp. 566-571.

Corcoran K. E.; Trzaska K. A.; Fernandes H.; Bryan M.; Taborga M.; Srinivas V.; Packman K.; Patel P. S. & Rameshwar P. (2008). Mesenchymal stem cells in early entry of breast cancer into bone marrow. *PLoS One*, Vol.3, No.6, pp. e2563.

Crisan M.; Yap S.; Casteilla L.; Chen C. W.; Corselli M.; Park T. S.; Andriolo G.; Sun B.; Zheng B.; Zhang L.; Norotte C.; Teng P. N.; Traas J.; Schugar R.; Deasy B. M.; Badylak S.; Buhring H. J.; Giacobino J. P.; Lazzari L.; Huard J. & Peault B. (2008). A perivascular origin for mesenchymal stem cells in multiple human organs. *Cell Stem Cell.*, Vol.3, No.3, pp. 301-313.

De Giorgi U.; Cohen E. N.; Gao H.; Mego M.; Lee B. N.; Lodhi A.; Cristofanilli M.; Lucci A. & Reuben J. M. (2011). Mesenchymal stem cells expressing GD2 and CD271 correlate with breast cancer-initiating cells in bone marrow. *Cancer Biol Ther*, Vol.11, No.9, pp. 812-815.

De Luca A.; Gallo M.; Aldinucci D.; Ribatti D.; Lamura L.; D'Alessio A.; De Filippi R.; Pinto A. & Normanno N. (2010). The role of the EGFR ligand/receptor system in the secretion of angiogenic factors in mesenchymal stem cells. *J Cell Physiol*, Vol.226, No.8, pp. 2131-2138.

De Wever O. & Mareel M. (2003). Role of tissue stroma in cancer cell invasion. *J Pathol*, Vol.200, No.4, pp. 429-447.

Dembinski J. L.; Spaeth E. L.; Fueyo J.; Gomez-Manzano C.; Studeny M.; Andreeff M. & Marini F. C. (2009). Reduction of nontarget infection and systemic toxicity by targeted delivery of conditionally replicating viruses transported in mesenchymal stem cells. *Cancer Gene Ther*, Vol.17, No.4, pp. 289-297.

Di Nicola M.; Carlo-Stella C.; Magni M.; Milanesi M.; Longoni P. D.; Matteucci P.; Grisanti S. & Gianni A. M. (2002). Human bone marrow stromal cells suppress T-lymphocyte proliferation induced by cellular or nonspecific mitogenic stimuli. *Blood*, Vol.99, No.10, pp. 3838-3843.

Ding D. C.; Shyu W. C. & Lin S. Z. (2011). Mesenchymal stem cells. *Cell*, Vol.20, No.1, pp. 5-14.

Direkze N. C.; Hodivala-Dilke K.; Jeffery R.; Hunt T.; Poulsom R.; Oukrif D.; Alison M. R. & Wright N. A. (2004). Bone marrow contribution to tumor-associated myofibroblasts and fibroblasts. *Cancer Res*, Vol.64, No.23, pp. 8492-8495.

dit Faute M. A.; Laurent L.; Ploton D.; Poupon M. F.; Jardillier J. C. & Bobichon H. (2002). Distinctive alterations of invasiveness, drug resistance and cell-cell organization in

3D-cultures of MCF-7, a human breast cancer cell line, and its multidrug resistant variant. *Clin Exp Metastasis*, Vol.19, No.2, pp. 161-168.

Dittmer A.; Hohlfeld K.; Lutzkendorf J.; Muller L. P. & Dittmer J. (2009). Human mesenchymal stem cells induce E-cadherin degradation in breast carcinoma spheroids by activating ADAM10. *Cell Mol Life Sci.*, Vol.66, No.18, pp. 3053-3065.

Dittmer J. (2010). Mesenchymal stem cells: "repair cells" that serve wounds and cancer? *ScientificWorldJournal*, Vol.10, pp. 1234-1238.

Dittmer A.; Fuchs A.; Oerlecke I.; Leyh B.; Kaiser S.; Martens J. W. M.; Lützkendorf J.; Müller L. & Dittmer J. (2011). Mesenchymal stem cells and carincoma-associated fibroblasts sensitize breast cancer cells in 3D cultures to kinase inhibitors. *Int. J. Oncol.* Vol.39, No.3, pp. 689-696.

do Amaral J. B.; Urabayashi M. S. & Machado-Santelli G. M. (2010). Cell death and lumen formation in spheroids of MCF-7 cells. *Cell Biol Int*, Vol.34, No.3, pp. 267-274.

Dominici M.; Le Blanc K.; Mueller I.; Slaper-Cortenbach I.; Marini F.; Krause D.; Deans R.; Keating A.; Prockop D. & Horwitz E. (2006). Minimal criteria for defining multipotent mesenchymal stromal cells. The International Society for Cellular Therapy position statement. *Cytotherapy*, Vol.8, No.4, pp. 315-317.

Dontu G.; Abdallah W. M.; Foley J. M.; Jackson K. W.; Clarke M. F.; Kawamura M. J. & Wicha M. S. (2003). In vitro propagation and transcriptional profiling of human mammary stem/progenitor cells. *Genes Dev*, Vol.17, No.10, pp. 1253-12570.

Dvorak H. F. (1986). Tumors: wounds that do not heal. Similarities between tumor stroma generation and wound healing. *N Engl J Med*, Vol.315, No.26, pp. 1650-1659.

Dwyer R. M.; Potter-Beirne S. M.; Harrington K. A.; Lowery A. J.; Hennessy E.; Murphy J. M.; Barry F. P.; O'Brien T. & Kerin M. J. (2007). Monocyte chemotactic protein-1 secreted by primary breast tumors stimulates migration of mesenchymal stem cells. *Clin Cancer Res*, Vol.13, No.17, pp. 5020-5027.

Ehninger A. & Trumpp A. (2011). The bone marrow stem cell niche grows up: mesenchymal stem cells and macrophages move in. *J Exp Med*, Vol.208, No.3, pp. 421-428.

Fierro F. A.; Sierralta W. D.; Epunan M. J. & Minguell J. J. (2004). Marrow-derived mesenchymal stem cells: role in epithelial tumor cell determination. *Clin Exp Metastasis*, Vol.21, No.4, pp. 313-319.

Fillmore C. & Kuperwasser C. (2007). Human breast cancer stem cell markers CD44 and CD24: enriching for cells with functional properties in mice or in man? *Breast Cancer Res*, Vol.9, No.3, pp. 303.

Friedenstein A. & Kuralesova A. I. (1971). Osteogenic precursor cells of bone marrow in radiation chimeras. *Transplantation*, Vol.12, No.2, pp. 99-108.

Friedenstein A. J.; Chailakhyan R. K.; Latsinik N. V.; Panasyuk A. F. & Keiliss-Borok I. V. (1974). Stromal cells responsible for transferring the microenvironment of the hemopoietic tissues. Cloning in vitro and retransplantation in vivo. *Transplantation*, Vol.17, No.4, pp. 331-340.

Friedenstein A. J.; Piatetzky S., II & Petrakova K. V. (1966). Osteogenesis in transplants of bone marrow cells. *J Embryol Exp Morphol*, Vol.16, No.3, pp. 381-390.

Ginestier C.; Hur M. H.; Charafe-Jauffret E.; Monville F.; Dutcher J.; Brown M.; Jacquemier J.; Viens P.; Kleer C. G.; Liu S.; Schott A.; Hayes D.; Birnbaum D.; Wicha M. S. & Dontu G. (2007). ALDH1 is a marker of normal and malignant human mammary stem cells and a predictor of poor clinical outcome. *Cell Stem Cell*, Vol.1, No.5, pp. 555-567.

Gjerstorff M.; Burns J. S.; Nielsen O.; Kassem M. & Ditzel H. (2009). Epigenetic modulation of cancer-germline antigen gene expression in tumorigenic human mesenchymal stem cells: implications for cancer therapy. *Am J Pathol*, Vol.175, No.1, pp. 314-323.

Glennie S.; Soeiro I.; Dyson P. J.; Lam E. W. & Dazzi F. (2005). Bone marrow mesenchymal stem cells induce division arrest anergy of activated T cells. *Blood*, Vol.105, No.7, pp. 2821-2827.

Goldstein R. H.; Reagan M. R.; Anderson K.; Kaplan D. L. & Rosenblatt M. (2010). Human bone marrow-derived MSCs can home to orthotopic breast cancer tumors and promote bone metastasis. *Cancer Res*, Vol.70, No.24, pp. 10044-10050.

Grayson W. L.; Zhao F.; Izadpanah R.; Bunnell B. & Ma T. (2006). Effects of hypoxia on human mesenchymal stem cell expansion and plasticity in 3D constructs. *J Cell Physiol*, Vol.207, No.2, pp. 331-339.

Grisendi G.; Bussolari R.; Cafarelli L.; Petak I.; Rasini V.; Veronesi E.; De Santis G.; Spano C.; Tagliazzucchi M.; Barti-Juhasz H.; Scarabelli L.; Bambi F.; Frassoldati A.; Rossi G.; Casali C.; Morandi U.; Horwitz E. M.; Paolucci P.; Conte P. & Dominici M. (2010). Adipose-derived mesenchymal stem cells as stable source of tumor necrosis factor-related apoptosis-inducing ligand delivery for cancer therapy. *Cancer Res*, Vol.70, No.9, pp. 3718-3729.

Herberts C. A.; Kwa M. S. & Hermsen H. P. (2011). Evaluation of risk factors in the development of stem cell therapy. *J Transl Med*, Vol.9, No.1, pp. 29.

Hess D.; Li L.; Martin M.; Sakano S.; Hill D.; Strutt B.; Thyssen S.; Gray D. A. & Bhatia M. (2003). Bone marrow-derived stem cells initiate pancreatic regeneration. *Nat Biotechnol*, Vol.21, No.7, pp. 763-770.

Hombauer H. & Minguell J. J. (2000). Selective interactions between epithelial tumour cells and bone marrow mesenchymal stem cells. *Br J Cancer*, Vol.82, No.7, pp. 1290-1296.

Ishii G.; Sangai T.; Oda T.; Aoyagi Y.; Hasebe T.; Kanomata N.; Endoh Y.; Okumura C.; Okuhara Y.; Magae J.; Emura M.; Ochiya T. & Ochiai A. (2003). Bone-marrow-derived myofibroblasts contribute to the cancer-induced stromal reaction. *Biochem Biophys Res Commun*, Vol.309, No.1, pp. 232-240.

Ito T.; Suzuki A.; Imai E.; Okabe M. & Hori M. (2001). Bone marrow is a reservoir of repopulating mesangial cells during glomerular remodeling. *J Am Soc Nephrol*, Vol.12, No.12, pp. 2625-2635.

Jiang X. X.; Zhang Y.; Liu B.; Zhang S. X.; Wu Y.; Yu X. D. & Mao N. (2005). Human mesenchymal stem cells inhibit differentiation and function of monocyte-derived dendritic cells. *Blood*, Vol.105, No.10, pp. 4120-4126.

Kale S.; Karihaloo A.; Clark P. R.; Kashgarian M.; Krause D. S. & Cantley L. G. (2003). Bone marrow stem cells contribute to repair of the ischemically injured renal tubule. *J Clin Invest*, Vol.112, No.1, pp. 42-49.

Karnoub A. E.; Dash A. B.; Vo A. P.; Sullivan A.; Brooks M. W.; Bell G. W.; Richardson A. L.; Polyak K.; Tubo R. & Weinberg R. A. (2007). Mesenchymal stem cells within tumour stroma promote breast cancer metastasis. *Nature*, Vol.449, No.7162, pp. 557-563.

Kidd S.; Spaeth E.; Dembinski J. L.; Dietrich M.; Watson K.; Klopp A.; Battula V. L.; Weil M.; Andreeff M. & Marini F. C. (2009). Direct evidence of mesenchymal stem cell tropism for tumor and wounding microenvironments using in vivo bioluminescent imaging. *Stem Cells*, Vol.27, No.10, pp. 2614-2623.

Kidd S.; Spaeth E.; Klopp A.; Andreeff M.; Hall B. & Marini F. C. (2008). The (in) auspicious role of mesenchymal stromal cells in cancer: be it friend or foe. *Cytotherapy*, Vol.10, No.7, pp. 657-667.

Kim S. M.; Kim D. S.; Jeong C. H.; Kim D. H.; Kim J. H.; Jeon H. B.; Kwon S. J.; Jeun S. S.; Yang Y. S.; Oh W. & Chang J. W. (2011). CXC chemokine receptor 1 enhances the ability of human umbilical cord blood-derived mesenchymal stem cells to migrate toward gliomas. *Biochem Biophys Res Commun*, Vol.407, No.4, pp. 741-746.

Klopp A. H.; Gupta A.; Spaeth E.; Andreeff M. & Marini F., 3rd (2011). Dissecting a discrepancy in the literature: do mesenchymal stem cells support or suppress tumor growth? *Stem Cells*, Vol.29, No.1, pp. 11-19.

Klopp A. H.; Lacerda L.; Gupta A.; Debeb B. G.; Solley T.; Li L.; Spaeth E.; Xu W.; Zhang X.; Lewis M. T.; Reuben J. M.; Krishnamurthy S.; Ferrari M.; Gaspar R.; Buchholz T. A.; Cristofanilli M.; Marini F.; Andreeff M. & Woodward W. A. (2010). Mesenchymal stem cells promote mammosphere formation and decrease E-cadherin in normal and malignant breast cells. *PLoS One*, Vol.5, No.8, pp. e12180.

Klopp A. H.; Spaeth E. L.; Dembinski J. L.; Woodward W. A.; Munshi A.; Meyn R. E.; Cox J. D.; Andreeff M. & Marini F. C. (2007). Tumor irradiation increases the recruitment of circulating mesenchymal stem cells into the tumor microenvironment. *Cancer Res*, Vol.67, No.24, pp. 11687-11695.

Krabbe C.; Zimmer J. & Meyer M. (2005). Neural transdifferentiation of mesenchymal stem cells--a critical review. *Apmis*, Vol.113, No.11-12, pp. 831-844.

Krampera M.; Glennie S.; Dyson J.; Scott D.; Laylor R.; Simpson E. & Dazzi F. (2003). Bone marrow mesenchymal stem cells inhibit the response of naive and memory antigen-specific T cells to their cognate peptide. *Blood*, Vol.101, No.9, pp. 3722-3729.

Krinner A.; Hoffmann M.; Loeffler M.; Drasdo D. & Galle J. (2010). Individual fates of mesenchymal stem cells in vitro. *BMC Syst Biol*, Vol.4, pp. 73.

Kucerova L.; Matuskova M.; Pastorakova A.; Tyciakova S.; Jakubikova J.; Bohovic R.; Altanerova V. & Altaner C. (2008). Cytosine deaminase expressing human mesenchymal stem cells mediated tumour regression in melanoma bearing mice. *J Gene Med*, Vol.10, No.10, pp. 1071-1082.

Kurozumi K.; Nakamura K.; Tamiya T.; Kawano Y.; Kobune M.; Hirai S.; Uchida H.; Sasaki K.; Ito Y.; Kato K.; Honmou O.; Houkin K.; Date I. & Hamada H. (2004). BDNF gene-modified mesenchymal stem cells promote functional recovery and reduce infarct size in the rat middle cerebral artery occlusion model. *Mol Ther*, Vol.9, No.2, pp. 189-197.

Lee R. H.; Seo M. J.; Reger R. L.; Spees J. L.; Pulin A. A.; Olson S. D. & Prockop D. J. (2006). Multipotent stromal cells from human marrow home to and promote repair of pancreatic islets and renal glomeruli in diabetic NOD/scid mice. *Proc Natl Acad Sci U S A*, Vol.103, No.46, pp. 17438-17443.

Leung C. T. & Brugge J. S. (2009). Tumor self-seeding: bidirectional flow of tumor cells. *Cell*, Vol.139, No.7, pp. 1226-1228.

Li G. R.; Sun H.; Deng X. & Lau C. P. (2005). Characterization of ionic currents in human mesenchymal stem cells from bone marrow. *Stem Cells,* Vol.23, No.3, pp. 371-382.

Li N.; Yang R.; Zhang W.; Dorfman H.; Rao P. & Gorlick R. (2009). Genetically transforming human mesenchymal stem cells to sarcomas: changes in cellular phenotype and multilineage differentiation potential. *Cancer,* Vol.115, No.20, pp. 4795-4806.

Lin F.; Cordes K.; Li L.; Hood L.; Couser W. G.; Shankland S. J. & Igarashi P. (2003). Hematopoietic stem cells contribute to the regeneration of renal tubules after renal ischemia-reperfusion injury in mice. *J Am Soc Nephrol,* Vol.14, No.5, pp. 1188-1199.

Lin P. P.; Wang Y. & Lozano G. (2011). Mesenchymal Stem Cells and the Origin of Ewing's Sarcoma. *Sarcoma.,* Vol.407, No.4, pp. 741-746.

Lin S. Y.; Yang J.; Everett A. D.; Clevenger C. V.; Koneru M.; Mishra P. J.; Kamen B.; Banerjee D. & Glod J. (2008). The isolation of novel mesenchymal stromal cell chemotactic factors from the conditioned medium of tumor cells. *Exp Cell Res,* Vol.314, No.17, pp. 3107-3117.

Ling X.; Marini F.; Konopleva M.; Schober W.; Shi Y.; Burks J.; Clise-Dwyer K.; Wang R. Y.; Zhang W.; Yuan X.; Lu H.; Caldwell L. & Andreeff M. (2010). Mesenchymal Stem Cells Overexpressing IFN-beta Inhibit Breast Cancer Growth and Metastases through Stat3 Signaling in a Syngeneic Tumor Model. *Cancer Microenviron,* Vol.3, No.1, pp. 83-95.

Liu S.; Ginestier C.; Ou S. J.; Clouthier S. G.; Patel S. H.; Monville F.; Korkaya H.; Heath A.; Dutcher J.; Kleer C. G.; Jung Y.; Dontu G.; Taichman R. & Wicha M. S. (2011). Breast cancer stem cells are regulated by mesenchymal stem cells through cytokine networks. *Cancer Res,* Vol.71, No.2, pp. 614-624.

Liu S. & Wicha M. S. (2010). Targeting breast cancer stem cells. *J Clin Oncol,* Vol.28, No.25, pp. 4006-4012.

Locke M.; Feisst V. & Dunbar P. R. (2011). Concise review: human adipose-derived stem cells: separating promise from clinical need. *Stem Cells,* Vol.29, No.3, pp. 404-411.

Loebinger M. R.; Eddaoudi A.; Davies D. & Janes S. M. (2009). Mesenchymal stem cell delivery of TRAIL can eliminate metastatic cancer. *Cancer Res,* Vol.69, No.10, pp. 4134-4142.

Lu Y.; Cai Z.; Galson D. L.; Xiao G.; Liu Y.; George D. E.; Melhem M. F.; Yao Z. & Zhang J. (2006). Monocyte chemotactic protein-1 (MCP-1) acts as a paracrine and autocrine factor for prostate cancer growth and invasion. *Prostate,* Vol.66, No.12, pp. 1311-1318.

Mahmood A.; Lu D.; Lu M. & Chopp M. (2003). Treatment of traumatic brain injury in adult rats with intravenous administration of human bone marrow stromal cells. *Neurosurgery,* Vol.53, No.3, pp. 697-702.

Manabe Y.; Toda S.; Miyazaki K. & Sugihara H. (2003). Mature adipocytes, but not preadipocytes, promote the growth of breast carcinoma cells in collagen gel matrix culture through cancer-stromal cell interactions. *J Pathol,* Vol.201, No.2, pp. 221-228.

Mani S. A.; Guo W.; Liao M. J.; Eaton E. N.; Ayyanan A.; Zhou A. Y.; Brooks M.; Reinhard F.; Zhang C. C.; Shipitsin M.; Campbell L. L.; Polyak K.; Brisken C.; Yang J. & Weinberg R. A. (2008). The epithelial-mesenchymal transition generates cells with properties of stem cells. *Cell,* Vol.133, No.4, pp. 704-715.

Marchini C.; Montani M.; Konstantinidou G.; Orru R.; Mannucci S.; Ramadori G.; Gabrielli F.; Baruzzi A.; Berton G.; Merigo F.; Fin S.; Iezzi M.; Bisaro B.; Sbarbati A.; Zerani M.; Galie M. & Amici A. (2010). Mesenchymal/stromal gene expression signature relates to basal-like breast cancers, identifies bone metastasis and predicts resistance to therapies. *PLoS One*, Vol.5, No.11, pp. e14131.

Martin F. T.; Dwyer R. M.; Kelly J.; Khan S.; Murphy J. M.; Curran C.; Miller N.; Hennessy E.; Dockery P.; Barry F. P.; O'Brien T. & Kerin M. J. (2010). Potential role of mesenchymal stem cells (MSCs) in the breast tumour microenvironment: stimulation of epithelial to mesenchymal transition (EMT). *Breast Cancer Res Treat*, Vol.124, No.2, pp. 317-326.

May C. D.; Sphyris N.; Evans K. W.; Werden S. J.; Guo W. & Mani S. A. (2011). Epithelial-mesenchymal transition and cancer stem cells: a dangerously dynamic duo in breast cancer progression. *Breast Cancer Res*, Vol.13, No.1, pp. 202.

Medici D.; Shore E. M.; Lounev V. Y.; Kaplan F. S.; Kalluri R. & Olsen B. R. (2010). Conversion of vascular endothelial cells into multipotent stem-like cells. *Nat Med*, Vol.16, No.12, pp. 1400-1406.

Mei S. H.; Haitsma J. J.; Dos Santos C. C.; Deng Y.; Lai P. F.; Slutsky A. S.; Liles W. C. & Stewart D. J. (2010). Mesenchymal stem cells reduce inflammation while enhancing bacterial clearance and improving survival in sepsis. *Am J Respir Crit Care Med*, Vol.182, No.8, pp. 1047-1057.

Mendez-Ferrer S.; Michurina T. V.; Ferraro F.; Mazloom A. R.; Macarthur B. D.; Lira S. A.; Scadden D. T.; Ma'ayan A.; Enikolopov G. N. & Frenette P. S. (2010). Mesenchymal and haematopoietic stem cells form a unique bone marrow niche. *Nature*, Vol.466, No.7308, pp. 829-834.

Menon L. G.; Kelly K.; Yang H. W.; Kim S. K.; Black P. M. & Carroll R. S. (2009). Human bone marrow-derived mesenchymal stromal cells expressing S-TRAIL as a cellular delivery vehicle for human glioma therapy. *Stem Cells*, Vol.27, No.9, pp. 2320-2330.

Menon L. G.; Picinich S.; Koneru R.; Gao H.; Lin S. Y.; Koneru M.; Mayer-Kuckuk P.; Glod J. & Banerjee D. (2007). Differential gene expression associated with migration of mesenchymal stem cells to conditioned medium from tumor cells or bone marrow cells. *Stem Cells*, Vol.25, No.2, pp. 520-528.

Mi Z.; Bhattacharya S. D.; Kim V.; Guo H.; Talbot L. J. & Kuo P. C. (2011). Osteopontin Promotes CCL5-Mesenchymal Stromal Cell Mediated Breast Cancer Metastasis. *Carcinogenesis*, Vol.32, No.4, pp. 477-487.

Mishra P. J. & Banerjee D. (2011). Activation and differentiation of mesenchymal stem cells. *Methods Mol Biol*, Vol.717, pp. 245-253.

Mishra P. J.; Humeniuk R.; Medina D. J.; Alexe G.; Mesirov J. P.; Ganesan S.; Glod J. W. & Banerjee D. (2008). Carcinoma-associated fibroblast-like differentiation of human mesenchymal stem cells. *Cancer Res*, Vol.68, No.11, pp. 4331-4339.

Mohseny A. B. & Hogendoorn P. C. (2011). Concise review: mesenchymal tumors: when stem cells go mad. *Stem Cells*, Vol.29, No.3, pp. 397-403.

Molloy A. P.; Martin F. T.; Dwyer R. M.; Griffin T. P.; Murphy M.; Barry F. P.; O'Brien T. & Kerin M. J. (2009). Mesenchymal stem cell secretion of chemokines during differentiation into osteoblasts, and their potential role in mediating interactions with breast cancer cells. *Int J Cancer*, Vol.124, No.2, pp. 326-332.

Monneret G. (2009). Mesenchymal stem cells: another anti-inflammatory treatment for sepsis? *Nat Med*, Vol.15, No.6, pp. 601-602.

Motaln H.; Schichor C. & Lah T. T. (2010). Human mesenchymal stem cells and their use in cell-based therapies. *Cancer*, Vol.116, No.11, pp. 2519-2530.

Mueller M. M. & Fusenig N. E. (2004). Friends or foes - bipolar effects of the tumour stroma in cancer. *Nat Rev Cancer*, Vol.4, No.11, pp. 839-849.

Natsu K.; Ochi M.; Mochizuki Y.; Hachisuka H.; Yanada S. & Yasunaga Y. (2004). Allogeneic bone marrow-derived mesenchymal stromal cells promote the regeneration of injured skeletal muscle without differentiation into myofibers. *Tissue Eng*, Vol.10, No.7-8, pp. 1093-1112.

Noth U.; Osyczka A. M.; Tuli R.; Hickok N. J.; Danielson K. G. & Tuan R. S. (2002). Multilineage mesenchymal differentiation potential of human trabecular bone-derived cells. *J Orthop Res*, Vol.20, No.5, pp. 1060-1069.

Olumi A. F.; Grossfeld G. D.; Hayward S. W.; Carroll P. R.; Tlsty T. D. & Cunha G. R. (1999). Carcinoma-associated fibroblasts direct tumor progression of initiated human prostatic epithelium. *Cancer Res*, Vol.59, No.19, pp. 5002-5011.

Omatsu Y.; Sugiyama T.; Kohara H.; Kondoh G.; Fujii N.; Kohno K. & Nagasawa T. (2010). The essential functions of adipo-osteogenic progenitors as the hematopoietic stem and progenitor cell niche. *Immunity.*, Vol.33, No.3, pp. 387-399.

Onder T. T.; Gupta P. B.; Mani S. A.; Yang J.; Lander E. S. & Weinberg R. A. (2008). Loss of E-cadherin promotes metastasis via multiple downstream transcriptional pathways. *Cancer Res*, Vol.68, No.10, pp. 3645-3654.

Orimo A.; Gupta P. B.; Sgroi D. C.; Arenzana-Seisdedos F.; Delaunay T.; Naeem R.; Carey V. J.; Richardson A. L. & Weinberg R. A. (2005). Stromal fibroblasts present in invasive human breast carcinomas promote tumor growth and angiogenesis through elevated SDF-1/CXCL12 secretion. *Cell*, Vol.121, No.3, pp. 335-348.

Ortiz L. A.; Gambelli F.; McBride C.; Gaupp D.; Baddoo M.; Kaminski N. & Phinney D. G. (2003). Mesenchymal stem cell engraftment in lung is enhanced in response to bleomycin exposure and ameliorates its fibrotic effects. *Proc Natl Acad Sci U S A*, Vol.100, No.14, pp. 8407-8411.

Pantel K.; Alix-Panabieres C. & Riethdorf S. (2009). Cancer micrometastases. *Nat Rev Clin Oncol*, Vol.6, No.6, pp. 339-351.

Parekkadan B.; van Poll D.; Suganuma K.; Carter E. A.; Berthiaume F.; Tilles A. W. & Yarmush M. L. (2007). Mesenchymal stem cell-derived molecules reverse fulminant hepatic failure. *PLoS One*, Vol.2, No.9, pp. e941.

Park K. S.; Jung K. H.; Kim S. H.; Kim K. S.; Choi M. R.; Kim Y. & Chai Y. G. (2007). Functional expression of ion channels in mesenchymal stem cells derived from umbilical cord vein. *Stem Cells*, Vol.25, No.8, pp. 2044-2052.

Patel S. A.; Heinrich A. C.; Reddy B. Y.; Srinivas B.; Heidaran N. & Rameshwar P. (2008). Breast cancer biology: the multifaceted roles of mesenchymal stem cells. *J Oncol*, Vol.2008, pp. 425895.

Patel S. A.; Meyer J. R.; Greco S. J.; Corcoran K. E.; Bryan M. & Rameshwar P. (2010). Mesenchymal stem cells protect breast cancer cells through regulatory T cells: role of mesenchymal stem cell-derived TGF-beta. *J Immunol*, Vol.184, No.10, pp. 5885-5894.

Patki S.; Kadam S.; Chandra V. & Bhonde R. (2010). Human breast milk is a rich source of multipotent mesenchymal stem cells. *Hum Cell*, Vol.23, No.2, pp. 35-40.

Phinney D. G. (2002). Building a consensus regarding the nature and origin of mesenchymal stem cells. *J Cell Biochem Suppl*, Vol.38, pp. 7-12.

Pinzone J. J.; Hall B. M.; Thudi N. K.; Vonau M.; Qiang Y. W.; Rosol T. J. & Shaughnessy J. D., Jr. (2009). The role of Dickkopf-1 in bone development, homeostasis, and disease. *Blood*, Vol.113, No.3, pp. 517-525.

Pittenger M. F.; Mackay A. M.; Beck S. C.; Jaiswal R. K.; Douglas R.; Mosca J. D.; Moorman M. A.; Simonetti D. W.; Craig S. & Marshak D. R. (1999). Multilineage potential of adult human mesenchymal stem cells. *Science*, Vol.284, No.5411, pp. 143-147.

Ponte A. L.; Marais E.; Gallay N.; Langonne A.; Delorme B.; Herault O.; Charbord P. & Domenech J. (2007). The in vitro migration capacity of human bone marrow mesenchymal stem cells: comparison of chemokine and growth factor chemotactic activities. *Stem Cells*, Vol.25, No.7, pp. 1737-1745.

Prockop D. J. & Olson S. D. (2007). Clinical trials with adult stem/progenitor cells for tissue repair: let's not overlook some essential precautions. *Blood*, Vol.109, No.8, pp. 3147-3151.

Pulukuri S. M.; Gorantla B.; Dasari V. R.; Gondi C. S. & Rao J. S. (2010). Epigenetic upregulation of urokinase plasminogen activator promotes the tropism of mesenchymal stem cells for tumor cells. *Mol Cancer Res*, Vol.8, No.8, pp. 1074-1083.

Qiao L.; Xu Z. L.; Zhao T. J.; Ye L. H. & Zhang X. D. (2008a). Dkk-1 secreted by mesenchymal stem cells inhibits growth of breast cancer cells via depression of Wnt signalling. *Cancer Lett*, Vol.269, No.1, pp. 67-77.

Qiao L.; Zhao T. J.; Wang F. Z.; Shan C. L.; Ye L. H. & Zhang X. D. (2008b). NF-kappaB downregulation may be involved the depression of tumor cell proliferation mediated by human mesenchymal stem cells. *Acta Pharmacol Sin*, Vol.29, No.3, pp. 333-340.

Raffaghello L.; Bianchi G.; Bertolotto M.; Montecucco F.; Busca A.; Dallegri F.; Ottonello L. & Pistoia V. (2008). Human mesenchymal stem cells inhibit neutrophil apoptosis: a model for neutrophil preservation in the bone marrow niche. *Stem Cells*, Vol.26, No.1, pp. 151-162.

Ramasamy R.; Fazekasova H.; Lam E. W.; Soeiro I.; Lombardi G. & Dazzi F. (2007). Mesenchymal stem cells inhibit dendritic cell differentiation and function by preventing entry into the cell cycle. *Transplantation*, Vol.83, No.1, pp. 71-76.

Rasmusson I. (2006). Immune modulation by mesenchymal stem cells. *Exp Cell Res*, Vol.312, No.12, pp. 2169-2179.

Rasmusson I.; Ringden O.; Sundberg B. & Le Blanc K. (2003). Mesenchymal stem cells inhibit the formation of cytotoxic T lymphocytes, but not activated cytotoxic T lymphocytes or natural killer cells. *Transplantation*, Vol.76, No.8, pp. 1208-1213.

Rasmusson I.; Ringden O.; Sundberg B. & Le Blanc K. (2005). Mesenchymal stem cells inhibit lymphocyte proliferation by mitogens and alloantigens by different mechanisms. *Exp Cell Res*, Vol.305, No.1, pp. 33-41.

Rattigan Y.; Hsu J. M.; Mishra P. J.; Glod J. & Banerjee D. (2010). Interleukin 6 mediated recruitment of mesenchymal stem cells to the hypoxic tumor milieu. *Exp Cell Res*, Vol.316, No.20, pp. 3417-3424.

Rhodes L. V.; Antoon J. W.; Muir S. E.; Elliott S.; Beckman B. S. & Burow M. E. (2010). Effects of human mesenchymal stem cells on ER-positive human breast carcinoma cells mediated through ER-SDF-1/CXCR4 crosstalk. *Mol Cancer*, Vol.9, pp. 295.

Rhodes L. V.; Muir S. E.; Elliott S.; Guillot L. M.; Antoon J. W.; Penfornis P.; Tilghman S. L.; Salvo V. A.; Fonseca J. P.; Lacey M. R.; Beckman B. S.; McLachlan J. A.; Rowan B. G.; Pochampally R. & Burow M. E. (2009). Adult human mesenchymal stem cells enhance breast tumorigenesis and promote hormone independence. *Breast Cancer Res Treat*, Vol.121, No.2, pp. 293-300.

Riggi N.; Suva M. L.; Suva D.; Cironi L.; Provero P.; Tercier S.; Joseph J. M.; Stehle J. C.; Baumer K.; Kindler V. & Stamenkovic I. (2008). EWS-FLI-1 expression triggers a Ewing's sarcoma initiation program in primary human mesenchymal stem cells. *Cancer Res*, Vol.68, No.7, pp. 2176-2185.

Ritter E.; Perry A.; Yu J.; Wang T.; Tang L. & Bieberich E. (2008). Breast cancer cell-derived fibroblast growth factor 2 and vascular endothelial growth factor are chemoattractants for bone marrow stromal stem cells. *Ann Surg*, Vol.247, No.2, pp. 310-314.

Rojas M.; Xu J.; Woods C. R.; Mora A. L.; Spears W.; Roman J. & Brigham K. L. (2005). Bone marrow-derived mesenchymal stem cells in repair of the injured lung. *Am J Respir Cell Mol Biol*, Vol.33, No.2, pp. 145-152.

Romieu-Mourez R.; Francois M.; Abate A.; Boivin M. N.; Birman E.; Bailey D.; Bramson J. L.; Forner K.; Young Y. K.; Medin J. A. & Galipeau J. (2010). Mesenchymal stromal cells expressing ErbB-2/neu elicit protective antibreast tumor immunity in vivo, which is paradoxically suppressed by IFN-gamma and tumor necrosis factor-alpha priming. *Cancer Res*, Vol.70, No.20, pp. 7742-7747.

Rosland G. V.; Svendsen A.; Torsvik A.; Sobala E.; McCormack E.; Immervoll H.; Mysliwietz J.; Tonn J. C.; Goldbrunner R.; Lonning P. E.; Bjerkvig R. & Schichor C. (2009). Long-term cultures of bone marrow-derived human mesenchymal stem cells frequently undergo spontaneous malignant transformation. *Cancer Res*, Vol.69, No.13, pp. 5331-5339.

Ryniers F.; Stove C.; Goethals M.; Brackenier L.; Noe V.; Bracke M.; Vandekerckhove J.; Mareel M. & Bruyneel E. (2002). Plasmin produces an E-cadherin fragment that stimulates cancer cell invasion. *Biol Chem*, Vol.383, No.1, pp. 159-165.

Sacchetti B.; Funari A.; Michienzi S.; Di Cesare S.; Piersanti S.; Saggio I.; Tagliafico E.; Ferrari S.; Robey P. G.; Riminucci M. & Bianco P. (2007). Self-renewing osteoprogenitors in bone marrow sinusoids can organize a hematopoietic microenvironment. *Cell*, Vol.131, No.2, pp. 324-336.

Sanchez C.; Penfornis P.; Oskowitz A. Z.; Boonjindasup A. G.; Cai D. Z.; Dhule S.; Rowan B. G.; Kelekar A.; Krause D. S. & Pochampally R. R. (2011). Activation of Autophagy in Mesenchymal Stem Cells Provides Tumor Stromal Support. *Carcinogenesis*, Vol.32, No.7, pp. 964-972.

Sasser A. K.; Mundy B. L.; Smith K. M.; Studebaker A. W.; Axel A. E.; Haidet A. M.; Fernandez S. A. & Hall B. M. (2007a). Human bone marrow stromal cells enhance breast cancer cell growth rates in a cell line-dependent manner when evaluated in 3D tumor environments. *Cancer Lett*, Vol.254, No.2, pp. 255-264.

Sasser A. K.; Sullivan N. J.; Studebaker A. W.; Hendey L. F.; Axel A. E. & Hall B. M. (2007b). Interleukin-6 is a potent growth factor for ER-alpha-positive human breast cancer. *Faseb J*, Vol.21, No.13, pp. 3763-3770.

Schor S. L.; Schor A. M. & Rushton G. (1988). Fibroblasts from cancer patients display a mixture of both foetal and adult-like phenotypic characteristics. *J Cell Sci*, Vol.90, No.Pt 3, pp. 401-407.

Seeberger K. L.; Dufour J. M.; Shapiro A. M.; Lakey J. R.; Rajotte R. V. & Korbutt G. S. (2006). Expansion of mesenchymal stem cells from human pancreatic ductal epithelium. *Lab Invest*, Vol.86, No.2, pp. 141-153.

Selmani Z.; Naji A.; Zidi I.; Favier B.; Gaiffe E.; Obert L.; Borg C.; Saas P.; Tiberghien P.; Rouas-Freiss N.; Carosella E. D. & Deschaseaux F. (2008). Human leukocyte antigen-G5 secretion by human mesenchymal stem cells is required to suppress T lymphocyte and natural killer function and to induce CD4+CD25highFOXP3+ regulatory T cells. *Stem Cells*, Vol.26, No.1, pp. 212-222.

Shin S. Y.; Nam J. S.; Lim Y. & Lee Y. H. (2010). TNFalpha-exposed bone marrow-derived mesenchymal stem cells promote locomotion of MDA-MB-231 breast cancer cells through transcriptional activation of CXCR3 ligand chemokines. *J Biol Chem*, Vol.285, No.40, pp. 30731-30740.

Sonabend A. M.; Ulasov I. V.; Tyler M. A.; Rivera A. A.; Mathis J. M. & Lesniak M. S. (2008). Mesenchymal stem cells effectively deliver an oncolytic adenovirus to intracranial glioma. *Stem Cells*, Vol.26, No.3, pp. 831-841.

Sotiropoulou P. A.; Perez S. A.; Gritzapis A. D.; Baxevanis C. N. & Papamichail M. (2006). Interactions between human mesenchymal stem cells and natural killer cells. *Stem Cells*, Vol.24, No.1, pp. 74-85.

Spaeth E. L.; Dembinski J. L.; Sasser A. K.; Watson K.; Klopp A.; Hall B.; Andreeff M. & Marini F. (2009). Mesenchymal stem cell transition to tumor-associated fibroblasts contributes to fibrovascular network expansion and tumor progression. *PLoS One*, Vol.4, No.4, pp. e4992.

Spaggiari G. M.; Capobianco A.; Abdelrazik H.; Becchetti F.; Mingari M. C. & Moretta L. (2008). Mesenchymal stem cells inhibit natural killer-cell proliferation, cytotoxicity, and cytokine production: role of indoleamine 2,3-dioxygenase and prostaglandin E2. *Blood*, Vol.111, No.3, pp. 1327-1333.

Stoff-Khalili M. A.; Rivera A. A.; Mathis J. M.; Banerjee N. S.; Moon A. S.; Hess A.; Rocconi R. P.; Numnum T. M.; Everts M.; Chow L. T.; Douglas J. T.; Siegal G. P.; Zhu Z. B.; Bender H. G.; Dall P.; Stoff A.; Pereboeva L. & Curiel D. T. (2007). Mesenchymal stem cells as a vehicle for targeted delivery of CRAds to lung metastases of breast carcinoma. *Breast Cancer Res Treat*, Vol.105, No.2, pp. 157-167.

Studeny M.; Marini F. C.; Dembinski J. L.; Zompetta C.; Cabreira-Hansen M.; Bekele B. N.; Champlin R. E. & Andreeff M. (2004). Mesenchymal stem cells: potential precursors for tumor stroma and targeted-delivery vehicles for anticancer agents. *J Natl Cancer Inst*, Vol.96, No.21, pp. 1593-1603.

Sun B.; Roh K. H.; Park J. R.; Lee S. R.; Park S. B.; Jung J. W.; Kang S. K.; Lee Y. S. & Kang K. S. (2009). Therapeutic potential of mesenchymal stromal cells in a mouse breast cancer metastasis model. *Cytotherapy*, Vol.11, No.3, pp. 289-298.

Sun B.; Yu K. R.; Bhandari D. R.; Jung J. W.; Kang S. K. & Kang K. S. (2010). Human umbilical cord blood mesenchymal stem cell-derived extracellular matrix prohibits metastatic cancer cell MDA-MB-231 proliferation. *Cancer Lett*, Vol.296, No.2, pp. 178-185.

Theillet C. (2010). What do we learn from HER2-positive breast cancer genomic profiles? *Breast*, Vol.12, No.3, pp. 107.

Tlsty T. D. & Coussens L. M. (2006). Tumor stroma and regulation of cancer development. *Annu Rev Pathol*, Vol.1, pp. 119-150.

Tocci A. & Forte L. (2003). Mesenchymal stem cell: use and perspectives. *Hematol J*, Vol.4, No.2, pp. 92-96.

Toma C.; Pittenger M. F.; Cahill K. S.; Byrne B. J. & Kessler P. D. (2002). Human mesenchymal stem cells differentiate to a cardiomyocyte phenotype in the adult murine heart. *Circulation*, Vol.105, No.1, pp. 93-98.

Tondreau T.; Lagneaux L.; Dejeneffe M.; Massy M.; Mortier C.; Delforge A. & Bron D. (2004). Bone marrow-derived mesenchymal stem cells already express specific neural proteins before any differentiation. *Differentiation*, Vol.72, No.7, pp. 319-326.

Uccelli A.; Moretta L. & Pistoia V. (2008). Mesenchymal stem cells in health and disease. *Nat Rev Immunol*, Vol.8, No.9, pp. 726-736.

Visvader J. E. & Lindeman G. J. (2008). Cancer stem cells in solid tumours: accumulating evidence and unresolved questions. *Nat Rev Cancer*, Vol.8, No.10, pp. 755-768.

Walczak H.; Miller R. E.; Ariail K.; Gliniak B.; Griffith T. S.; Kubin M.; Chin W.; Jones J.; Woodward A.; Le T.; Smith C.; Smolak P.; Goodwin R. G.; Rauch C. T.; Schuh J. C. & Lynch D. H. (1999). Tumoricidal activity of tumor necrosis factor-related apoptosis-inducing ligand in vivo. *Nat Med*, Vol.5, No.2, pp. 157-163.

Wang J. S.; Shum-Tim D.; Chedrawy E. & Chiu R. C. (2001). The coronary delivery of marrow stromal cells for myocardial regeneration: pathophysiologic and therapeutic implications. *J Thorac Cardiovasc Surg.*, Vol.122, No.4, pp. 699-705.

Wang L.; Li Y.; Chen J.; Gautam S. C.; Zhang Z.; Lu M. & Chopp M. (2002). Ischemic cerebral tissue and MCP-1 enhance rat bone marrow stromal cell migration in interface culture. *Exp Hematol*, Vol.30, No.7, pp. 831-836.

Wexler S. A.; Donaldson C.; Denning-Kendall P.; Rice C.; Bradley B. & Hows J. M. (2003). Adult bone marrow is a rich source of human mesenchymal 'stem' cells but umbilical cord and mobilized adult blood are not. *Br J Haematol*, Vol.121, No.2, pp. 368-374.

Willis L.; Alarcon T.; Elia G.; Jones J. L.; Wright N. A.; Tomlinson I. P.; Graham T. A. & Page K. M. (2010). Breast cancer dormancy can be maintained by small numbers of micrometastases. *Cancer Res*, Vol.70, No.11, pp. 4310-4307.

Wislet-Gendebien S.; Hans G.; Leprince P.; Rigo J. M.; Moonen G. & Rogister B. (2005). Plasticity of cultured mesenchymal stem cells: switch from nestin-positive to excitable neuron-like phenotype. *Stem Cells*, Vol.23, No.3, pp. 392-402.

Xu J.; Lu Y.; Ding F.; Zhan X.; Zhu M. & Wang Z. (2007). Reversal of diabetes in mice by intrahepatic injection of bone-derived GFP-murine mesenchymal stem cells infected with the recombinant retrovirus-carrying human insulin gene. *World J Surg*, Vol.31, No.9, pp. 1872-1882.

Yagi H.; Soto-Gutierrez A.; Parekkadan B.; Kitagawa Y.; Tompkins R. G.; Kobayashi N. & Yarmush M. L. (2010). Mesenchymal stem cells: Mechanisms of immunomodulation and homing. *Cell Transplant,* Vol.19, No.6, pp. 667-679.

Yang B.; Wu X.; Mao Y.; Bao W.; Gao L.; Zhou P.; Xie R.; Zhou L. & Zhu J. (2009). Dual-targeted antitumor effects against brainstem glioma by intravenous delivery of tumor necrosis factor-related, apoptosis-inducing, ligand-engineered human mesenchymal stem cells. *Neurosurgery,* Vol.65, No.3, pp. 610-624.

Yen B. L. & Yen M.-L.-. (2008). Mesenchymal Stem Cells and Cancer - for Better or for Worse? *J Cancer Molecules,* Vol.4, No.1, pp. 5-8.

You M. H.; Kim W. J.; Shim W.; Lee S. R.; Lee G.; Choi S.; Kim D. Y.; Kim Y. M.; Kim H. & Han S. U. (2009). Cytosine deaminase-producing human mesenchymal stem cells mediate an antitumor effect in a mouse xenograft model. *J Gastroenterol Hepatol,* Vol.24, No.8, pp. 1393-1400.

Zhao M.; Dumur C. I.; Holt S. E.; Beckman M. J. & Elmore L. W. (2010). Multipotent adipose stromal cells and breast cancer development: Think globally, act locally. *Mol Carinogenesis,* Vol.49, No.11, pp. 923-937.

Zielske S. P.; Livant D. L. & Lawrence T. S. (2009). Radiation increases invasion of gene-modified mesenchymal stem cells into tumors. *Int J Radiat Oncol Biol Phys,* Vol.75, No.3, pp. 843-853.

Zuk P. A.; Zhu M.; Ashjian P.; De Ugarte D. A.; Huang J. I.; Mizuno H.; Alfonso Z. C.; Fraser J. K.; Benhaim P. & Hedrick M. H. (2002). Human adipose tissue is a source of multipotent stem cells. *Mol Biol Cell,* Vol.13, No.12, pp. 4279-4295.

Permissions

The contributors of this book come from diverse backgrounds, making this book a truly international effort. This book will bring forth new frontiers with its revolutionizing research information and detailed analysis of the nascent developments around the world.

We would like to thank Prof. Dr. Mehmet Gunduz, for lending his expertise to make the book truly unique. He has played a crucial role in the development of this book. Without his invaluable contribution this book wouldn't have been possible. He has made vital efforts to compile up to date information on the varied aspects of this subject to make this book a valuable addition to the collection of many professionals and students.

This book was conceptualized with the vision of imparting up-to-date information and advanced data in this field. To ensure the same, a matchless editorial board was set up. Every individual on the board went through rigorous rounds of assessment to prove their worth. After which they invested a large part of their time researching and compiling the most relevant data for our readers. Conferences and sessions were held from time to time between the editorial board and the contributing authors to present the data in the most comprehensible form. The editorial team has worked tirelessly to provide valuable and valid information to help people across the globe.

Every chapter published in this book has been scrutinized by our experts. Their significance has been extensively debated. The topics covered herein carry significant findings which will fuel the growth of the discipline. They may even be implemented as practical applications or may be referred to as a beginning point for another development. Chapters in this book were first published by InTech; hereby published with permission under the Creative Commons Attribution License or equivalent.

The editorial board has been involved in producing this book since its inception. They have spent rigorous hours researching and exploring the diverse topics which have resulted in the successful publishing of this book. They have passed on their knowledge of decades through this book. To expedite this challenging task, the publisher supported the team at every step. A small team of assistant editors was also appointed to further simplify the editing procedure and attain best results for the readers.

Our editorial team has been hand-picked from every corner of the world. Their multi-ethnicity adds dynamic inputs to the discussions which result in innovative outcomes. These outcomes are then further discussed with the researchers and contributors who give their valuable feedback and opinion regarding the same. The feedback is then collaborated with the researches and they are edited in a comprehensive manner to aid the understanding of the subject.

Apart from the editorial board, the designing team has also invested a significant amount of their time in understanding the subject and creating the most relevant covers. They scrutinized every image to scout for the most suitable representation of the subject and create an appropriate cover for the book.

The publishing team has been involved in this book since its early stages. They were actively engaged in every process, be it collecting the data, connecting with the contributors or procuring relevant information. The team has been an ardent support to the editorial, designing and production team. Their endless efforts to recruit the best for this project, has resulted in the accomplishment of this book. They are a veteran in the field of academics and their pool of knowledge is as vast as their experience in printing. Their expertise and guidance has proved useful at every step. Their uncompromising quality standards have made this book an exceptional effort. Their encouragement from time to time has been an inspiration for everyone.

The publisher and the editorial board hope that this book will prove to be a valuable piece of knowledge for researchers, students, practitioners and scholars across the globe.

List of Contributors

Judith C. Keen
University of Medicine and Dentistry of New Jersey, USA

Tania Benatar, Yutaka Amemiya, Wenyi Yang and Arun Seth
Division of Molecular and Cellular Biology, Sunnybrook Research Institute, Department of Anatomic Pathology, Sunnybrook Health Sciences Centre, Department of Laboratory Medicine and Pathobiology, University of Toronto, ON, Canada

Emilie Bana and Denyse Bagrel
Université Paul Verlaine – Metz Laboratoire d'Ingénierie Moléculaire ET Biochimie Pharmacologique, France

Siddik Sarkar and Mahitosh Mandal
School of Medical Science and Technology, Indian Institute of Technology Kharagpur Kharagpur, West Bengal, India

Seyed Nasser Ostad and Maliheh Parsa
Faculty of Pharmacy, Tehran University of Medical Sciences, Tehran, Iran

Farshad H. Shirazi
Department of Pharmaco-Toxicology, SBMU Pharmacy School, Tehran, Iran
SBMU Pharmaceutical Research Center, Tehran, Iran

E.A. García-Zepeda
CBRL, México
Departamento de Inmunología, Instituto de Investigaciones Biomédicas, Universidad Nacional Autónoma de México, México

J. Valdivia-Silva
Life Science & Astrobiology Division, NASA Ames Research Center, Moffett Field, CA, USA

J. Franco-Barraza and E. Cukierman
Cancer Biology Program, Fox Chase Cancer Center, Philadelphia, PA, USA

Patricia J. Simpson-Haidaris
Department of Medicine, University of Rochester School of Medicine and Dentistry, USA

Brian J. Rybarczyk
Department of Biology, University of North Carolina at Chapel Hill, USA

Abha Sahni
Aab Cardiovascular Research Institute, University of Rochester School of Medicine and Dentistry, USA

Nicholas J. Sullivan
The Ohio State University, Columbus, Ohio, USA

Caitlin Ward and Patrick G. Telmer
London Regional Cancer Program, London Health Sciences Center, Victoria Hospital, London ON, Canada

Catalina Vasquez
London Regional Cancer Program, London Health Sciences Center, Victoria Hospital, London ON, Canada
Dept. of Medical Biophysics University of Western Ontario, Canada

Cornelia Tolg
London Regional Cancer Program, London Health Sciences Center, Victoria Hospital, London ON, Canada
The Hospital for Sick Children, Toronto ON, Canada

Eva Turley
London Regional Cancer Program, London Health Sciences Center, Victoria Hospital, London ON, Canada
Dept. of Oncology, University of Western Ontario, London ON, Canada
Dept. of Biochemistry, University of Western Ontario, London ON, Canada

Fengyan Yu, Qiang Liu, Yujie Liu, Jieqiong Liu and Erwei Song
Department of Breast Tumor Center, Sun Yat-Sen Memorial Hospital, Sun Yat-Sen University, Guangzhou People's Republic of China

Deepak Kanojia and Hexin Chen
University of South Carolina, USA

Jürgen Dittmer, Ilka Oerlecke and Benjamin Leyh
Clinic for Gynecology, University of Halle, Germany